Praise for *Childhood Cancer Survivors*

"Keene, the mother of a leukemia survivor, and nurse practitioners specializing in pediatric oncology explain the long-term challenges that patients will face. They discuss issues such as growth problems, fertility, discrimination in the workplace and in obtaining insurance, and the emotional aspects of surviving cancer. This is a very useful book for both survivors and their families."

—*Library Journal*
#5 Best Consumer Health Book of 2000

· · · · ·

"This extraordinary book speaks to all ages as it describes the world of childhood cancer and provides information vitally needed by survivors, families, and medical teams. In an easy-to-read and well-organized format, the book is packed with facts about the emotional upheavals and drastic changes in both mental and physical health of young patients during treatment and long after the cancer has been cured."

—*Surviving: A Cancer Patient Magazine*
Stanford Hospital and Clinics

· · · · ·

"This book is a survivor's dream! It draws heavily on survivor talk. My response was quick and extremely positive, as it made me feel this was 'our' book, not something written for doctors or nurses, but for us. It talks our talk, deals with our issues, and faces reality head-on with the gutsy manner of survivors themselves. There's plenty of accurate and understandable 'technical' info, but there's plenty of heart as well, which is precisely what we haven't had in resources for us to date. No sugar-coating here. For that, I take my hat off to the authors. Thank you for having the courage to call us by our names and call all our difficulties out by name. I really feel that after publication of this book, I will no longer struggle with what to give patients I work with regarding late effects, or what to give new-survivor friends who are interested and need to know this. The book addresses the issues in the gentle yet straightforward method that is needed. That's what I call a success."

—Kimbra Wilder Gish, Hodgkin lymphoma survivor
Biomedical librarian

· · · · ·

"*Navigating our current healthcare system in the hope of optimizing one's health requires an educated and empowered survivor. This book will fill a critical educational gap by providing childhood cancer survivors practical and up-to-date information regarding their cancer and treatment. Perhaps of equal value are the many poignant vignettes that describe the trials and victories of the cancer experience. I consider this book a 'must read' for the survivors followed in our long-term follow-up program.*"

—Kevin C. Oeffinger, M.D.
Director, Living Beyond Cancer: A Program for
Adult Survivors of Pediatric Cancer
Memorial Sloan-Kettering Cancer Center

· · · · ·

"Childhood Cancer Survivors *and its companion website are clearly an ongoing labor of love by three experts and advocates in the area of childhood cancer survivorship. These publications unmistakably communicate the expectation that childhood cancer survivors can and should take charge of their health to live long and well after they overcome their disease. This is a relatively new message; however, it is one that is becoming increasingly important to individuals and society as survival rates improve and the population of childhood cancer survivors expands. I highly recommend this book for childhood cancer survivors and their families, as well as for oncology, general pediatric, and adult practitioners who care for them.*"

—Sheila Judge Santacroce, APRN, Ph.D.
Associate Professor, The University of North Carolina
at Chapel Hill Chapel Hill, NC

· · · · ·

"*There is a paucity of guides for both health care providers and patients that address the special issues of childhood cancer survivors. This important book was written to fill this void and empower survivors. The topics in the beginning of the book range from relationships with families and friends to discrimination at jobs to health insurance issues. Subsequent sections deal with specific childhood cancers and long-term health effects from cancer treatments and recommended follow-up tests. Each organ system is addressed with a discussion of the possible late effects, their detection, and management. Throughout the book, stories of childhood cancer survivors personalize the text.* Childhood Cancer Survivors *contains a wealth of important information that will benefit survivors for years after their treatment of cancer. It also contains a listing of service organizations, books, and online resources. It is clearly a 'must have' reference for both healthcare professionals and childhood cancer survivors. OncoLink gives this book its highest recommendation."*

—www.oncolink.com
University of Pennsylvania Cancer Center

· · · · ·

"This is a wonderful resource for childhood cancer survivors—a complete, concise guide to potential health problems that can occur following treatment for cancer in childhood. With information comes power, and with the information in this book, childhood cancer survivors will be empowered to take an active role in their life-long medical follow-up. In some cases, this information could be life-saving!"

—Wendy Landier, PhD, RN
Clinical Director, Center for Cancer Survivorship
City of Hope Comprehensive Cancer Center

· · · · ·

"This is a vitally important book for anyone who has had cancer or been touched by cancer in a child, spouse, parent, sibling, loved one, or friend. That's just about everyone. Many of these people may feel that, once treatment has ended, especially after the magic 5 years have passed without incident, it is nonproductive to think about the cancer anymore. Dwelling on one's past is, of course, going too far, especially if it prevents one from moving on to the many adventures awaiting him or her. And a parent's efforts, however well intended, to keep a child forever cognizant of the past cancer can make that child unnecessarily fearful. But if knowledge is power, then ignorance is just plain dumb and can even be harmful. This book treads a fine middle ground by advocating education, providing information on all the potential late effects, some of which have a strong probability of appearing and many of which have very little probability of occurring, and, most important, encouraging those affected to advocate for themselves and to educate others, especially their doctors."

—Kathryn, mother of Casey, 7-year survivor
of osteogenic sarcoma

· · · · ·

"This book is an extraordinary resource for survivors of childhood cancer, as well as for their families, caregivers, and friends. It provides clear answers to the important medical, psychosocial, and financial questions that young survivors raise during and after cancer treatment."

—Barbara Hoffman, J.D.
Editor, *A Cancer Survivor's Almanac: Charting Your Journey*

. . . . .

"This book is a must for any parent or adult survivor of childhood cancer who is seeking to understand real and potential late effects of cancer therapy—both physical and psychosocial. It is also a valuable resource for healthcare professionals involved in pediatric oncology. The chapters about specific childhood cancers and body systems affected by therapy are comprehensive and detailed. The chapters dedicated to survivorship, relationships, and emotions capture the positives and negatives of the double-edged sword of survivorship. The many personal quotes interspersed throughout the book provide a personal link to which most, and possibly all, families affected by childhood cancer can relate. After reading this book, there can be no question about the necessity of specialized long-term follow-up for survivors. The practical chapters on insurance and follow-up describe how to best obtain this care."

—Mary Nelson, M.S., R.N., CPNP
Imaging Services & Anesthesia
Children's Hospital Los Angeles

. . . . .

"There is compelling evidence in the scientific literature to support continued follow-up for childhood cancer survivors. If all survivors were followed in a comprehensive late effects clinic, this book might not be necessary. However, we are a mobile society with variable medical care and insurance practices. Ensuring that survivors themselves understand the late effects associated with their individual therapy is probably the most important means to obtain compliance with follow-up. Providing survivors with information necessary to monitor for late effects of therapy allows them to advocate for their own healthcare. This book will prove to be an important resource for survivors as they navigate various healthcare systems."

—Cindy Proukou, PNP
Long-term Childhood Cancer Survivors Program
Golisano Children's Hospital at Strong
University of Rochester Medical Center

. . . . .

"I think this book is terrific. It is clear, direct, and contains valuable information and advice. It will surely be an excellent resource for survivors and their families. I will certainly recommend it to patients I see."

—Mary Rourke, Ph.D.
Assistant Professor, Widener University
Previously was Psychologist, Children's Hospital of Philadelphia

· · · · ·

"Congratulations on being a survivor of childhood cancer. Cancer and its therapy can be associated with short- and long-term effects on your health. We want you to focus now on a happy and healthy life. It is important to protect your health by learning as much as you can about the type of cancer you had, the treatment you received, and the best medical follow-up. This book will give you the information to bring back to your healthcare providers to help them provide the best possible healthcare for you. You will learn invaluable information about possible delayed effects of cancer and its treatment, health and wellness promotion, recommendations for follow-up, and prevention strategies. Curing your cancer was important to us—now we want you to join us by reading this book and becoming an active partner with us in your ongoing healthcare needs."

— Debra L. Friedman, M.D.
Director, Pediatric Hematology-Oncology
Medical Director, REACH for Survivorship Program
Vanderbilt-Ingram Cancer Center
Nashville, Tennessee

· · · · ·

"Every childhood cancer survivor and family member of a survivor, should have a copy of Childhood Cancer Survivors—*it is that good! This is the book that you read all the way through when you first get it, then keep nearby as a ready reference. Each medical late effect is discussed clearly, with details on risk factors, signs and symptoms, and medical management. Frank discussions of education, insurance, and disability issues empower survivors and guide them through the complex maze of policies and agencies that can help them. But that's not all: I love the personal stories that are included throughout the book; it is so friendly and readable. And the third edition has been updated with current information on late effects, including references to journal articles.* Childhood Cancer Survivors *is one of a kind, the only book written specifically for the survivors and their families. I highly recommend it."*

— Patty Feist, M.S.
Mother of a long-term survivor of childhood cancer
Organic Chemist
Webmaster, Pediatric Oncology Resource Center
www.ped-onc.org

Childhood Cancer Survivors

A Practical Guide to Your Future

Nancy Keene, Wendy Hobbie,
and Kathy Ruccione

Childhood Cancer Guides
www.childhoodcancerguides.org

Childhood Cancer Survivors: A Practical Guide to Your Future, Third Edition
by Nancy Keene, Wendy Hobbie, and Kathy Ruccione

Copyright © 2012, 2007, 2000 Childhood Cancer Guides. All rights reserved.
Printed in the United States of America.

Published by Childhood Cancer Guides
P.O. Box 31937, Bellingham, WA 98228

Distributed by O'Reilly Media, Inc.
1005 Gravenstein Highway North, Sebastopol, CA 95472

Library of Congress Cataloging-in-Publication Data

Keene, Nancy.

Childhood cancer survivors : a practical guide to your future / Nancy Keene, Wendy Hobbie, and Kathy Ruccione. -- 3rd ed.

    p. cm.

Summary: "A resource for survivors of childhood cancer and their families that includes information about medical late effects of treatment, necessary follow-up care, emotional aspects of survivorship, navigating the healthcare system, ways to maximize heath, a survivor's treatment record, and a list of helpful organizations"-- Provided by publisher.

Includes bibliographical references and index.

ISBN 978-1-941089-10-1

1. Cancer in children--Popular works. 2. Cancer in children--Treatment--Complications.
3. Cancer in children--Social aspects. 4. Cancer in children--Psychological aspects. I. Hobbie, Wendy, 1959- II. Ruccione, Kathy, 1946- III. Title.

RC281.C4K44 2012

618.92'994--dc23

2012012549

 This book uses RepKover™, a durable and flexible lay-flat binding.

For all survivors and those who love them.

Table of Contents

Foreword

ENORMOUS PROGRESS HAS BEEN MADE in treating children with cancer in the last half century. This period is emphasized because it has been 50 years since the beginning of modern pediatric oncology. One hundred years ago, the only effective means of treating any patient with cancer was to remove the growth surgically. In the early decades of the 1900s, radiation therapy was developed and local control of the disease was improved. But neither surgery nor irradiation was of much value to patients in whom the malignant cells had already spread beyond the original site of involvement. Means of controlling cancer growing in more distant sites were needed. Those means were sought and were first found 50 years ago in drugs that destroyed leukemia cells. Since then, effective chemical agents have been developed to control virtually every form of childhood cancer, resulting in steadily improving survival rates.

Even in the early years of this century, however, physicians were already aware that achieving cure today had its tomorrows. That is, whatever form of treatment was used, be it surgery alone or with radiation therapy, long-term disabilities and complications could arise at some later date. Those associated with surgery were obvious and well-known because the immediate and long-term consequences of radical surgery had been known for centuries. Those associated with radiation therapy were studied as early as 1905, when a German investigator irradiated one of the two wings of chicks and saw that the irradiated side failed to grow normally. This gave rise to research by radiologists to find ways to minimize the disruptions in normal growth and development that treatment can cause.

Recital of history is important because it demonstrates the interest physicians have had for decades concerning these aspects of pediatric oncology. Such concerns were, however, the least of the worries assailing the physicians confronted with children and cancer five decades ago. The survival of patients with leukemia was measured in weeks, very rarely in months, and never in years. To even discuss treatment-related problems that might arise 5 years after the diagnosis was to live in a dream world.

Still, the pioneers persisted. As survival rates climbed in the affluent countries, the proportion of young adults who were survivors of childhood cancer rose concomitantly. That proportion is now estimated to be 1 in 750 20-year-olds. This is not very different from the incidence of heart disease in that age group, to give some perspective. Chronic illnesses among long-term survivors, if not prevented or at least managed well, could therefore become a national health problem in nations like the United States. It is thus important to make every effort to ensure that the cured child of today does not survive only to become the disabled, incapacitated adult of tomorrow. To quote the motto of pediatric oncology, "Cure is not enough."

There is an appropriate and continuing research effort by physicians around the world to identify the long-term complications—the so-called late effects—associated with the use of surgery, radiation therapy, and chemotherapy alone and in their various combinations. More than that, there has been an increasing research emphasis on the psycho-socio-economic impacts of the disease. These studies have encompassed not only the patient at the time of diagnosis and thereafter, but the whole family.

The care of the patient and the family by the healthcare team does not end with the last dose of chemotherapy. Nor does it end 3 or 5 years later when the chance for recurrent disease in children with cancer becomes very low. Rather, there are persisting emotional and psychological overlays that affect all members of the family.

These aspects of pediatric oncology and the information concerning late effects gathered over the years have been distilled in the pages of this volume. The authors have succeeded in this ambitious endeavor by careful organization of their voluminous material. The various malignant diseases of childhood are described, the treatments used are explained, the normal functions of vital organs are detailed, and then the untoward possible late effects of anticancer treatment are documented. This is done in easily understood language without confusing technical jargon. The specific types of problems that can arise are exemplified by numerous capsule case histories recounting, in their own words, the personal experiences of patients and their families. These graphic and often poignant recitals make important points in unforgettable ways. Finally, recommendations for follow-up are provided according to the particular malignant disease and the specific form of treatment.

This volume will benefit the long-term survivors of childhood cancer and their families. Not only they will be helped, however. The book will be of great value to all physicians, few of whom are conversant with the various malignant diseases of childhood. Yet, the average family physician can expect, as part of his or her daily practice, to see more and more patients with this past history. Guidance is needed. Indeed, even pediatric oncologists will find recommendations concerning long-term surveillance extremely helpful and should have this book on their shelves for ready reference.

The authors are to be congratulated for having helped to achieve one of the major goals of pediatric oncology in this way. They have written a uniquely comprehensive review of the late effects problem while providing a manual of how to look after the long-term survivor. In doing so, they are making an important contribution to the years after cure—that is, to securing as much as possible a healthy and productive future for the adult who was cured of cancer as a child.

—Giulio D'Angio, M.D.
Professor Emeritus, Radiation Oncology
University of Pennsylvania

Preface

SURVIVORS OF CHILDHOOD CANCER are considered to be society's "miracles." Because the cure rates have risen so dramatically in just two generations, it is still hard to believe that so many children survive cancer. Survivors, their families, and their doctors and nurses rejoice at this good fortune. But, as Dr. Giulio D'Angio noted in a historic article many years ago, "Cure is not enough."

A 2003 report from the Institute of Medicine estimated that more than 270,000 survivors of childhood cancer live in the United States. Since then, the estimate has risen to more than 325,000. This book was written to empower survivors to act on their own behalf to obtain excellent follow-up care. To take action, they must have knowledge. For instance, thousands of young women who had chest radiation do not know of their increased risk for breast cancer. Many survivors who were given certain chemotherapy drugs are at risk for heart problems later in life. In addition, information about possible late effects is still being learned long after survivors are no longer seen at the children's hospitals that treated them.

Survivors sometimes face difficulties obtaining adequate insurance. Some encounter job discrimination due to their health history. And many survivors describe social and emotional upheavals at different points after cancer. If people know of these potential problems, they can take steps to identify, cope with, or treat them early if they do develop. We wrote this book to help survivors make the most of their lives after "cure."

What this book offers

This book is not just about science but about the experience of survivorship. It blends basic technical information in easy-to-understand language with stories and advice from more than a hundred survivors and parents of young survivors. The stories share emotions, fears, thoughts, and triumphs. We wanted to explore the richness and variety of the survivorship experience and help survivors feel less alone in their journeys.

One of the beauties of including true stories throughout the book is that we are able to present late effects that often are not well represented in the scientific literature such as immune problems and fatigue. It also allows us to put a face on the suffering that many survivors experience by not being believed and thus not treated appropriately. We are really saddened by how many people with radiation-induced heart problems are told they are short of breath from anxiety or asthma, or survivors whose spleen has been removed who don't know they are at risk for massive infections. We want survivors with late effects to take this book to their healthcare provider and say, "I think the symptoms I'm having may be from my cancer treatment years ago," so that together they can make a plan for care.

This book does not minimize or sugarcoat the reality of late effects. We lay out what is known and what is not known and let survivors and their healthcare providers determine what applies. We hope to educate both survivors and healthcare providers by clearly explaining the most common medical, psychological, and social late effects. Survivors can then use the great strength they used to beat cancer to face any problems that may develop months or years after cure.

Many survivors are thriving. They share great insights into life and are wonderfully deep in the way they look at the world, but there are still cues, memories, and experiences that can remind them of cancer. It's a double-edged sword. There are often very positive things that arise from surviving cancer treatment, but we need also to recognize and acknowledge the difficult aspects and discuss ways to cope with them.

The huge numbers of young adult survivors are a legacy to the hard work of hundreds of physicians, nurses, and other members of the healthcare team. But the next challenge is to help survivors make the most of the lives they have won. Our hope is that survivors who read this book will find medical facts simply explained and advice that eases their daily life so they will feel empowered to be strong advocates for themselves.

The stories in this book are all true, although some names have been changed to protect privacy. Every word has been spoken by survivors, parents, or siblings. They wanted to share their stories to provide reassurance, information, and a sense of community for other survivors. As so many survivors said, dealing with late effects can be difficult, but having a life in which to address them is a gift.

How this book is organized

We have organized the book sequentially in an attempt to parallel the survivorship journey. We start at the end of treatment with its celebrations and fears. We deal with the challenge of finding comprehensive care and how to get the best medical follow-up available. We discuss the emotions of survivors at different points after treatment and relationships with parents, siblings, friends, and spouses. Because schooling, insurance, and jobs are often affected by a cancer history, we examine ways to navigate the system.

The second half of the book deals with the medical aspects of survivorship. It begins with Chapter 6, *Diseases*, which briefly describes types of childhood cancer and their treatments. Chapter 6 has tables at the end that list various treatments and some recommended follow-up tests to monitor your long-term health. By screening for problems that may occur, you can quickly identify and treat them.

The remainder of the book is divided into body systems and the late effects that can develop in each. The body systems chapters include identical sections: organ damage, signs and symptoms, screening and detection, and medical management. Throughout the book, helpful organizations and websites are listed in the text. Their addresses and telephone numbers can be found in Appendix B, *Resources*.

Because approximately half of survivors are male and half female, we did not adopt the common convention of using only masculine personal pronouns. Because we do not like using he/she, we have alternated personal pronouns within chapters. This may seem awkward as you read, but it prevents half of the readers from feeling that the text does not apply to them.

Many of the people who read this book are adult survivors of childhood cancer, and many are the parents of survivors. In some cases, parents are addressed and, in others, adult survivors are the focus. Again, this can make reading the book feel as if it is not directly aimed at you. However, we adopted this method because survivorship deeply affects both individuals and families.

All of the medical information contained in this second edition is current for 2012. As knowledge about the medical and psychological after-effects of cancer treatment is constantly evolving and improving, there will inevitably be changes. You can use the information in this book as a map that will have more detail filled in as knowledge of late effects increases.

Much of the information in this book is about problems that can arise after treatment for childhood cancer. All people, whether they had cancer or not, face challenges and find ways to incorporate what they learn into the rest of their lives. The survivors interviewed for this book are thrilled to be alive. They talk of how they cherish each day and the valuable lessons they learned from cancer. To balance the problems described in the text, we invited survivors to describe a bit of the rest of their lives. With warmth and humor, they did so. Appendix A, *Survivor Sketches*, will give you a glimpse of the richness and wonder of life after cancer.

To give you more places to find help, we included Appendix B, *Resources*, which lists books, organizations, and online resources. We provided a section called *References* that provides sources for facts cited in the text. Finally, we have included an indispensable health record to be filled out at the end of treatment and copied and given to each subsequent caregiver for the rest of your life. This personal long-term follow-up guide will inform your healthcare providers about the types of treatment you had and the follow-up schedule necessary to maintain optimum health.

How to use this book

Survivors' needs for information vary according to coping styles and where they are on their survivorship journey. If you just ended treatment and are seeking ways to find a new normal, you may not want to read about potential late effects. Instead, you may need to hear about how other people your age coped with the end of treatment. You may be a college student who no longer goes to the doctor but is getting more concerned about your health. What you might want from this book is a method to locate a healthcare provider who can give you great medical care. Or you may be a survivor of 30 years who is bedeviled by increasing numbers of physical ailments, all possibly related to the high-dose radiation you received as a child.

Because the needs of survivors are so diverse and change over time, this book is full of stories from more than 100 survivors and parents of survivors. These snapshots in time cover the greatest joys to moments of despair. Some of these may be hard to read, especially for those who have just completed treatment. Here are our suggestions for positive ways to use the information contained in this book:

- Consider reading only sections that apply to the present or immediate future. Reading about disclosure of cancer history makes sense for a young adult who is dating, but not for the parent of a preschooler who just finished cancer treatment.

- Recognize that your need for information may change. Survivors range from infants to baby boomers, and the late effects of treatment can be none to debilitating. Every survivor has a different need for information, and this can change over time.

- Consider all of the body system chapters to be references. Dig into those chapters for specific information about your particular situation on a need-to-know basis. If you read straight through all of these chapters, you may feel overwhelmed.

- Realize that only a fraction of the late effects described in the book apply to you. This book contains information that pertains to a large group of people, but every survivor is different: some have no late effects, some have only a few, and some have life-changing problems. Take the information in this book to your healthcare provider to figure out your unique situation. Learn what you are at risk for and what you shouldn't worry about. Devise a strategy to screen for potential late effects and develop a plan to stay healthy and fit.

- Recognize that knowledge of late effects from cancer treatment, both psychological and medical, is growing daily. The impact of today's treatments will unfold over the next 10 to 20 years. This book describes what is known now. You will need to form a relationship with a knowledgeable healthcare provider to keep abreast of new information as it becomes available.

- We have struggled to keep each chapter short and the technical information easy to read. If you want to delve into any topic in greater depth, Appendix B, *Resources*, is a good place to start. It contains a list of books, organizations, and online resources for survivors of all ages.

- If you wish to, share the book with family and friends. Often they want to understand and help but just don't know how.

This book contains not only medical information but the thoughts and feelings of dozens of children, teens, and adults who have survived childhood cancer. Reading their stories may help you feel part of a growing community of people who faced, and beat, childhood cancer.

Acknowledgements

We would like to thank our families for their patience and encouragement as we wrote each edition of the book. Nancy's children, who were in elementary school when the first edition was published, are now young adults in college. Big hugs and thanks to both of them for helping Nancy keep the cancer part of our lives in perspective, and the laughter and joy part of our lives center stage.

Special thanks to Kathy's son, Daniel, for being her best teacher. Facing daunting challenges himself with humor and sensitivity, he has shown her that life can be full and fun even when the deck seems to be stacked against you. To Kathy's professional "family" at the Children's Hospital of Los Angeles, thanks for being endlessly supportive and enthusiastic about the book even though it has meant adding one more ball to the daily juggling act.

Wendy would like to thank her husband, Dan, for his unending support and encouragement, and Jon and Sarah, her children, who are daily reminders that healthy children are a gift. And a special thank you to her Children's Hospital of Philadelphia survivorship family, who care for hundreds of survivors with patience and a deep understanding of their special needs. Finally, thanks to Nancy, whose passion and tireless efforts makes this book better with each edition.

We deeply appreciate Scott Odom for allowing us to use his high school basketball portrait for the cover of this book. It makes the book real. Also, thanks to Cook Children's Medical Center, for giving us permission to use the photo, which was first reproduced in *Children's Promise* magazine, Fall 1999.

Unending gratitude to Patty Feist, who read every word of this edition with the eye of a parent of a childhood cancer survivor, a scientist, and an editor. Her suggestions make each edition better. Special thanks to our copyeditor, Sarah Farmer, and graphic designer Susan Jarmolowski. They both are tremendously talented and their suggestions help make the book both appealing and professional. Huge thanks to Alison Leake who proofread every word. And special thanks to Tim O'Reilly for believing in and supporting Childhood Cancer Guides.

All three editions of this book have been true collaborations between survivors and medical professionals. Many well-known and respected members of the pediatric oncology community, as well as survivors and their parents, carved time out of busy schedules to make invaluable suggestions and catch errors. Thank you: Erin Armideo, MSN, PNP; D.B. Bass, MD; Sarah Bottomley, MSN, CRNP; Colleen Callahan MSN, FNP; Concetta DiDomenico, MSN, PNP; Patty Feist, MS; Dominic Femino, MD; Daniel Fiduccia, BA; David Freyer, DO, MS; Debra Friedman, MD; Jill Ginsberg, MD; Ernest Katz, PhD; Kimbra Wilder Gish, MS; Linda Goettina, DMH; Mark Greenberg, MD; Jeanne Harvey, MSN, CPNP; Kathryn Havemann, JD; Andrea Hinkle, MD; Barbara Hoffman, JD; F. Leonard Johnson, MD; Anne Kazak, PhD; Wendy Landier, PhD, RN; Missy Layfield, PT; Ellen Levy, MSN, PNP; Marcio Malogolowkin, MD; Anna Meadows, MD; Kathleen Meeske, PhD, RN; Grace Monaco, JD; Mary Nelson, MS, RN, CPNP, CPON; Jan Ober; Kevin Oeffinger, MD; Sue Ogle, MSN, CRNP; Cindy Proukou, RN, CPNP; Ralph Richardson, PhD; Kim Ritchey, MD; Mary Rourke, PhD; Jennifer Saggio, MSN, CRNP, CPON; Sheila Santacroce, PhD, APRN, CPNP; Lisl Schweers, MSW; Ami Shah, MD; Charles Sklar, MD; Bea Smith, AuD; Anne Spurgeon; Theresa Sweeney, MD; Kristina Tarczy-Hornoch, MD, DPhil; Karla Wilson, RN, MSN, FNP-C, CPON; Anne Wohlschlaeger, MSN, PNP; Catherine Woodman, MD; Brad Zebrack, PhD.

To all of the survivors and those who love them, whose words form the heart and soul of this book, thank you: Andrea; Rene; Zach; Kerryn (mum of Terri); Noreen (Coley's mom); B. Jared Akers; Karen Akers; Christine Aney (Sarah's mom); Mark B.; Ann Bagley; B. Elisabeth Bain; Jan Barber; Shirley Barkley; Kathleen Barry; Naomi Bartley; Barbara Bradley; Dottie Bradford Buttafogo; Ricky Carroll; Lori Cox; Claire Diamond; Wendy Corder Dowhower; Anne S. Draghi; Lisa Ellis; Patty Feist-Mack; Ardeth Saunders Files; Carol A. Foreman; Kimbra Wilder Gish; Roxie Glaze; Deborah K. Gominiak; Kevin Grant; L. Grimes; Kathryn G. Havemann; Denise Glassmeyer Hendler; Paul Honsinger; Mary Hubbell; Margie Huhner; Chris and Marge Hum; Cheryl Putnam Jagannathan; Erin Jordan; Pagie and Susan Kalika; Teresa Kluey; Rima Lang; Joel Layfield; Missy Layfield; E.J. Lemky; Connie Luck; Dawn MacIntosh; Sharon Filer Maerten; Beth McQuin; Lori Michelle Miller; Marilyn Brodeur Morin; Jan Ober; Leah Paley; Clare Patterson; Trevor and Vicki Pogue; Thomas H. Prader; Susan D. Prince; Linda R.; Laura Randall (Matthew's mom); Mary C. Riecke, Pharmacist; Patricia Dane Rogers; Jennifer Marie Rohloff; Jennifer Rutkowski; Steve and Shirlene S.; Teri San Souci; Mark and Judith Schumann; Laura Myers Sechier; Susan Sennett; Erin Shanahan; Lynnette Shanahan; Cathy Shilling; Lori Shipman; Barb Skogstad; Gilbert (Gib) Smith, JD; Anne Spurgeon; Jenny Swink; Teresa K. Tanoos; Jennifer M. Thompson, MD; Jennifer Thompson; Lisa Tignor; Laura Todd-Pierce; Jackie Trzyna; Elaine Vizena; Ralene Walls; D. Walters; Tami Watchurst; Kerri Weisenberger; Sheri and Greg White (parents to Matthew); Helen Wilder; Jan Williamson; Laurie English Winans;

Carol Jean Maresic Worra; Linda Zame; Steve Zielinski; and those who wish to remain anonymous.

Special thanks to Linda Zame, who suggested adding the survivor sketches section. Hearing the rest of the story adds balance and depth, and we are grateful that she shared her wisdom with us.

Despite the inspiration and contributions of so many, any errors, omissions, misstatements, or flaws are entirely our own.

Chapter 1

Survivorship

*From the time of discovery and for the
balance of life, an individual diagnosed
with cancer is a survivor.*

—National Coalition for
Cancer Survivorship

MANY OF the 12,400 children and adolescents (under age 20) diagnosed each year with childhood cancer can now be cured. Survivors of childhood cancer often find that the illness and its treatment changed their lives in many powerful, and often positive, ways. There is much to celebrate.

However, long-term survivors of childhood cancer face an uncertain future. The surgery, radiation, chemotherapy, and stem cell transplants used to cure children sometimes affect growing bodies and developing minds. Complications from these treatments may occur later in life and are known as late effects. In addition, some survivors encounter job discrimination, difficulties obtaining insurance, and emotional or social difficulties.

During your (or your child's) journey through the many phases of survivorship, you may find yourself educating your family, friends, and healthcare providers about your physical and psychological responses to treatment and its aftereffects. Knowing about your disease, its treatment, and potential late effects will help you advocate for the care you need to maximize your health and well-being.

This chapter discusses some of the many facets of survivorship. It covers the transition from active treatment to going off treatment. It also discusses the shift from childhood to the independence of adulthood. To take charge of your health, you need to collect information about your treatment and then assemble a team to help chart your medical course. This chapter discusses ways to find the best healthcare providers for your unique needs.

Survivorship

You are part of a growing community of children, teenagers, and adult survivors of childhood cancer who are pioneers in the post-treatment journey into adulthood. In the months and years after treatment ends, you may encounter physical late effects, emotional upheaval, and unexpected benefits. Your journey may be easy or hard. It may take surprising turns and dips and reach dizzying heights. Although thousands of others are making the same journey, your path is unique.

> *I'm a long-term survivor of Hodgkin's disease. I think you have to recognize the cancer as part of your history, absorb it into yourself, and hopefully grab some of the good things it has given you—a feistiness, a capacity for great compassion. You also have to be able to not let it overwhelm you with fear and anxiety so that it's all you can think about. How do you walk this line? If you don't think about it and don't let yourself be identified as a cancer survivor, then you can't protect yourself if you go in with late effects. You have to be able to say, "I may only be 28 years old, but I had radiation to my chest when I was 15 and I'm at risk for heart disease now." But then, you also don't want to become so obsessed that you start to define yourself as a cancer patient rather than a person who just happened to have had cancer. It's sometimes hard to strike that balance.*

Life for all people is sometimes rocky and sometimes smooth. Being a survivor may throw a few unexpected stones in your path or may pave the way to new opportunities. Many survivors talk about how cancer opened their eyes and left them with an appreciation for life. They are able to shake off the small stuff and focus on the important things in their lives. They feel as if the cancer gave them perspective, and that this is a great gift. Others feel that the cancer was one small part of their lives and they prefer not to think about it. As time goes by, your feelings about the experience may change.

> *We are all walking down the same path, but we are at different places on it. The first few months after treatment, I had a deep feeling of gratitude for every day that I was alive. I did reach a point, however, when I had to let myself be thoroughly pissed off at the trauma from the diagnosis, treatment, and recovery. I am coming to realize that these negative thoughts are normal and are due us from time to time. I am learning to walk the middle of the road, to not be such a perfectionist. That is coming with time. I have been on the elated end of the spectrum, and I have also spent many days in the basement of life (generally while returning to "normal life" post-treatment). It is a humbling, enlightening, lively experience.*

· · · · ·

I think that everyone should try to learn from every experience in their life. But being a survivor is not the whole part of my being. I am also a student, a teacher, a daughter, a granddaughter, a girlfriend, a visionary, a historian, and a sugar addict (among many other things). But sometimes people see you as just a survivor and nothing else. I want to be a survivor. I just want to be Andrea as well.

· · · · ·

I've never really dealt with having cancer. I really didn't want to think about it. I felt like it was a defense mechanism because I didn't have the physical energy to deal with it. I went to a support group meeting once and felt like it was getting thrown in my face when I just wanted to forget. I feel bad sometimes because I think I should be giving back in some way, but I'm just not strong enough.

· · · · ·

I had a brain tumor when I was 10. I'm pretty short (4'6") and skinny. I'm in a wheelchair. I can feel my lower body, but I can't walk. Sometimes it bothers me. It was bad enough to have cancer, but then to be in a wheelchair too. I used to love to dance and I can't do that anymore. It's hard when I go to weddings. But my dad always told me to have a positive attitude. He said it could always be worse—I could be in bed all of the time. So basically I have a positive attitude and think good things can come out of it.

· · · · ·

I had leukemia when I was 15, over 20 years ago. I feel like it put me on a fast track and that I missed a lot, but I gained a lot too. I missed quite a bit of high school and lost lots of friends. I became very serious and matured quickly. I had different interests and just didn't communicate the same as the high school kids. But I graduated, went to college and graduate school. I made friends with people who are goal-oriented but relaxed. I have a wonderful wife, three healthy kids (19 months apart— no fertility problems there!), and lots of good friends. I have a sense for how fragile life is and I make the most of it.

Part of surviving childhood cancer is dealing with and educating medical personnel, family, friends, and loved ones about the medical and emotional aspects of survivorship. You may find that family members want to pretend that it never happened. You may be told to put it all behind you. Or you may find people treating you as if you are a fragile piece of glass. Deciding what parts of your cancer history to explain and what parts to ignore may take some reflection, and will certainly involve planning how to communicate your thoughts and needs to loved ones. This topic is discussed more in Chapter 2, *Emotions*, and Chapter 3, *Relationships*.

> *I have had so many people say to me, "Why don't you put it behind you and get on with your life? You're done with that now." Am I? Am I really done with that? You're going to tell me I'm done with that when every day of my life when I'm getting dressed I have to look at that laparotomy scar. I have to take all kinds of pills daily. I need to prevent and immediately treat infections because I don't have a spleen. The radiation killed my thyroid. If I get the flu, it might just be the flu, but we have to treat it with aggressive antibiotics and supportive therapy because it could be a lethal post-splenectomy infection, and those kill within hours. Pretty hard to ignore.*

$$\bullet \quad \bullet \quad \bullet \quad \bullet \quad \bullet$$

> *Is the cup half empty or half full? I fully believe it is half full. I live each day thankful that my son is here, thankful that there is a treatment for his cancer, because if this were the year 1949 instead of 1999, he would be dead. This is so scary, it always makes my heart skip a beat and my eyes tear and my mouth go dry. And it makes me go in the next room to look at him, to make him smile, to run my eyes over this marvel that is him. And it makes me wonder why any of us are alive, so I think of things that are beautiful as I go through my day: my lovely chaotic daughter, my clowning stable husband, my furry soft cat, my old and very sweet dog, my young and full-of-life puppy, the cool-looking clouds in the sky, the way the bare branches of the trees are outlined against the pink sky at sunset or the pale blue winter day sky, the sound of my favorite songs, the feel of my sweat and my muscles when I work out, the warm shower and good-smelling soap, fresh bread coming out of the oven, the banter of my family as we gather in the living room before dinner.*

> *And in an odd way I am thankful that something woke me up to the wonder that is life. I am only so sad and angry that that something was cancer.*

$$\bullet \quad \bullet \quad \bullet \quad \bullet \quad \bullet$$

> *We choose life and not what might come with the future. Even though I'm currently disabled by the late effects of treatment, I don't waste time regretting the decisions that my parents and I made in 1972. We made the best-informed decision at the time, and for most of the 28 years post-treatment I've been very healthy.*

$$\bullet \quad \bullet \quad \bullet \quad \bullet \quad \bullet$$

> *My 8-year-old daughter Katherine is more than 5 years out from a bone marrow transplant. She had juvenile chronic myelogenous leukemia. She*

has some very manageable long-term effects from total body radiation (cataracts, subtle learning disabilities, sterility). For the most part she is a normal, happy, active girl who along with her brothers is the joy of my life.

· · · · ·

I have been told many times that I had a "good" cancer; one doctor even went so far as to say my cancer was a "cupcake." No cancer is a good cancer, and no treatment is without its harmful effects. But in my mind having a "good" cancer meant that the treatment couldn't have been so very bad and certainly that it didn't carry any long-term risks. Since I wanted to believe, needed to believe that I had emerged unscathed, I blithely went along with this version of reality. Trying to make light of cancer by calling one or another of the curable cancers a "good" cancer does a disservice to me and my physicians. It disarms us in the face of potential late effects and makes us less effective in monitoring our health.

Transitions

According to Webster's *New Collegiate Dictionary*, transition is a "passage from one state, stage, place, or subject to another." This definition expresses very well the road that survivors of childhood cancer travel, from active treatment to off treatment, and then from off treatment to long-term survival. The definition also fits because "place" changes as the adolescent moves from pediatric healthcare overseen by parents to self-designed and self-monitored adult healthcare. These periods of change can evoke anxiety and require a period of adjustment. For survivors, transitions involve medical, psychological, social, and educational changes.

People cope better with transitions if a period of planning occurs before the change happens. The transition from cancer patient to survivor should be acknowledged by all healthcare providers, and the psychosocial and educational aspects of survival should be addressed. For instance, if a teen's medical care shifts from a pediatric clinic to an adult clinic without discussions about his understanding of his disease, he may still have only the information that was given to him when first diagnosed as a young child. This is hardly the amount or depth of information needed by a survivor entering adulthood who will have to advocate for his own healthcare and make wise lifestyle choices.

The following sections discuss going off treatment and moving from teen to adult healthcare.

End of treatment

The last day of treatment is a time for both celebration and fear. The protocol schedules and frequent appointments provided reassurance and structure. While most families are thrilled that the days of pills and procedures have ended, some fear a future without powerful medicines to keep the disease away. Concerns about relapse are an almost universal response, and family members often feel vulnerable after active treatment ends.

Many parents and survivors describe ending treatment as almost as wrenching an experience as diagnosis. Families begin to experience the gamut of emotions—from elation to terror—months before the final day.

> I had a lot of anticipatory worry—it started about 6 months before ending treatment. By the last day of treatment I had been worrying for months, so it was just a relief to quit.

· · · · ·

> I expected to feel a profound sense of relief when treatment ended. The 6 months prior to ending treatment I felt almost euphoric. But when she was finally finished, I began to be unexpectedly fearful. I just started to worry. I didn't really relax until she was a year off treatment. Now weeks go by without me thinking of relapse, although I still think of the years of treatment frequently.

· · · · ·

> We were thrilled when treatment ended. I knew many people who felt that celebrating would jinx them; they just didn't feel safe. Well, I felt that we had won a big battle—getting through treatment—and we were going to celebrate that. If, heaven forbid, in the future we had another battle to fight, we'd deal with it. But on the last day of treatment, we were delighted.

Survivors and their parents should anticipate that after months or years spent going through the rigors of treatment, they will have lost the feeling of a "normal" life. They may experience relapse scares, and they may need to call the doctor to describe the symptoms and be reassured.

> Several months after my son ended treatment, I was driving down the street, and I started to worry that he seemed excessively tired lately. I started to feel my throat constricting, and tears sprang to my eyes. I had to pull over because I literally couldn't breathe. I had to force myself to calm down, breathe slowly, and realize that I was just having a normal attack of being petrified that he would relapse.

With diagnosis came the awareness that life can be cruel and unpredictable. Because many parents and children feel that treatment is keeping the cancer away, the end of treatment sometimes leaves families feeling exposed and vulnerable. When treatment ends, survivors and their parents must find ways to live with uncertainty, to find a balance between hope and reasonable worry.

People forget sometimes that the toughest part of being off treatment is being off treatment! You aren't doing anything active to nail any microscopic tumor—no drugs, no zaps, no cutting, just sitting. And that can be terrifying.

· · · · ·

I was told nothing about late effects when I was treated for Hodgkin's as a teen. The good part of that was that I had no excess anxiety. I see people come out of treatment now and they go from mentally fighting the disease to being very fearful and anxious. That's a very difficult thing. But then my ignorance caused a lot of other suffering when I tried to get good care for my late effects. Finding a balance is a very complex thing, and the way the doctor handles it from the beginning sets the tone.

Meeting with doctors and nurses

Doctors and nurses can help with the transition to survivorship by having a meeting with the family before the end of treatment. You may have to suggest the meeting to your child's medical team, although at many centers these meetings are routine. Many families make a separate appointment for this discussion so that it will not be on the actual last day of treatment. The appointment should be long enough to allow a lengthy conversation. Topics discussed during this meeting might include:

- The disease, the treatment, and possible late effects.

- When and who to call with specific questions and concerns, including a written list of symptoms that should prompt a call.

- A detailed discussion of the next steps: which healthcare providers will see your child, the appointment schedule, the follow-up schedule, when the central line will be removed, and what (if any) immunizations to get.

- A document (such as the one at the back of this book) that includes the name of the disease, date of diagnosis, place of treatment, total dosages of drugs, amounts of radiation, and necessary follow-up. This document will help survivors provide all future healthcare providers with comprehensive information about their unique medical histories.

- An explanation of how to notify the treatment center of any change in address and/or how to share results of tests performed outside of the treatment center.

- A realistic, but hopeful, portrayal of the future.
- Praise for the child or teen for handling a very difficult time in her life with grace (or courage, or whatever word is appropriate).
- Recognition of all of your family's hard work.
- A chance to give the healthcare team feedback and thanks.
- An acknowledgment that you may be relieved but also fearful of the future.
- A discussion of any concerns.

If any of these items are not mentioned in the last meeting, ask to have another meeting or phone call to address these or any other questions or concerns you may have.

Celebrations—or not

Some families enjoy having ceremonies to mark the end of cancer treatment. For younger children in particular, who have spent much of their lives taking pills and having procedures, ceremonies can help them grasp that the most active phase of treatment is truly over and the important transition to life as a survivor is about to begin. Following are ideas from many families about how to commemorate this important occasion.

- Take pictures of the hospital and staff.
- Take a picture of your child or teen taking his last pill.
- Give trophies to your child and any siblings.

> We had a big party during which my husband, Scott, stood up and called for everyone's attention. He gave a talk about how proud we were of Jeremy and handed him a big trophy. It had the victory angel on top and was engraved with "Jeremy, we are so proud of you and your victory. Love, Mom and Dad." We gave a plaque to his brother, Jason, for being the world's most supportive brother.

- Throw a party for friends and family.
- Have friends and family send cards or messages of congratulations.
- Go on a trip or vacation to celebrate.
- If consistent with your beliefs, have a religious ceremony of thanksgiving.
- Organize a party at your child's school.

> When Joseph finished treatment he was in kindergarten, but the kids had gone through almost an entire year with him, and they had known

all about his treatments and frequent hospitalizations and had talked as a group about it when we made a presentation to the class. It seemed appropriate to have an "all done with treatment" celebration. We even had his two best friends who go to different schools come over to join us, and his big brother came down from his class to share in the fun.

It was a very joyous occasion, and we made it as much like a birthday party as we could. I made cupcakes and juice, and we played games. A friend who leads the story hour at our children's bookstore came and did some songs and stories with the kids, and I even sent each classmate home with a treat bag. At the end, right before time to go home, Joseph pulled out several cans of his favorite hospital discovery, and the kids took turns blasting a shower of Silly String® on everyone else! We all clapped and cheered, and Joseph's wonderful teacher and I had a chance to have a good celebratory cry while the kids put on their things to go home. Clean-up wasn't too darn bad, and it meant a lot to all of us.

There's still a tiny remnant of green Silly String® on one of the fluorescent light fixtures, and my big second grader likes to go down and admire it when he visits his old kindergarten teacher.

The decision of what to do with remaining medical supplies can be problematic. Some families get rid of them immediately, some keep them until they feel more like it is really over, and others keep them forever.

I didn't give away or throw away the formula for Tim's nasogastric tube until it expired—almost 1 year after we got it. He only had that tube in for 24 hours, but I was terrified that if we got rid of the formula he'd have to have it again. I've kept all his supplies, too. Maybe I'll get rid of them when we hit the 5-year mark. I know it is "magical thinking," but a relatively harmless thing.

The parents I know have been more upset over end of treatment than they have been relieved. The "protection" of the chemo is gone. The weekly or biweekly visits are reduced to monthly. Also, for me, I kept my emotions in check so I could function during treatment. When treatment ended, there was enough "safe time" for it all to come out.

• • • • •

I couldn't get rid of those medical supplies fast enough. I boxed them up and wanted them out of the house now. I was afraid that keeping them in the house would mean that we would need them again.

I was the same way when it came to having Elizabeth's central line removed. Nurse Linda told me there had been a mix-up in the surgery schedule and they were going to have to postpone Elizabeth's surgery. My hands started shaking and I began to cry. I was afraid that if it stayed in for even 1 more week, Elizabeth's cancer would come back. Irrational, I know. Somehow they squeezed Elizabeth into the original surgery date.

As you will discover in this book, every child, parent, and relative reacts differently to the phases of treatment and survivorship. The differences do not matter. What is important is that you recognize that all of the above feelings are normal. Whether you feel joyful, relieved, fearful, or terrified, the end of treatment evokes strong emotions in every member of the family.

Return to normal

After years of treatment, families grapple with the idea of returning to normal. Unfortunately, most families don't really know what "normal" is any longer. Parents and children realize that returning to the innocent pre-cancer days is unrealistic, that life has changed. The constant interaction with medical personnel is ending, and a new phase is beginning in which routines do not revolve around being sick, taking medicines, and going to the hospital. Although it is true that the blissful ignorance of the days prior to cancer are gone forever, a different life, a new, normal one—often enriched by friends and experiences from the cancer years—begins.

> *I try hard to believe in the "happily ever after." But I also try very hard to keep at least one foot firmly planted in reality. That way if that 2x4 ever takes another swing at me, I have a fairly good chance of being able to duck. That 2x4 packs quite a wallop!*

Parents and survivors need to talk to one another, examine their emotions, decide what course they want to chart, and work together toward a healthy life after cancer, recognizing that the journey will have twists and turns and ups and downs.

> *Many of us get pressure from family/friends/institutions to just "move on" or to "get over it." From my perspective as a cancer mom 6 years past my child's bone marrow transplant, I can tell you that moving on is relative.*
>
> *We have definitely moved on from the day-to-day struggle of current treatment. We don't have to juggle a normal family life around treatments and treatment side effects. Our stress level is definitely less than a family on current treatment. Six years out, we also rarely worry about relapse. That day-to-day fear is gone. Of course the relapse monster raises its ugly head when there are fevers or unexplained tiredness, but these are few and far between.*

We do deal with our daughter's treatment-induced learning disabilities. But even these are mundane and such a part of our lives to be considered normal (at least normal for us).

From the outside, it would seem that we should move on. However, nearly losing my child 6 years ago has changed me forever. This illness nearly ruined us financially, nearly ruined our marriage, had lasting effects on the psyches of our healthy children, and shook the very core of my spiritual and emotional self. I will never be the same. I will never be the innocent I was before. I now know that no matter how good, how bad, how smart, how stupid one is, your child can die. Because of that, I can't totally move on to the "normal" world. These feelings aren't with me every moment of every day, but they pop up enough to know I view life differently.

Since this experience is a journey, I will feel differently in 1 year and 5 years from now. I only know where I am right now.

· · · · ·

I realize that, in many ways, we have been lucky regarding our battle with cancer. Tim is still here (that is the big one). And his late effects have been much less than many kids I know of. Still, if we were really lucky, we would never have had to be in this battle at all. And I am all too aware that we are far from out of the woods. We keep reshaping our dream of what our child's life can be, grieving as we have to let go of the dream that was, and fearing for what reshapings may need to come.

· · · · ·

Joseph turned 8 a month ago and as of this morning is officially a third grader! He's quite a contrast to the kid who felt lucky to be in kindergarten 50 percent of the time, bald and skinny and barely able to climb the stairs to get to his classroom. He's dealing with some residual effects of those huge vincristine doses, but his newly restarted occupational therapy is helping a lot, and I only wish we'd done more in the past 2 years since he's been off treatment. The radiation to his right eye has caused a massive cataract, which has left him able to use only his left eye, but we're going to schedule cataract surgery in a few months and take care of that as well.

We have moved into a version of normal that certainly isn't the same as before, but it's a lovely place to be. It's sweeter, if shakier, and has a much better perspective on what's important and what the heck isn't. We're all more accepting and more relaxed. In the new normal, if it ain't bad news, then it's just fine with us. I ditched years of work and a Ph.D. dissertation to spend a year in the hospital with my kid and another year recovering, and I've kept expecting to feel slighted, but it just hasn't happened.

As survivors grow and mature, their understanding of what happened to them when they had cancer unfolds and expands. They are also ready for, and often desire, more detailed and current medical information concerning their diagnoses and treatments. The past is viewed from the perspective of an older individual with a broader world view, more education, and firmer values. They ask more questions of parents and medical personnel to more fully understand the past and its implications for the future. They will struggle to cope with, or make their peace with, any late effects from treatment that arise. And they do this on top of all the usual developmental challenges of growing up.

It's so hard to tell what life experiences are related to cancer and what aren't. It's really hard to tell if a difficulty has anything to do with my cancer history or if it's something that everybody is going through. And does that distinction even matter? I'm trying to decide now whether to drift away from my many cancer-related activities. Should I stop going to the support group? Should I spend more time with my non-cancer friends? Have I gotten everything that they can give me? And have I given enough back? I've become almost like a mentor to the other survivors. I've become a big support to many of them and at times it's stressful.

• • • • •

Elizabeth was 3 when diagnosed. In the beginning I don't think she realized she was different. Sort of like losing a tooth: it happens to everyone eventually, but somebody has to be first. During that short period of time her innocence was intact. Then the reality hit that it wasn't going to happen to everyone, she could die. Then Chelsea did die; Sam lost her arm; Sammie died. Her innocence is now gone.

In many ways she is different from the other kids. I remember when I was young, death was this vague thing that just didn't seem real, it only happened to old folks. Elizabeth doesn't have that view. Some things in life she takes very seriously. Safety issues, smoking, eating healthy, recycling, are all things that she can be quite vehement about. That is what makes her different. Her cancer experience has given her a maturity that she would not have had otherwise. And there are times when I am sad for what she has lost. But in so many more ways I'm so proud of the person she is turning into. She will be much stronger, more outspoken, more aware than I ever was.

All of that said, Elizabeth is also still very much a child. She still thinks the word "fart" is the funniest thing she has ever heard. Boys either have cooties or are her latest flame. Sleepovers are for giggling until midnight. Everything in the world should be either purple or pink. She loves to run through the woods, swing as high as the swing set will go, do flips on the monkey bars, swim until the skin threatens to peel off, and cuddle and tickle with her mom. Her world is still filled with laughter, ponytails, popsicles, and hugs. She is very much a child enjoying her childhood.

From child to adult

The passage from adolescence to adult life may be a stormy one. The maturing teen must gradually separate from the protection of parents and home and become self-reliant and independent. This process is difficult for many teens and their parents. For survivors of childhood cancer, this task can be complicated by uniquely strong ties forged with parents or complex family dynamics that grew out of the turmoil of cancer treatment. However, the progress through adolescence into young adulthood is fairly normal for most survivors. Parents show great variability in how they feel as their teens begin to think about leaving home.

> *My son left for college this week and I feel great. I was really worried about it before he left. But he's happy and he comes home weekends. He should be making friends, I guess. I talked about this with him—I asked point-blank: "Do you need friends?" and he said no, not really. He has acquaintances in his classes and I know he will be well-liked. But I said, "Well, they probably just party and drink all weekend," and he said, "Well, they drink and party all week!" So actually I'm relieved that he comes home.*

· · · · ·

> *I'm having a hard time letting go of my 18-year-old daughter. I spent so many years and so much energy keeping her alive. I was so fearful of losing her. She's a miracle. But now she needs her own life and can't continue to be tied to cancer. She wants to leave it behind and she needs to move on. Part of me also wants that for her, while another part is screaming, "I can't lose you." Thinking of her leaving is the only thing that makes me sob, and I'm always surprised at how long the sobbing lasts.*

Teens and young adults also show a mixed response to leaving the security of home for the first time.

> *In some ways, I was so mature so fast, and in other ways I was too dependent. For instance, I didn't even have my driver's license until I was 20. I really didn't drive much until I was 25. I know the social workers thought everything went seamlessly and, on the outer surface, that was so. There were many hesitancies. I stayed close to home for college. I didn't want to leave the clinic or my parents. In some ways, I feel like I'm still making the transition to adulthood, even though I'm 25 and*

married. I work with a lot of people around my age, and I'm envious. They don't have to worry about insurance or late effects from cancer, or friends who die. So in some ways I feel like I have a normal life, and in other ways I feel quite different.

· · · · ·

I had leukemia 30 years ago when I was in high school. My mother was a rock. She said, "We are going to attack this and you are going to live. Where there's a will, there's a way." My grandmother was very positive too. They pounded that into me. And I'm still here. My mother was way cool about independence. She had remarkable foresight. Here I was, a teenager, sick and dependent. She taught me to drive and let me drive to doctor appointments by myself. She gradually let me go so by the time I was leaving for college, she was treating me like an adult. And I felt ready to go and mature beyond my years.

· · · · ·

My transition was normal because I went away to college—4 hours from home. I don't think that my folks thought I would leave. I didn't show a lot of academic ambition, so it surprised them. But one day, I just decided I wanted to go and I applied to five schools. I did end up at the same college as my brother, and we even lived in the same dorm one year. In college, I made a big, fresh, new start. College was a wonderful experience for me. I had been socially awkward in grade school and high school, but in college, I made lots of friends and tried many new things. I was on cloud nine.

One aspect of transitioning to adult life is assuming control of medical decision-making. Teens change from pediatric to adult healthcare when they leave home to enter college or take a job. Many young adults do not seek out comprehensive healthcare, and for healthy individuals, this is often not a problem. But for survivors of childhood cancer who are at risk for possible late effects, difficulty in obtaining access to adult healthcare services can be serious.

I've always been very conscientious about my follow-up care. When I took a job far from home after college, I wanted to find a specialist to provide skilled follow-up care. I heard about a doctor from my hematologist and some friends who have had good experiences with him. I wrote a letter explaining my Hodgkin's history and saying that if he was accepting new patients, I'd like to set up an appointment.

Well, at my first appointment, I was delighted. He knocked, instead of walking right in, introduced himself (without the Dr. in front of his name), and sat down to take the history while I was still in my regular clothes. We went over exactly what things we needed to be concerned about at this point and what I needed to do in terms of screening, *infection prevention, etc., in a very reassuring, non-scary way. The way he individualized everything just felt so comforting.*

· · · · ·

I'm not on my parent's insurance anymore since I'm out of college. So I don't go to the clinic. I don't even have a regular doctor. I'm supposed to get tests like an echo every year, but I just don't. I guess if I get sick, I'll find a doctor.

By taking responsibility for your adult life, you can integrate the physical, emotional, intellectual, spiritual, and social parts of your life. In decades past, you might have been referred to as a "cancer victim." Now you can view yourself as someone who was victorious over cancer.

I'm an adult survivor of childhood cancer. I think you reach a point in your life where you need to integrate the experience so you are not just a cancer survivor, but a person who had cancer and learned something from it. I know people who still harbor a lot of anger or use the cancer history as a crutch. I still feel some pain for the part of my childhood that I lost, but I try not to let it get out of hand. I've realized that all humans face different crises and struggles in their lives, so my cancer experience doesn't make me special. It should help make us more under-standing of other people's struggles. I'm old enough to realize that it wasn't just about me. Everyone in my family was in the experience and changed by it. I like to turn it around in my mind and view it as some-thing that gave me strength.

Working with healthcare providers

All survivors need a long-term relationship with a knowledgeable and atten-tive healthcare provider (physician or nurse practitioner) whom they trust. If you are a cancer survivor, the provider you choose should oversee all of your medical care and refer you to specialists as the need arises. The provider should either specialize in treating survivors of cancer or be willing to work with you to keep up with the latest research and recommendations for care. Follow-up care for survivors of childhood cancer is lifelong. It is an invest-ment in your future health, and perhaps your life, to spend time finding a healthcare provider who is capable of taking care of your particular needs.

Your treatment

The first thing you share with a healthcare provider is your medical history, which includes your cancer diagnosis and treatment. Many of the 325,000 survivors of childhood cancer in North America do not know the specifics of their treatments.[1] Some do not even know they had cancer. If you don't have a detailed treatment summary, go back to your treating institution and get this important information. The more time passes, the harder it may be to track down the specifics of your treatment.

The easiest way to get a record of your treatments is to take the personal health history document in the back of this book to the healthcare providers who treated you when you had cancer and ask them to fill in the information. This health history will become an indispensable part of your medical records for the rest of your life. It should be kept in a safe place, and a copy should be given to each of your healthcare providers. When you leave home to begin your adult life, this document should go with you.

If you do not have a copy of your health history document, have a doctor or nurse at the institution that treated you write down the following important information:

- Name of disease
- Date of diagnosis and relapse, if any
- Place of treatment
- Dates of treatment
- Clinical trial protocol number and name, if applicable
- Names of attending oncologist and nurse practitioner
- Names and total dosages of chemotherapy drugs used
- Name of radiation center
- Dates radiation was received
- Amount of radiation and to what body part (for example, whole body, cranial, pelvis)
- Date and type of any surgeries
- Date and type of stem cell transplant(s), if any
- Any major treatment complications
- Any persistent side effects of treatment
- Recommended medical follow-up
- Contact numbers for treating institutions

It is also a good idea to obtain copies of key x-rays and scans. It is also important to get copies of the reports for x-rays, scans, and major surgeries that were part of your treatment. Hospitals and clinics may not retain these or they may be put in storage and be difficult to track down at a later date. You may be charged for copies, but it is well worth the price for the peace of mind that comes from having your own set of records. If you develop late effects from treatment, these early records are crucial for your current healthcare providers to review.

If late complications arise, the current doctors want to and need to see complete medical records. For instance, in my case they would have a much better idea of how extensive the heart muscle damage is if they could see the radiation records that don't exist anymore. I have spent the last year chasing medical records. It just never occurred to me that I would need them or that they would in the end be unobtainable.

· · · · ·

I'm a social worker now, and I recently moved to a big city. I called the pediatric oncology clinic at the children's hospital to ask about follow-up and was told they only follow kids who were treated there. They didn't have a recommendation for me. Then I called the women's hospitals, and they seemed to be most familiar with breast or ovarian cancer survivors—not childhood leukemia. Then I contacted the cancer society's facilitator of young adult survivor programs. She gave me the name of a nurse, who recommended a doctor. I made an appointment with the doctor and told her that it had taken a long time to find her, but I didn't know if I was in the right place. She told me I was. And it's been perfect since then.

Follow-up programs

In the past, survivors of cancer were often on their own after treatment ended. With increasing numbers of long-term survivors, it became apparent that these young men and women faced complex medical and psychosocial effects from their years of treatment. Fitzhugh Mullan, M.D., co-founder of the National Coalition for Cancer Survivorship, said, "It is as if we have invented sophisticated techniques to save people from drowning, but once they have been pulled from the water, we leave them on the dock to cough and sputter on their own in the belief that we have done all we can."[2]

Some institutions, realizing the need for long-term services for survivors, started comprehensive programs. Other institutions have difficulty obtaining support and the financial resources to start and maintain follow-up programs.

You wouldn't believe the problems survivors have with the medical community. Some doctors, acknowledging the rapidly growing body of biomedical literature demonstrating late effects as a major problem of "cure," are managing it very well. And some are playing ostrich, sticking their heads in the sand and pretending it isn't happening. The ostrich approach could cost us our lives. Ironically, I see the same set of responses from survivors themselves. We need to recognize that this isn't time for us to panic or do the ostrich thing, but a time for us to face reality with all the courage we summoned up for that first battle. Then we can find the strength to deal with this.

I'm glad my doctor isn't in the ostrich group. He deals with late effects realistically as things that may never happen to me, but problems that we simply need to keep a watchful eye out for, "just in case," so they could be treated as early as possible. I think that the state of healthcare for long-term survivors is very much like the Titanic: those in charge of our care have stayed calm and complacent for far too long. We survivors don't expect miracles, just the truth.

History of follow-up care

In 1996, the International Society of Pediatric Oncologists developed guidelines for the care of childhood cancer survivors and stressed the importance of psychological support and the education of patients about a healthy lifestyle. They stated, "We advocate the establishment of a specialty clinic oriented to the preventive medical and psychosocial care of long-term survivors . . . The goal is to promote long-term physical, psychosocial, and socioeconomic health and productivity, not merely to maintain an absence of disease or dysfunction."[3] In 2003, the Institute of Medicine published a book called *Childhood Cancer Survivorship: Improving Care and Quality of Life*, which stressed the importance of follow-up programs. The Children's Oncology Group then published follow-up guidelines in 2004 to help survivors and the healthcare providers who treat them (*www.survivorshipguidelines.org*). In addition, the American Academy of Pediatrics published guidelines in 2004 for pediatric cancer centers, which stressed the importance of long-term follow-up with "An established program designed to provide long-term, multidisciplinary follow-up of successfully treated patients at the original treatment center or by a team of healthcare professionals who are familiar with the potential adverse effects of treatment for childhood cancer."[4]

As a result of these recommendations and a growing awareness of the needs of survivors of childhood cancer, some institutions began follow-up clinics using a multidisciplinary team to monitor and support survivors. The nucleus of the team usually includes a nurse coordinator, pediatric oncologist, pediatric nurse practitioner, social worker, and psychologist. They have a close working relationship with cardiologists, endocrinologists, orthopedic surgeons, and other specialists whose services are needed by some survivors.

> *Every patient at our facility has a family care coordinator, which for us has been great. Before they started this program, every time we called we got a different nurse. Since my daughter has all sorts of late effects—seizures, brittle bones, a feeding tube, cognitive problems—trying to explain over and over again was difficult. Now we call and we always get our coordinator.*

A nurse practitioner who runs a large, well-established follow-up clinic said:

> *We really need to educate the community of healthcare providers. We have problems with healthcare workers who are attributing medical problems to cancer treatment that have nothing to do with the survivor's cancer treatment. The opposite problem happens, too. Many physicians and nurses miss obvious and sometimes life-threatening late effects. For instance, women who had high-dose radiation to the chest may develop heart disease at a young age. They are too often diagnosed with asthma or anxiety, when they really have restrictive pericarditis.*

Comprehensive follow-up care

Follow-up programs usually provide a review of treatments received, counseling about potential health risks, and any necessary diagnostic tests such as cardiac evaluations, hormonal studies, psychological evaluations, or testing for learning disabilities. These follow-up clinics not only provide comprehensive care for long-term survivors, but also participate in research projects that track the effectiveness of, and side effects from, various clinical trials. In addition, members of the follow-up clinic team act as advocates for survivors with schools, health insurance agencies, and employers. The focus of these programs should be to educate survivors about strategies to maximize their health and well-being.

> *I had neuroblastoma at age 9 months and I'm now 34. What they do in the long-term follow-up clinic is take an abdominal and chest x-ray and blood work. They ask how I am feeling, and then I leave. It is staffed by the oncologist I saw for treatment. They don't even do a physical exam. I never have been cautioned about any behaviors that increased my risk for late effects. There is never a mention of eating, drinking, sex, or sun exposure. Nothing. I'm now on a committee to change that because a teenager is not going to volunteer information during a medical appointment. If we create a comfortable climate and give out brochures about potential problems and how to take care of your health, maybe our survivors will get better care.*

• • • • •

My daughter had high-risk ALL (acute lymphoblastic leukemia) and has numerous late effects including learning disabilities, endocrine problems, hypothyroidism, osteopenia, and others. We go to an excellent follow-up program that not only provides thorough physical evaluations, but also discusses in a caring way what we may face in the future. They also talk with my teenage daughter about why doing illegal drugs, smoking, or having unsafe sex is riskier for her than for other teens. They have a whole group of specialists that we see during the same visit. The nurse practitioner writes summaries and sends them to my daughter's pediatrician and us. And they help us educate the school, her doctors, and her therapists. They are wonderful.

Finding follow-up care

Many cancer centers see long-term survivors, but do not have a comprehensive program. Others have excellent follow-up clinics. A group of parents and professionals called more than 300 institutions in the United States and Canada that treat children with cancer to assess the services each provides for survivors. The results of this survey (which is updated periodically) are on the Internet at *www.ped-onc.org/treatment/surclinics.html*. To assess the programs nearest to you, you can ask the following questions:

• How do you provide follow-up for childhood cancer survivors?

• Who is in charge of the program (doctor, nurse practitioner)?

• What is your experience in treating the late effects of childhood cancer?

• Which other professionals are part of the team?

• What is a typical visit to the follow-up clinic like?

• What transition services from child to adult care do you provide?

• Are there support groups or mentoring programs available?

The children's hospital that treated my daughter has no follow-up program. So I did some research and now we fly 1,000 miles every year to the closest good program. The appointments last a couple of hours. We see the attending physician who specializes in late effects, a social worker, and an educational specialist. A pediatric radiologist reviews her bone age x-rays, and she has blood work done that is ordered by the pediatric endocrinologist there. They also do all of the recommended screenings that she needs such as an echo every 2 years and a bone density test every 3 years. They are very helpful and thorough.

I was diagnosed with retinoblastoma in both eyes in 1956 when I was 23 months old. Both eyes were removed and I had radiation. My mother took me back for checkups, but they ended when I was 5 years old. I've basically lived a normal life. I had no recurrence. The rehab agency sends me to a normal doctor every so often for a checkup. He looks and says, "Everything seems okay," but I wouldn't call it a thorough evaluation by any means. No one's ever really followed my other late effects: hearing loss, dental problems, and sensitivity to the sun.

Comprehensive follow-up not only improves the health and quality of life for survivors, but also helps physicians evaluate the long-term effects of cancer therapies and develop safer therapies for newly diagnosed children. Advocating for comprehensive follow-up not only helps you as an individual, but may help children who will be diagnosed in the future.

I think one of the most difficult issues surrounding late effects is that some doctors want to minimize their importance and get you to focus on the "big picture," that you still have a living child. I think I can appreciate what the chemo and radiation did for my child and still get serious about getting him help to minimize the effects they will have on him as he grows older. Also, I find our oncologist to be much more straightforward about accepting and dealing with the clear-cut physical late effects of treatment. He is willing to talk very matter-of-factly about the destruction of my son's tear ducts and the large cataract caused by high-dose radiation treatments, but he has been more hesitant to help us look into the neuromuscular issues caused by chemo that are harder to diagnose and more complicated to treat. Ultimately, though, when I persisted in asking him about what looked like pretty major deficits, he referred us to a terrific occupational therapist, and my son is making good progress.

Richard Klausner, M.D., former director of the National Cancer Institute, wrote, "We must move away from the 'take no prisoners' theory of cancer care and begin considering the sequelae of the treatment we are giving patients. We have to overhaul our programs so that we can follow survivors, ask the questions, and get the answers we need to evaluate the effects of cancer treatment on long-term health."[5]

Our children's hospital doesn't have a follow-up program. Your child just sees whatever fellow happens to be there. There are no referrals, no discussion of what to watch out for. Basically it's a CBC (complete blood count) and a physical exam. I really think part of the problem in establishing these programs is that the doctors don't really want to learn about all of the late effects. I think they really feel a lot of satisfaction about curing so many kids (and we are grateful!), but knowing the price the survivors and their families sometimes pay can be very painful. That's why I think there should be a completely different program with attending physicians who specialize in late effects seeing the survivors.

It is sometimes difficult to leave your treating physician and staff for new healthcare providers. Often, the deep trust and strong ties you feel for the staff are hard to give up. However, sometimes continuing to see your treating oncologist for follow-up can create barriers to communication. Many survivors don't want to disappoint their doctors. They feel that discussing their complex feelings after treatment is not "worthy" of the doctor's time. Survivors are frequently reminded how lucky they are to be alive. Often gratitude for their life is the only socially acceptable emotion for survivors. The lack of support from society and the medical community for the difficulties that survivors often face can increase distress and frustration.

Well, we had our checkup yesterday, and our nurse practitioner gave us some good news. We will be transferring to the long-term effects clinic after our next appointment in 6 months. The long-term clinic focuses not so much on possible relapse, but on the long-term effects of childhood cancer. The clinic is run by an oncologist and a nurse. I was very happy to hear this. It really feels like we are putting this phase of our life on the back burner. I know it will never completely come off the stove, but knowing it is just simmering will be wonderful.

Some survivors feel that to express their resentment or anger will make the doctor think they are ungrateful. If you go to the oncology clinic and wait for your appointment with patients who are on treatment, you may feel that your problems are too insignificant to mention. And healthcare providers who treated you are sometimes—perhaps unconsciously—unwilling or unable to elicit all of the late effects information necessary to give good follow-up care. If you go to a specialist in late effects who was not involved in your treatment, you will not be invested in trying to protect your former healthcare provider's feelings. These problems do not arise at institutions in which treatment teams work closely with late effects specialists. At these locations, survivors get the benefits of seeing both kinds of healthcare providers without having to choose between them.

I know that they had to do the treatments to save my life, but these treatments have lots of long-term effects. I think doctors who give front-line treatment have a moral and ethical responsibility to ensure that any child or teen they treat gets educated about the risks and steered toward a place where they can get comprehensive follow-up services. The harm that has been done in saving lives needs to be addressed. We can all have more than one feeling about this. Survivors are grateful for their lives, yet sad/angry/grieving about the price they paid. Doctors can be happy to cure the kids and be disappointed or pained or angry that late effects resulted. But let's not use the difficult feelings to erect barriers to follow-up. Let's work together to address the issues.

• • • • •

I think emotionally it's very difficult for healers to deal with late effects. They do cure lots of children with cancer these days, but often at great cost. It's sometimes difficult for both survivors and treating doctors to face and discuss the physical, psychological, and social late effects. It reminds me of the line from the musical "The Wiz": "Don't nobody bring me no bad news."

Creating your own follow-up team

If you do not live near a comprehensive follow-up clinic, you will need to assemble a team of healthcare providers in your community. The first and most important member of the team is a primary care provider. This could be an internist, pediatrician, nurse practitioner, or women's health specialist (gynecologist). You may need to interview several healthcare providers to find the best fit.

I have multiple late effects and see many specialists. I don't have a family doctor who looks at all of me. So I call my GI (gastrointestinal) doctor my "triage doctor." He is the one who discovered my heart problems. Whenever I see him I ask him to look over my whole body, but I'll only make him care for the GI problems. We are a good team.

• • • • •

I was treated by an adult oncologist when I had Hodgkin's and have continued to see him for 22 years. We never needed a follow-up schedule because I have so many late effects. I've seen him every 3 or 4 months since I was diagnosed. Thank heaven for my doctor. When I'm sick, I can call him up and he believes what I tell him. I don't have to march my sick body down there every time to make sure I'm telling him the truth. We really trust one another and I've had great care.

The most important qualities to look for in your primary care provider are the abilities to care about you, listen to you, work with you to assemble a team, and read the literature about late effects. The provider should refer you to specialists as needed, organize your healthcare, and function as your medical case manager.

I like being followed at a teaching hospital. I just don't think most doctors have time to keep up with the literature. I think that's why the conscientious ones go to seminars so they can get a bunch of information in a hurry. There is a lot for each doctor to know. So it does place responsibility on the patient. When you have an unusual pattern going on, have several doctors look at you. Go for that second opinion so you get more information. I don't expect doctors to know everything, but I do wish that more were intellectually curious. Those are the ones who have helped me the most with my multiple late effects.

Try to find someone who is willing to work with you to address any health problems that arise and do thorough checkups to find any problems early. You need someone who listens, provides plenty of time, and is interested in working with you to make a long-term health plan. If your current healthcare provider stands with one hand on the doorknob while you are asking questions, it may be time to look elsewhere.

I was diagnosed in 1976 with leukemia (ALL). After 5 years of treatment, I maintained contact and had annual checkups with my cancer clinic as well as the family pediatrician. Clinic visits included blood tests and physicals, as well as psychosocial adjustment and learning patterns. During high school, I continued with checkups; during college, I may have missed a year.

In graduate school, I fell out of follow-up. This was due to many factors, including living out of state, no longer being covered under my parents' insurance, and not really understanding the need to go back to the childhood cancer clinic. I really didn't fit in there anymore. I did get a copy of my records and gave a copy to my general practice doctor. This was just in the nick of time as my hospital was bought out and closed down.

Then about 3 years ago, I moved to a large city, and after much struggle, I found a doctor who specialized in long-term cancer follow-up and late effects at a university hospital. I now see her annually as well as a general practitioner and a gynecologist.

The more informed you are about your own risk profile, the better you can advocate for appropriate care. For example, if you know you are at risk for thickening of the wall of the heart and you are having chest pains, you can ask your primary healthcare provider for a referral to a cardiologist. If you then tell the cardiologist your history, symptoms, and what you are at risk for, you are much more likely to be properly diagnosed. Spending the time to find a caring healthcare provider to whom you can go and say, "I'm having these symptoms," is well worth it. Together you can work toward a healthy life.

I had Wilms tumor in 1962 when I was 2 years old. I have no late effects other than slight scoliosis (curvature of the spine). I went for yearly checkups with an obstetrician but never had a primary doctor until recently. I had had joint swelling off and on for years and had been to several doctors who all blew me off. I found a really great primary care doctor, and she sent me to a rheumatologist who found swollen lymph nodes. So I was sent to an oncologist for a thorough evaluation. It was not cancer, but I was very glad my primary care provider sent me to see the specialists.

After you have educated yourself about your history and risks, do not hesitate to be a friendly advocate. Explain (in person, on the phone, or by email) your position and concerns, and state what you would like to have happen.

Our transplant center was relatively new (my daughter was their 21st patient) and thus inexperienced at follow-up. My daughter wasn't growing and I pushed for an appointment with an endocrinologist. I knew she'd have endocrine problems because the tumor was right next to her pituitary gland and she got a lot of radiation there. After seeing the local endocrinologist, I told my oncologist that I didn't have a lot of confidence in the endocrinologist. He said there were only a handful of doctors in the country who were experienced in what my daughter was going through. I researched the literature and went to get a second opinion from one of the leading pediatric endocrinologists in the country. He explained clearly what was known and what was not. It was reassuring to talk with him.

· · · · ·

I am a big fan of second opinions. They either reassure that you are on the right treatment plan or tell you are on the wrong treatment plan and explain why. What makes more sense than that?

The following are some ways to advocate for the best possible medical care:

- Use the personal health record at the back of this book to educate your primary healthcare provider and all specialists about your treatments.

- Refer to the Children's Oncology Group's recommendations for follow-up care.

- Keep files containing copies of key x-rays, diagnostic tests, and reports.

- Keep your healthcare provider updated about any health concerns or symptoms you have. A nurse practitioner from a busy follow-up clinic said:

I've been taking care of survivors for 18 years. Many of them apologize for "bothering me" when they call with a question or concern. Almost always they are calling with good questions about appropriate issues. Even if you think it is insignificant, if it bothers you, discuss it with your healthcare provider by phone, email, or during an appointment.

- Find a resource person at a comprehensive follow-up clinic whom your healthcare provider can call for specialized information or advice. Phone consultations are common.

- Based on an accurate understanding of your treatment, know what medical services you require and what type of monitoring you need, and ensure that these are provided by your healthcare team. If you are not getting the follow-up you need, consider having a frank discussion about your concerns or locating a primary care provider with a better understanding of survivorship.

I have been a Hodgkin's survivor for 33 years. I recently asked my husband what his strongest memory about my health problems is. He said when I became proactive and insistent about my care 4 years ago. It changed my healthcare completely. Survivors need to get second opinions and insist on tests if they think something is going on. This reduces your anxiety as well as minimizes risks. I think we will educate the doctors, one by one, by providing them with information on survivorship that they don't have. We all need to develop a partnership mentality. We survivors are on the leading edge of these changes. Doctors are strong team members with information and skills that we need. We, however, bring to the partnership knowledge, information, and late effects that the doctor may not have seen.

- Learn what you need to know, surround yourself with knowledgeable professionals, and live your life to the fullest.

Information is a double-edged sword. There is considerable relief in knowing what the future might hold. But often when we are told we are cured, we go into magical thinking that it is over. It is not for most of us. Reading a book about late effects may bring grief. You may realize that life has been forever changed. But grieving the losses and even what the future may hold is a way of deepening your life.

Chapter 2

Emotions

*It has done me good to be somewhat parched
by the heat and drenched by the rain of life.*

—Henry Wadsworth Longfellow

IMPROVEMENT IN TREATMENT for childhood cancer is a huge success story in modern medicine. It is now known, however, that survivors and their families often face many physical and psychological challenges after cure. You may be dealing with late effects from treatment, as well as struggling to find a new "normal" in your life. You will probably experience a range of strong emotions as you adjust to your after-cancer life; these can include fear of recurrence, anxiety, guilt, and grief, as well as gratitude and joy. Some survivors experience these reactions even if they remember very little—or even nothing—about their cancer experience. Knowing that other survivors and members of their families share these emotions can help you feel less alone.

Fears of recurrence

Survivors and their parents experience a whole spectrum of feelings about possible relapse. Some people say they never think about it. They acknowledge it could happen, but they say, "I'll deal with it if it happens." It no longer seems to be a part of their daily, weekly, or monthly reality. Many feel anxious when an anniversary date approaches or it is time for a medical checkup. And some, even many years after treatment, still have nightmares or anxiety attacks that may interfere with daily life.

> *Matthew has his first post-treatment scans in 12 hours. I'm freaked out and can't sleep. Every time I think about it, I feel the bile rising. I have been watching his every little move and complaint, and each time I'm convinced that it must be a relapse. If he walks in saying, "Mommy, my toe hurts!" I think, "Oh, no, relapse!" But then I have to stop myself, calm down, and recognize that it's only a stubbed toe. Then I count how many bruises he has—how many are just from playing outside and how many are from low platelets? I even checked his temperature yesterday*

because I was convinced that he had a fever—it was 98.2°. He was cold. I think I'm going nuts!

This is really hard, being off treatment. I feel like I'm just waiting...waiting...waiting...and holding down the vomit. Of course some members of my family say these great things like, "I'm sure it will be just fine," or "You just aren't accepting the fact that he is a normal, healthy kid now." How am I going to even make it through the day? How do I respond when the scans come back clear? Will I scream for joy? Cry? Laugh? Oh God, what if they aren't clear?

• • • • •

It's been 4 years since my osteosarcoma was diagnosed and I don't even think about relapse. Relapse happens most often in the first year, so the farther out I get the less likely it is to occur. But, honestly, I never really worried about it.

You may be surprised to find that your feelings about recurrence vacillate over time. You may go through a period of fearfulness, followed by a long time when you do not think about cancer. One mother said, "Funny how you think you've got the fear under control, then something happens and you again feel your head swimming, stomach churning, and your legs becoming spaghetti." It's normal to be at different places on this spectrum at different times.

I was just thinking that this state of vigilance and worry never seems to go away. I know that parents of kids who are years out of treatment seem to do better with this, but it's not easy. Even when things are going well and you're sure it's just a cold, that worry is there. The thought in the back of your head says, "What if it isn't just a cold?" I look forward to the day when that thought in the back of my head is not my first thought when my son is sick. I know it will come.

In the last week, my teenage son, who is 3 months off treatment, has had a decreased appetite and has been very tired. I know he's worried about the "what if" question, but hasn't voiced it. He's just extra quiet, so we've mentioned that he probably just has a cold or "bug" that's going around and needs more sleep (what teenager doesn't?). But we all know that somewhere in all of our heads, there are bells ringing. I know, in my head, that this is just a cold. But my heart whispers, "What if?"

• • • • •

My daughter is 12 years out from a diagnosis of average risk ALL (acute lymphoblastic leukemia). She is doing just great. But last week I noticed bruises on her legs and I flipped right back into that fear and panic. I thought, "Oh, my God, it's back."

· · · · ·

Seven years ago my daughter was diagnosed with leukemia. I had panic attacks while she was on treatment, and periodically during the first year off treatment when she was most at risk to have a recurrence. But those fears gradually just faded off my radar scope. I don't think about it at all—it's just no longer part of my life. I realize there is a tiny chance it could come back, but it just doesn't concern me. If it happens, we'll deal with it—just like we did the first time.

· · · · ·

My AML (acute myelogenous leukemia) was cured 15 years ago with chemotherapy. There are good things and bad things that came out of it. I'm very careful when I drive because I know I can die. This is good. I also grew as a person, and also realize that cancer is not the only thing in life. I do not worry about getting it again.

· · · · ·

I'm 14 and had a brain tumor when I was 8. I never worry about it coming back, but I'm reminded of it almost every day when problematic situations arise due to my visual problems. The brain tumor caused my vision problem, but the vision impairment is the only thing that bothers me today.

You may not normally be bothered by fears of relapse—until your annual follow-up appointment draws close. Sometimes, visiting the hospital for blood work, x-rays, and an examination causes dormant feelings to surface. This is a very common phenomenon, and each survivor has individual ways of dealing with these normal feelings.

I was incredibly embarrassed the first time I walked into the follow-up clinic with my daughter. I hadn't been in a children's hospital for over 3 years, and I thought I had worked through all of my strong feelings about her treatment. But the first bald kid I saw crying about an "owie" caused me to just break down in tears. I felt all the craziness that I felt back then just well up and spill out. I could barely talk and I was mortified. The only person who seemed comfortable with my feelings was the social worker who told me that I was experiencing a perfectly normal post-traumatic stress reaction. My daughter just pretty much shut down and wouldn't talk to anyone. Afterwards, she just said, "Mom, let's walk around outside for a while and we'll both feel better."

Some survivors and some parents of survivors find that they continue to have deep fears of recurrence over an extended period of time. For others, fear and distress are less about recurrence and more about the emergence of late effects. If you find that any of these concerns interfere on a regular basis with your daily life, get some mental health support. Individual or family counseling and support groups help to reduce isolation, allow sharing of suggestions for dealing with survivorship issues, and can help channel strong feelings in constructive ways. Mental health professionals can help you prevent problems from arising or deal with them if they do appear.

> *The concerns about relapses haunted me through most of my young adult life, and it was only with outside help that I was able to put to rest the more troubling aspects of these worries. Psychotherapy gave me better coping mechanisms and made me a better advocate for my own healthcare. I got to be a better observer of my symptoms with a better balance between realistic health concerns and what I call my more neurotic concerns. I also was able to overcome my hospital and needle phobia, both of which developed during my initial treatment. Mastering those two fears was a wonderful thing, especially since my career has often found me in hospital settings.*

Anniversary reactions

Anniversaries can be times of pain or joy and sometimes an inexplicable mix of both. There are different anniversaries for everyone: for some it is the date of diagnosis, while for others it is the last day of treatment. Some survivors celebrate the 5-year remission date. Whether or not any of these anniversary dates are "marked," they are likely to touch off some kind of emotional reaction—and this is normal. One mother of a teen with cancer said, "I think that whenever we touch the same place in the circle of the year, we stop and look around us to see the different shapes and colors of reality. And it often takes our breath away."

For families of survivors with few or no long-term effects from their treatment for cancer, anniversaries are sometimes forgotten and sometimes celebrated. Some families file the memories away and skip rituals that tie them to the memories of hard times. Others remember and give thanks for their life and good health.

> *I was diagnosed a couple of days before my dad's birthday and had my port surgery on that day—February 7. But I don't think about that on his birthday anymore. My family actually celebrates a "cancer-free" day every year on the date of my last chemotherapy. Now that I'm in college, they usually send me flowers. I also send an email out to all my friends that says something like, "Three years—Yay Erin." I get lots of congratulations emails back.*

············

Some memories are so clear and just never fade with time. I was diagnosed with Hodgkin's disease in 1972. I can remember exactly what I was doing when I found the enlarged lymph node that led to my diagnosis. And I remember exactly what I was wearing when the doctors told me I had HD. And I remember exactly what my fiancé said after we walked out of the doctor's office. And what my parents' faces looked like when they came out of the office and walked back across campus with us. So when Christmas rolls around I find myself with thoughts that stray to these very vivid memories. Hard not to.

Families of survivors with numerous or serious late effects from treatment may have more evident daily reminders of their anniversaries. They often struggle with the urge to be grateful for life, but grieve the many losses.

I guess it's not surprising or novel that I have mixed emotions about this anniversary. First and foremost I am out of my mind joyful that he is still here with me, cancer-free, able to talk and walk and sing and do every little thing that I will never take for granted again.

But then there are the constant reminders of all that he has lost, and I know I need to somehow and finally come to grips with those losses, but I don't have the capacity to do that yet, it seems. When we are in a crowd, and maybe he is 5 feet from me, and he looks around for me, I know he can't see, because he doesn't know which person is me until I say his name and wave. This is unbearably sad for me.

My son was singing songs at 6 months old, a leader in his day care, the biggest, most advanced kid in any group of peers, running laps at 20 months. And today people see this big kid who looks older than he is and who acts kind of clingy, limps, seems a bit slow, doesn't look you in the eye, doesn't pay attention, can't catch a ball or run. I just still want to grab the world by the lapels and shake it and scream.

But because it's cancer, I'm supposed to be just completely happy with the situation (which I am, at the same maddening time). But if my son had been hit by a drunk driver or in a hit and run, I would be allowed my rage. I'd be validated in my hatred for the person who caused this ruin in our lives.

Are these anniversary rantings? Oh, I think they're everyday rantings, but because it's anniversary time, they're just so much more intense. I'm beginning to think that anniversaries just sharpen the point of the pencil, and make the lines finer and the words sharper.

Sometimes it is not a specific date, but an entire month or season that is fraught with significance.

> Before 1988, our family had good associations for the month of August. Kimbra and all her cousins were born in August, and each of their dads was born in August. Each year we would have our big family picnic and celebrate everyone's birthday. My grandparents also had their wedding anniversary in August.

> In 1988, Kimbra was diagnosed with cancer. She had chemotherapy, radiation, and surgery. We got bad news on her birthday and her dad's birthday, so August now has some bad memories. However, the important thing is that we have August days to celebrate her still being with us. When the anniversary dates evoke bad memories, we try to cancel them out with lots of big hugs.

Cancer affects everyone in the family—often in different ways. It helps if family members share their feelings so they can create their own rituals to cope with or celebrate anniversaries. And each family should decide for itself when it is time to continue the tradition or let it fade into the past.

> My daughter is 7 and was diagnosed at age 3 with Wilms tumor. We celebrate her remission date every year. This year, we went to the hospital to say thank you to her doctors, then met some TV people who did a piece on childhood cancer, and then to Chuck E. Cheese®. It was a full, happy day. I wondered if I shouldn't just let the memories slip away and stop celebrating. I asked my daughter what she thought, and she said, "So many people worked so hard to save me that I think it is important to remember."

· · · · ·

> The diagnosis anniversary has always been hard for me. The way I deal with it—at least since I figured out what the problem was—is to try to cut myself some slack for those days. I eat my favorite meals, watch favorite movies plus ones I want to see for the first time, spend a lot of time basically just doing what I want when I'm not at work. I consider it my way of celebrating the fact that I'm still here after 10 years and of "defying" Hodgkin's—blowing raspberries, if you will!

> The more you try to deny your feelings about it, the worse it is. Give in and you might be surprised at how much better you feel. I cry less when I let myself do what I want instead of holding myself to the same standards as the rest of the year.

Grief and loss

Although survivors were able to grab the ultimate "gold ring"—life—they often suffer losses in the process. Losses come in all shapes and forms and may emerge or continue to exist for many years, or even a lifetime. A universal loss is the sense that the world is a safe place. Childhood cancer robs the entire family of that blissful belief in the natural order of things—that children will have happy and carefree childhoods and that children never die before their parents.

Treatment for childhood cancer also can result in the loss of abilities, life prospects, skills, or body parts. A star baseball player can be relegated to the bench. A skier might lose his leg. An "A" student might discover when she returns to school that she is no longer gifted in mathematics. And grief over the loss of normal development opportunities, such as missing the time when teens start to date or play competitive sports on organized teams, are common. These losses put survivors out of step with their peer groups, which in turn limits opportunities to develop friendships. Thus, survivors must cope not only with physical changes, but also with the alteration of their self-image.

> I was 16 years old and on the national championship hockey cheerleading team when I was diagnosed with osteosarcoma. I never went back to high school, and I'll never cheerlead again. I had an allograft and a total knee replacement. I can't kneel, sit cross-legged, or bend my knee all the way.

The feelings most often associated with the normal grieving process are denial, anxiety, fear, guilt, depression, and anger. These completely normal feelings are sometimes viewed by others as a problem when they are actually a natural response to a life-changing event. It is important and necessary to acknowledge these feelings in order to deal with what cannot be changed and to make the most of your life, even if it has changed.

> In the hubbub of packing this week for vacation, I came upon Nicholas playing in his room with Mr. Potato Head® and his potato head pals. The Big Spud was lying down, without arms or feet, and Nick was crying. I asked what was wrong, and Nicholas said he and the little pals were crying because "Mr. Potato Head® died since his bone marrow transplant didn't work right." Damn, a 5-year-old's play pals shouldn't be dying from failed bone marrow transplants. I hate this disease.

Part of coping with grief involves sharing it with loved ones. In our society, expressing these feelings is often socially unacceptable. Survivors and parents struggle to balance gratitude for life with sadness over the losses. However, parents and survivors may not view these issues in the same way, and conflicts may arise, creating an inability to rely on each other for support.

> I feel that having a life-threatening illness, being treated for it and surviving, can trigger strong emotions—anxiety, fear, anger, and sadness. If these feelings aren't acknowledged, addressed, and treated, they can over time evolve into more chronic problems like panic disorders and depression.

> Most of the psychosocial literature says that survivors as a group are pretty well adjusted, that we marry, work, and raise children if we can have them. And that most of us seem to have come to some terms with our illness. But I have to say that my experience, both personal and from having talked with so many survivors, differs. It is not that we aren't well adjusted, but that we have paid an emotional price for surviving and that we seldom meet non-survivors who get it. To the world of non-survivors, we present a face that is strong, mostly good natured, thankful, and grateful. With other survivors we are able to articulate our fears, anger, and sadness.

Relatives, friends, and professionals who work with families of people who have survived childhood cancer need to recognize that grief over loss is very similar to the grief one feels when a loved one dies. They need to listen, understand, and support the legitimacy of these feelings. Suffering is diminished when it is shared.

Parents of children who were treated at a very young age have a need to grieve about things their children may not even be aware of.

> I think the little kids with significant side effects soon learn they are different but don't remember who they were. Well, we do. We remember those carefree days with kids who glowed with health and good spirits. We know the price we paid, and it's incredibly painful. Yet we also know how lucky we are and feel that we should be grateful instead of grieving. It's a hard road.

In some cases, radiation at a young age can cause a change in personality and capabilities, so it may seem as if the child you knew and loved disappeared, and a new child replaced him.

It's so hard to talk about losing part of who your child was. I keep feeling I should be grateful for her life, but I'm grieving—by myself—for her losses. And it's not getting any easier. I have huge worries about whether she will ever be able to live independently. And I've never talked to anyone about it, nor have they asked. I mean, what a thing for a parent to deal with. We went from having a bright kid full of promise to a kid with major problems with basic life skills. I dreamed she'd go to college, maybe get married, move away, take care of herself. And now I don't know what's going to happen.

· · · · ·

My son has several disabilities from his treatment for a brain tumor. I don't know how much will improve or get worse. I lost the child I had before. I told a friend once that the child I brought into the hospital was a different one than the one I brought home. It shocked her, but I realized I really needed to grieve that loss. I'm not saying that I love him less, just that we all suffered a big loss.

You may find that at different ages, you view and feel your losses differently. A child of 10 may understand that his learning disabilities were the price he paid for cure from cancer, but a 20-year-old in college will probably have very different feelings as he is making career choices that may be affected by his disabilities. Similarly, a teenage girl may view potential infertility differently than an adult woman in love who is discussing marriage and contemplating having a family.

You can grieve fully, but later, still be stunned on occasion by a wave of grief. Everyone gets blindsided by a reminder of the loss. Stressors that can cause feelings to erupt include anniversaries, routine medical tests, or even a smell. Returning to the clinic for an appointment, developing an illness, or discovering a late effect can arouse strong feelings. The upsurge of physical or emotional responses doesn't mean you have to go through the whole process again, but it can feel overwhelming.

Survivors and their families describe a multitude of ways to work through the grief associated with childhood cancer. Some talk with family members and friends; others share their emotions by asking for hugs or a shoulder to cry on. Some join support groups (in person or online) to talk about their feelings with others in similar circumstances. Others prefer individual, private counseling to discuss their grief and feelings of loss. Some survivors describe taking better care of themselves or doing pleasurable activities whenever they felt sad about the changes in their lives. Others talk about the importance of their faith or religion in getting them through the tough spots. You can also ask loved ones for help during difficult times.

Anger

In addition to the emotional reactions already discussed, many survivors and their families experience feelings of anger in the years after treatment ends. It is not unusual for survivors or family members to feel robbed of a "normal" life when they experience reminders of the costs of cancer and treatment. Adolescents just understanding the ramifications of their physical differences, for example, might feel anger that waxes and wanes over several months as they deal with questions like: "Why did this happen to me?" "When will I just be a normal kid?" "What do you mean this won't ever really be over with?" Parents, too, might feel bursts of anger as they watch their children continue to struggle with late effects of treatment. One father disclosed, for example, that even 20 years after his daughter's successful treatment for a brain tumor, he has weeks when he is incredibly angry that the possibility of independent living has been stolen from her, and that he must continue to worry about who will provide for his child when he is no longer able to do so.

> My wife got sad, but I got very angry and have stayed that way in the years since my son was diagnosed. I feel like the disease stole his childhood and stole part of my life as a parent. It took away some of his abilities and wrecked his friendships. The disease is rotten, the treatment is rotten, and I get furious just thinking about it.

It is important to keep in mind that feeling angry is a normal, healthy reaction to the losses caused by cancer. You are most likely to feel bursts of anger at times when life changes or developmental demands remind you of the things you have lost to cancer. This might mean that you are angry a year after cancer, or even 20 years after cancer. These feelings might occur with other feelings or might occur by themselves. You might find that your anger, or that of your child, parent, sibling, or partner, is expressed through behavior such as tantrums or angry, destructive actions.

When these angry periods come up, it is best to recognize them for what they are—normal reactions to an unusual life situation—and to express that anger as best you can to those with whom you are close. If that is not possible, or if angry feelings or behaviors get in the way of doing what you want to do in your life or affect your relationships, seek support from a mental health professional, support group, nurse, nurse practitioner, or physician. Survivors and their family members have reported that once they feel supported in putting cancer and its inevitable effects in their place, they are able to more comfortably manage the anger without letting it derail them.

I was amply informed about anger as a normal emotion I might experience, but it really didn't surface for me until about 3 years after the end of treatment for Hodgkin's. Then it came out fighting and grew. I was mainly angry about how many friends I began losing to cancer, especially a so-called good kind like Hodgkin's. But as time passed, I became very angry about the ways in which cancer has influenced my life choices. I can't simply take a semester or year off to travel or do whatever like many of my colleagues have—there's the insurance coverage to consider. It makes me really angry when others try to tell me how I should feel, reminding me how much others have achieved after cancer and how grateful I should be just to be alive. Give me a break!

One thing that does help with the anger is channeling it into a constructive form. For example, anger over the deaths of my friends and over my own experiences led me to write an application piece to be a delegate from my state to The March in September 1998. I was indeed chosen, and even asked to speak before our representatives' and senators' assistants. It was an incredibly emotional experience, but one of the best I've ever had. Some of the audience members began crying as I spoke. It was a wonderfully fulfilling experience that grew out of my own anger and frustration.

Anxiety and depression

Anxiety and depression can be seen as two sides of the same coin. For many survivors, anxiety is fear related to losses that may occur in the future, while depression is sadness related to losses that occurred in the past. Both of these emotions are a normal part of anyone's life, but both can become troublesome for survivors.

In the case of anxiety, survivors can become focused on the fear of a relapse or fear of late effects. If the anxiety grows too large, it may compromise a survivor's ability to seek appropriate healthcare. In essence, the survivor becomes afraid of knowing. Sometimes survivors become embarrassed or ashamed of their concerns about their health and body. After all, young adults aren't generally worried about things such as cancer or heart problems. So normal health concerns for survivors may make them feel strange and out of step with their peers.

Just before the 11-year anniversary of my Hodgkin's diagnosis, I began seeing a psychologist who specializes in young adults with chronic and life-threatening illnesses. It has truly been the best decision I've ever made, and I'm glad that I was able to ignore the stigma enough to realize that there is nothing wrong with some good old-fashioned talk therapy.

I have friends and family, but there are some things you just can't say to them no matter how close you are. In working with my psychologist, I've rediscovered a lot of the best parts of my pre-cancer self, worked out a lot of my stressors, and just vented my spleen (or should I say the area where my spleen would be?) about issues. It has truly helped me feel less stressed, more at peace, and—well, there's no truly good word for the feeling. I wish this was something I could have started years ago.

Some survivors worry that they are hypochondriacs—that they are overly concerned about their health. They become fearful that their doctors will view them as complainers or find their health worries crazy. This type of anxiety can interfere with getting good, thorough follow-up care. Anxiety that interferes with life in this way can be crippling and detrimental. Survivors who feel extreme anxiety should seek help from a professional. There are many ways to reduce anxiety and not allow it to overwhelm your life.

Depression should be distinguished from the normal sadness about the real losses that can occur from treatment. Sadness can arise from temporary losses, such as the loss of hair, to permanent losses, such as the loss of fertility or mobility. Depression takes over normal sadness when a person is only able to focus on the losses and can no longer find any pleasure in life. It can become crippling and prevent the survivor from seeking and getting appropriate care and from enjoying the positive aspects of life.

When people are profoundly depressed, they may feel life is not worth living, or that they are not worthy of care and help. They often lack the energy to participate in activities that used to interest them, and they may withdraw from important relationships and social interactions. These feelings make it especially hard for them to get the help they need, both physically and emotionally. No one should have to suffer alone through depression; it can be successfully treated with counseling and/or medications.

There was a time after I finished treatment when my sadness and grief had clearly turned to depression. I found that life was bitter and sour, and I couldn't find joy or relief anywhere. I could identify reasons that this was so: Concerns about my health, my infertility, a marriage that had been strained beyond the saving point by my anxieties about a relapse. The reasons for the depression were everywhere I looked, and although I could identify the reasons, know what they were, I could not alter the depression.

In this case, I would say that things that I did and should feel naturally sad about had become twisted into something more than sadness, had become depression. And my internal world was bleak and dark, despite the fact that there were many fine and wonderful things in my external world.

This is when I sought out psychotherapy. I knew I was no longer able to help myself and disentangle the strands that had me caught in such a dark state. And it helped.

Survival guilt

Some survivors feel guilty that they survived when so many others did not. Sometimes they feel life is going to be short, so they must push themselves very hard. Because they feel they don't have much time, they want to squeeze in as much as possible.

The thing that I wrestle with all the time is survivor guilt. When children I know die, I almost can't look their parents in the face. I know in my head that it's not my fault, but it never feels like enough. I feel like saying, "I'm sorry I am here and your daughter is not; I wish to God I could change it." The best that I can do is share something special that I remember. It's a poor comfort, but at least somebody remembers. There is a lot in the storyteller concept. There's a great line in Miss Rose White where she says, "If I forget, who will remember?"

· · · · ·

Survivor guilt is a real problem. Often I find myself caught between needing to share my concerns and feeling guilty because I'm alive, I'm doing well, and so many aren't. It's a tough line to walk. I have found a great deal of comfort from reading Holocaust literature. Presently I'm reading Night, by Elie Wiesel, which is absolutely gripping. Frankly, I think there are a lot of similarities.

One of the hardest things to learn to realize is that we can't change certain things. My life did not come at the expense of anyone else's. If I could do anything to save theirs, I would do so gladly.

· · · · ·

Five years ago today, I gave a mini-memorial-eulogy for my best friend, who died following a second BMT (bone marrow transplant) at the very medical center where I now work. She was a sweet and kind and gentle and bright young woman, and her death left me with so many questions. Five years later I still can't say I have all the answers, but I have come to some peace with matters. Not the wrong kind—the kind that becomes complacent with seeing these things happen—but the kind that lets me understand that I cannot hold myself responsible for them.

Another form of guilt that survivors with many late effects sometimes feel is related to the effect their limitations have on those they love.

> My survivor's guilt has a different cause. I feel guilty about how much my need for high maintenance affects and limits my husband's choices about work, life and health insurance, where we live, how much extra money there is for recreation, how he has to go to many things by himself, how many chores I have to leave for him because it's too heavy. The list goes on. I know he is also gaining some things, too, like gold stars and a pair of angel wings.

Some families have genetic forms of cancer that are passed from parent to child through genes. When a child develops cancer, some parents feel very guilty that their genes are the cause of their child's suffering.

> I had neuroblastoma, and my daughter was born with neuroblastoma. I was angry that I passed it on to her although I knew it wasn't my fault. At one point I made a comment to my minister about it, and he looked at me and said, "You didn't ask for your genes either, did you?" I realized he was right and that was the end of that.

Another variation on survivor guilt is that some survivors are burdened by what feels like extra-high expectations about what they will do with their lives and what they will achieve. They have the sense that they are expected to do more than the average person, because they survived cancer. And they may feel guilty about just wanting to be themselves without the added weight of super-size expectations.

Post-traumatic stress

During treatment, patients are engaged in an arduous battle against their cancer. They direct all of their time, energy, and strength toward dealing with immediate survival. But when the treatments stop, the drugs aren't necessary, and the scars heal, many survivors come to realize there is also an emotional price to pay and that being free of cancer does not mean their emotions are cancer-free.

Some feelings may be set aside while you cope with treatment, but when treatment ends, you are left to come to grips with the experience and what it means in your life. That process can be very difficult. Family, friends, and doctors may brush off your concerns, saying it's time to "get on with your life." You may think that ignoring the feelings will cause them to disappear. Unresolved emotions usually don't just vanish—they may even grow stronger and surface unexpectedly.

I had Hodgkin's when I was 15. I tried so hard as a freshman in college to put it behind me and get on with my life. It just didn't work. Next to treatment, that was the worst year of my life. It showed me that if I didn't deal with it consciously, I was going to deal with it subconsciously. I had nightmares every night. I'd wake up feeling like I had needles in my arms. Once I started dealing with it, things improved. I had a wonderful English composition teacher that year. I really spilled out my soul to him in writing that year, and he held it gently. I've just written him a thank-you note telling him that upon rereading my journal, I came to realize how much I put into his hands that year.

After people experience a traumatic event, they may have feelings of anxiety that persist over time. Just like soldiers returning from combat, survivors of childhood cancer and family members may experience symptoms of post-traumatic stress. Some of the most common symptoms are:

• Avoiding people, places, and thoughts that remind you of treatment.

• Being hypervigilant (feeling constantly "on alert").

• Difficulty falling or staying asleep.

Other symptoms include irritability or angry outbursts, difficulty concentrating, or having an exaggerated startle response. Some people tend to have intrusive recollections or dreams of the event, or feelings that the trauma is recurring (flashbacks). Survivors and their family members may have only some of these symptoms of post-traumatic stress, or they may have enough symptoms to meet the criteria for a diagnosis of post-traumatic stress disorder (PTSD).

I had cancer when I was 19, and it recurred at 21. I have frequent nightmares. I sit up in my sleep screaming. My fiancé tells me about them in the morning—I usually don't remember. I also wake up if any sound reminds me of the hospital. For instance, that crinkly sound the hospital beds make when you move reminds me of getting transfusions. If I hear any crinkly sounds in the night, I wake up really scared. This Halloween I went into a haunted house and had an anxiety attack. The flashing lights disoriented me, and I felt like I was in the hospital on Ativan®. I started breathing fast and my heart raced. I had to leave and go home.

• • • • •

About 2 a.m., I woke up and my husband was sitting on the edge of the bed crying. I asked him if everything was okay and he said yes, so I drifted off again. A little while later he woke me up and asked me to stay awake with him. He was sweating, breathing fast, and his heart was racing. He said he had had a flashback about our son's cancer and was afraid he was losing his mind. I just held him and told him that our son was okay. In about half an hour he was calm again and we both went to sleep. The last few weeks it's been pretty obvious that he was suffering from other than ordinary stress, and we've been discussing him getting some help. My gut tells me this is urgent.

· · · · ·

A year or so after treatment, I was watching one of those St. Jude specials (I avoid them now). When one of the children's IV (intravenous) pumps beeped, all the blood left my head, I got terribly dizzy, and I almost passed out. What a visceral reaction! And I thought I had adjusted well.

Rates of PTSD among survivors and their parents are generally low, but many survivors and their parents have some symptoms of post-traumatic stress.[1,2] The good news is that treatments are available to help people recover from PTSD or manage post-traumatic stress symptoms.

Networking for support

You don't feel alone when you have close relationships with people who have walked the same path. Exchanging information, experiences, and thoughts with others who have similar life experiences forges close ties. Even survivors with close families and friendships often seek out peer support. Support networks can help you regain control of some aspects of your life and learn how others have coped with similar problems, as well as vent feelings that are shared by other members of the group. The sense of community can help dispel the isolation felt by too many survivors. Support can profoundly affect the way you view yourself and how you manage your life after cancer. Appendix B, *Resources*, contains lists of organizations and online sites that provide ways to network for support.

Our children's hospital organized a get-together for all the families of children with brain tumors. It was so nice to learn that the things we thought only happened to us were issues that all the other families were struggling to cope with. For instance, problems with reading and writing were widespread, and I just was not aware of that. I felt so much less alone. It opened another door for us.

· · · · ·

After I survived cancer in my teens, I became an outsider. I looked at life in a completely different way. I just couldn't relate to other teenagers. I felt like I had the mind of an 85-year-old woman. What saved me was the close friendships I formed with five other teens on treatment at the same time as I was. I'm the oldest now at 21 (5 years off treatment), and the youngest is 17. We all survived, and we talk all the time. They have been my biggest support. Even our parents are close.

Networking for support can occur in many ways: talking with a fellow survivor, attending survivor conferences and camps, joining a survivor support group, organizing or attending educational workshops, or participating in an Internet discussion group.

I had neuroblastoma when I was 9 months old and leukemia when I was 3. In my teens, I just wanted to move on. In my 20s, I concentrated on career and relationships. In my 30s, I wanted to give back. So a friend who is a medulloblastoma survivor and I started a group called Rebounders for adult survivors of childhood cancer. We connected a group of survivors from the '60s and '70s generation. Some of the group's members had pretty much had their social abilities wiped out. So we all gathered and talked for an entire weekend. We have an active group, and some people's social abilities have increased tenfold. I also sit on several committees to advocate for survivor needs. We distribute brochures and a newsletter. We organize fundraising events.

I personally hate the politics, but my friend is the goal setter. His motto is, "Nothing can't be done." We are now working to create a long-term follow-up package for our province. We hope to have a clinic, a book on how to take care of your healthcare needs, and a traveling medical passport. My work for survivors has been a very satisfying achievement.

Some survivors and family members feel so strongly about the lack of support in their lives that they volunteer with an existing group or organize their own group to address the needs of those treated for childhood cancer.

After Paige was diagnosed at 6 months old with retinoblastoma, it was 2½ years before we met any other cancer families. Her first treatment was surgery, then we went home. We were a family that fell through the cracks. It was a terrible loss. That's why I volunteer so much with Childcan (organization in Ontario, Canada), because I am concerned that no one else fall through the cracks. You need to meet other families to feel normal. It lifts a weight right off your shoulders.

An increasingly popular type of support system for survivors is Internet peer groups. Any time of the day or night, support is just a keystroke away. The Internet is a great leveler—it doesn't matter what you look like or what challenges you have—you will be accepted for your thoughts and words.

Thousands of survivors and their family members use this system to link up with others traveling the same emotional path, but who live around the world. Discussing their concerns, fears, and triumphs helps them make sense of what has happened to them, heal, and move on with their lives.

> *I had both eyes removed in 1956 to treat my bilateral retinoblastoma. Until a year ago, I didn't know any other survivors. I was a little ignorant about it. I happened to be on an Internet list for the National Alliance of Blind Students and a young lady said, "Hey, I've got retinoblastoma and am going to start a list. If you are interested, join me." So I did. Ever since I got on the list, I've learned so much. I'm very glad. Now I am cognizant of the possible secondary effects, and I am so thankful that I've finally run into people who make the whole thing real.*

Support groups for parents are also widely used. A parent of a child who was treated with a bone marrow transplant (BMT) explained:

> *The BMT-TALK discussion list [www.acor.org] has been my main lifesaver. When you get home there is nobody else to talk to who understands. I felt very isolated until I found the list on the Internet. It does have a downside—you can't get away from the BMT experience and you hear about all the relapses. But the upside is that whenever anything happens or I have a question, I post a question and one or more people have had that experience. When she had the kidney problems, there were people who knew all about it. When she needed hormones, there were lots of people who had already been through that. It helps to keep me from panicking to hear that those things are common.*

The need many survivors have for support from fellow survivors changes over time. They work through their emotions, give back to the community, and sense the need to move on.

> *I still know a couple of kids who had treatment at the same time that I did. I used to go to support group meetings. I'm off it now as I get ready to start high school. I have mixed feelings about these meetings, as sometimes they are helpful, but at other times it gets kind of annoying to go there and reflect on the past. Every time I had to tell my story, and I'm tired of telling my story. I want to solve problems by taking action rather than talking about them.*

Anytime medical information is shared in support groups—in person or online—remember that it could be accurate or totally wrong. Before acting on medical information obtained from a layperson, check with your healthcare provider.

Emotional expression and health

Emotions—of all kinds—are inevitably part of experiencing cancer and cancer survivorship. Being able to recognize your feelings and find healthy ways of expressing, channeling, and learning from them are keys to a balanced life. Not having tools for managing emotions can make life more difficult. Research has shown that survivors with high levels of psychological distress are more likely to engage in risky health behaviors such as smoking cigarettes and drinking alcohol. Obviously, unhealthy habits can complicate and worsen late effects from cancer treatment. So, in addition to the value of seeking support from healthcare professionals and networks of people with similar experiences, some of the other tools you may find helpful in dealing with strong emotions include blogging or journaling, physical activity, meditation, and yoga. Chapter 5, *Staying Healthy*, includes more information about this topic.

Future planning

Cancer treatment forces many children and their families to drop their plans for the future to focus on surviving the present. When treatment ends, an adjustment in mindset occurs. Some survivors resume working toward their pre-cancer goals—athletics, studies, relationships. Others find that they avoid thinking about the future because expectations of a long, healthy life have been changed by the cancer diagnosis. Commitment to a relationship or a long-term goal may be difficult. Thinking about having children may become more complicated. If future planning has become a daunting task, joining a support group or getting counseling may help you cope with altered perceptions of your future.

> *After my daughter's transplant we all felt like she had beaten the cancer. We did know many children who died—but there were reasons why we thought their situation differed from ours. For instance, we knew babies didn't do as well, so when a baby died, it didn't shake our optimism. But she befriended another teen who had a transplant for AML who really wanted to live. He was a great kid and they became close. When he passed away, it really hit us hard. She said, "Everything he felt, I feel too. I might really die from this disease." We had to rethink a lot of things.*

> *When she had to write an essay on what she would do if she won the monetary prize at a piano competition, she wrote, "I will use the money for a music camp or college, if I go." When I asked her if she was talking about if she lived that long, she said, "Yes." She doesn't say a lot about her concerns, but it's her reality. But we are learning to live in spite of that.*

Even now, 20 years later, I have a sense that I'll never get old. I just believe that I am going to die young. So I really don't plan for the future. It's too much of an unknown. I don't know if the left ventricle of my heart will continue to deteriorate. Or if my liver will hold up. There are too many things that I just don't know.

Sometimes survivors have to alter their life plans because cognitive or physical disabilities truly limit future possibilities. It can be very difficult for survivors, their families, and friends to accept that the price they paid for life has irrevocably changed the future.

In contrast, sometimes the cancer experience provides different views of the future. For example, cancer often gives children or teens their first glimpse of the medical world. Exposure to the helping professions and the medical world sometimes sparks an interest in youngsters that blossoms into a career.

I became a nurse as a result of having Wilms tumor when I was 2 years old. I had so much contact with the medical field that I became fascinated with it. I started out in adult intensive care, and then did pediatric home healthcare. One of the great things about nursing is that you can jump around and do all sorts of different things.

· · · · ·

My cancer changed my career aspirations. When I was a teenager I wanted to be a cop, but after cancer I decided to be a doctor. Treatment expanded my horizons by plopping me right into the middle of exciting times in the scientific community. I was diagnosed with ALL 25 years ago and was one of the first to get treatments that resulted in survival. Once I went to college, I was enjoying life too much to really focus and concentrate on getting into medical school, so I became a physician assistant.

The silver lining

In the past, most studies of the effects of the cancer experience on survivors have focused on negative effects. More recently, the existence of positive impact after cancer is also being recognized. Although no one would volunteer for the cancer experience, many survivors and their families find great meaning from their suffering. They tell heartwarming stories about the positive effects on their lives. Often, they discuss in reassuring and hopeful terms a renewed appreciation for life and an awareness of the value of each day.

Oh, there are a ton of benefits. While I don't think cancer is the best thing that ever happened to me (although I have a friend who says this), I do have a clarity I didn't have before. I know myself so much better. I know I can face anything since I beat cancer. I am very proud of myself for facing it and surviving. I've met a wonderful group of friends. And I'm much closer to my family than I was before the cancer.

· · · · ·

Today the director of personnel of our company came down to announce we would be selling our Gulf of Mexico assets and closing this office. Oddly, the human relations guy wondered why I took the news so well. Heck, I am thrilled at Garrett's test results and happy after a great family weekend. This is just a job. Last I heard they can't kill me or eat me. I guess that kind of perspective is one of the good things that have come from this cancer experience. (But I would never, ever recommend it!)

A teenager whose brother donated the bone marrow that cured her of AML said:

My brother and I were always really close, but his sharing his bone marrow bonded us forever. There is a part of him in me that will always live on in me. That's an amazing thing to have. He saved my life.

Having watched others battle cancer, and after fighting the disease myself, I have come to realize how very fortunate I am. The most important life lessons that I hold as daily guidance are the ones I learned at a very young age. I learned to never give up, and to keep striving no matter what the circumstance. I remember vividly one night when I was in the hospital. I decided that I had experienced enough, and was ready to give up. My mom, however, never lost hope. She bundled me up in my wheelchair, took me out of the hospital illegally, and we cruised around the streets of Toronto in the middle of winter. From that moment on, I looked at life in a different light. I saw how precious life was, and no matter how tough times might seem, there is always hope. Now, 12 years later, when I encounter difficulties, I know that I can make it through, because I made it through much worse.

And her mother speaks with wonder and gratitude about the bond her children share:

My daughter is great—a very positive and mature person. She has always loved her brother deeply, but they now have a bond that transcends any sibling relationship that I know. It's really quite moving watching them interact. She flew to New York for his birthday, and the woman who picked her up at the airport commented on them interacting when they saw each other. He throws his arms around her, protects her, etc. She said that she actually felt like she was intruding on a very magical relationship.

Many survivors, even very young ones, become deeply compassionate as a result of their cancer experiences.

There is a young boy on our street (moved in 1 week before the beginning of school) and he has a very bad lisp and appears to be a little slow. (He talks slow, walks slow, does things very slowly.) But because the other kids have not had an opportunity to be around this kind of person before, they shunned him. But not my Lizzy. She said, "Just because someone looks different or talks different or wears different clothing, it does not make them an animal. They are still human beings, and Robert from across the street will be my friend. He's okay, you know, Mom?" I did know that.

We have since found out that Robert from across the street was involved in a very horrible car accident when he was little, and hence the speech problem and slowness. Too bad we can't all get past our prejudices the way Lizzy has.

· · · · ·

As we approach the 3-year mark, I marvel at my son's ability to proceed with his life. He doesn't talk about his leukemia. He doesn't use it as an excuse, no matter how valid it might be. He's busy being a 17-year-old boy going into his senior year. Stand back please.

A week from today he and I, along with some friends, will leave for our annual bike ride across Iowa. This ride has been a symbol of his recovery for me for the last 2 years. He was diagnosed in July 1995. He rode 450 miles in July 1996 and again in 1997. Once more this year, as he climbs on his bike and heads down the road, I will give thanks that he is here to participate, just as I will when he runs onto the football field this fall. I am proud not only of his physical abilities, but of his resolve and courage. I am also proud of his compassion and sensitivity to other people, which has become so obvious over the last 3 years.

Our experience with leukemia has led us, child and parent, to grow in ways we never would have guessed. My first coherent thought in the hospital room 3 years ago after hearing the word leukemia was: "Our lives will never be the same again." I was right, but at the time, I had no idea of the many ways—some of them good—that leukemia would change us.

Other survivors stress the positive aspects of treatment for cancer.

> I've gained a lot of self-confidence from the cancer experience. Whenever there is a challenging obstacle to confront, I convince myself that if I survived the brain tumor, this is nothing! I've definitely become a much stronger person.

· · · · ·

> As horrible as it was, I wouldn't change the experience for anything. There were a lot of blessings that came out of it. It's given me a much more optimistic outlook on life. I don't think my family has ever laughed so much or so hard as those 3 years when I was on treatment. Now I laugh all the time—it's really improved my sense of humor.

> There are numerous people who helped my family while I was on treatment whom I probably would not have met otherwise. The track my life has taken has changed. I wouldn't have pursued art if not for the cancer. I don't think I would have been involved in crew in college if not for it. And winning the national championship was very rewarding. The people I've met on treatment and while working as a camp counselor for kids with cancer mean so much to me. It really changed my life.

Some family members express relief that it's over.

> Looking back on all that has happened is hard, but for now life is good, so that is what we concentrate on, squeezing every last drop out of all the good times. Treatment is like banging your head against a brick wall: wonderful when it stops!

Others simply say that their entire view of the world has shifted forever.

> I do wonder what he would have looked like if he hadn't had to go through treatment for cancer, but this really doesn't make me sad, nor do I reflect on it often. The whole cancer experience has changed my outlook so much that I know these things are not important. I laugh at my old ideas, how frivolous I was! Who can even imagine that looks are important at all in the large scheme of things?! I feel I had the luxury back then to be frivolous and petty and, well, lighthearted. I am no longer lighthearted, but my heart has grown so very much that I would not trade my old life for my new. I only wish my son hadn't had to have cancer for me to "see the light."

· · · · ·

> It's sad to say, but I think my daughter and I are better people for having survived the cancer experience. I've learned to appreciate things more.

It reminds me of the story about a wheel that lost a wedge out of it. It was no longer a perfect circle, so it was only able to roll very slowly. But because of its slow speed, it could smell the flowers and enjoy the beauty of the world around it. Later, the wheel found its missing piece and repaired itself. Being whole again it was able to roll much faster. At the faster speed, though, it wasn't able to notice the beauty around it. So it took the wedge back out.

Chapter 3

Relationships

Love looks not with the eyes,
but with the mind.

—Shakespeare
A Midsummer Night's Dream

THE TIME AFTER TREATMENT ENDS can involve tumultuous changes in relationships. Every survivor has stories to tell of lost or strained friendships and altered relationships with family members. Yet we are social creatures, reliant on a web of love and support from family, friends, and neighbors.

Cancer is a life-changing experience, and family dynamics inevitably shift during and after treatment. This chapter begins with a discussion about survivors' relationships with their loved ones. It then covers lost friendships, how survivors make and keep new friends, and romantic relationships. Dating opens up new worlds and sometimes old wounds. Rejection due to health history or altered appearance can occur, but deeply satisfying romantic relationships can develop. This chapter also contains many stories of how and when survivors disclosed their medical history to friends and partners. Finally, the chapter looks at marriage, fertility, health of offspring, and adoption.

Relationships with parents

Cancer is a family crisis. At diagnosis, the family system undergoes intense stress and reorganization. Roles and responsibilities are adjusted as parents struggle to balance taking care of their ill child with the needs of the rest of the family. Major financial decisions often need to be made; one parent sometimes must quit a job to help the child through treatment. Parents struggle to find ways to support one another emotionally and manage their own strong feelings of fear and uncertainty.

Interactions between parents and a child with cancer also dramatically shift. Family rules may change to adapt to behaviors caused by medication or emotional reactions. Sometimes children with cancer are too weak to perform chores. Parents need to become the medical overseers for their child—monitoring temperatures, side effects, and reactions to medication. When treatment ends, families often find that roles have permanently shifted.

> The cancer has made my dad and me closer. He lost his job shortly before I was diagnosed, so he was at the hospital every day and at home with me all day every day through treatment. It really made a difference because we had never spent time together. My mom told me that he was really upset when I was diagnosed. He said, "If she doesn't get through this you'll have no regrets, because you did all those fun things with her and I never had time." Now my dad and I do lots of stuff together.

· · · · ·

> I kind of incorporated the chemotherapy into my growing independence. When I first got my license, I asked to drive out to the doctor's office and get the treatment. My mom said, "Hey, that's no problem. I'll go with you the first couple of times, get you settled, then you can go on your own." It gave me so much confidence. My mom is a rock. She was always very positive. She's a real "Where there's a will there's a way," type of person. My mom told me we needed to attack this thing, and that there was no doubt that I'd get over it. This was in 1973 when very few kids survived ALL (acute lymphoblastic leukemia), and I was high risk. If it hadn't been for her attitude, it would have been a completely different ball game.

Cancer in adolescents may disrupt their normal developmental processes. At a time when they are gradually withdrawing from the family and beginning to function autonomously, they suddenly become dependent upon medical personnel to save their lives and on their parents to provide emotional and physical support. This can add considerable stress to the already turbulent teen years. After treatment ends, some parents continue to feel protective and have difficulty when their teens resume their journey toward independence.

> I was diagnosed with ALL when I was 12. My mom and I were extremely close, and our relationship just improved. She always stayed with me in the hospital. I was never alone. Extended family—grandparents, great-aunts and uncles—all pitched in. After treatment my mom became very protective. I just wanted to be a normal kid and hang out with my friends. I didn't want to worry about the cancer. Finally by senior year she conceded and let me be more normal. She was still worrying in her mind, but let me enjoy my last year in high school. She gradually went through the process of letting go.

• • • • •

I was diagnosed with cancer as a teen and had always had a lousy home life. My stepfather was a demanding alcoholic who resented the time my mom spent with me in the hospital. My cancer caused a lot of problems between them. The minute I was 18 I moved out, got three jobs, and a place to stay. I was determined to do it on my own. I really wanted to go to college to be a nurse, and asked my parents to sign a form explaining that they didn't have enough money to send me so that I could apply for a scholarship. They refused. So I never did go to college, but it's still a dream of mine.

• • • • •

When my daughter was having her bone marrow transplant, I felt like we were in the trenches in Vietnam. We formed a bond that is superhuman, magical, surreal, almost holy. People who haven't experienced it simply cannot understand the strength of that bond. It's impossible to describe how strongly I love her. When she is criticized I get an upsurge of strong emotions—almost a fight-or-flight response.

• • • • •

I had Hodgkin's when I was 14. I don't know what the doctors told my parents about possible late effects. My parents told me nothing. They didn't know if I'd live long enough to get married or have kids, so they just wanted me to have fun. As a result, they didn't give me any guidance or enforce any rules. I went into a bad marriage. I really didn't become a thinking, independent person until I was 25 or so.

Parents and their survivor children often have different views about what life after cancer should be like. Some surviving teens and young adults want to leave the cancer behind and get on with their lives. If their parents share this view, a smooth transition to adulthood can occur. If the parent has established deep ties in the cancer community, he or she may have difficulty accepting the child's decision to relegate the disease to the past. On the other hand, some parents want the child to pretend the cancer never happened or accept that it is over now and time to move on.

My mother and I have always been close, but as I've gotten older we've had more problems. We have very different ideas about survivorship. Some things that I do scare the daylights out of my mom. She wants me to put it behind me—that there is magic in moving on with my life. But I think the magic, if there is any, is in discussing it, reading about it, giving back. Our definitions of how you get on with your life are different. I noticed that when I was going to the survivors group, she'd tell people that I went to encourage others. I have to cut in and say, "Mom, I also go to get some help myself."

Being diagnosed with cancer—whether you are a toddler or a young adult—is a horrifying experience. But sometimes people do really nice things for you, like bring presents, or grant you a special wish, or have parties for you. It really makes you feel so loved and so special, and you save up those moments in your head because you know there will be bad days when you'll need them. And sometimes even after treatment, on days when you really aren't feeling well and wonder if you'll ever feel healthy again, one of those memories will fill you up and suddenly you feel just a little bit better. And during treatment, thinking about camp or a wish can get you through chemotherapy, radiation, or surgery.

So you finish treatment. Maybe you even have a party to celebrate. But you still have to go to the hospital and get needle sticks, only without your port or line. You may still have to take medications.

Once you're back at school, everyone may be nice, but there's no one you can talk to. Your friends are tired of hearing about it. Your brothers or sisters or both are really tired of it! If you try talking to your parents or other adults, they may remind you of how great you're doing and that you can get on with your life now. You see a lot less of the nice people at the hospital who helped you talk about it, like your child life therapist, social worker, nurses, chaplain.

If the special things still happen, sometimes those help. They may be the only contact you have with others who understand what you're dealing with. But when special things are also withdrawn, often there are few if any sources of support. This can be very discouraging—especially when children grow older and have to face frightening risks like secondary cancers and other serious effects. Your friends die and you miss them, but feel guilty that you are the one who survived, yet you're grateful that you did. You get confused and sad. You may be concerned about your future, about relationships and having kids and so forth. Every bug you catch means another round of antibiotics and a trip to the doctor because, although it's probably just a virus going around, it could be post-splenectomy sepsis. You may still lack the energy of your peers. And yet you're expected to forget it happened and return to the person you were before.

Parents' long-term responses to their children's survival vary widely and can fluctuate over time.

For the most part, my daughter is doing wonderfully. I know I should be grateful for so much, and I am. But I am having some problems. I started back to work in February of this year, but I can't hold a job. I have no patience whatsoever with other people and their way of life. The way they whine over such trivial things drives me nuts. I ended up working at a bank that dealt with mortgages, and the pressure was great. But I didn't feel the pressure the way others did. I told my boss, "These are just numbers we are dealing with and they can wait till tomorrow." Then I went home to my kids. I just can't cope with what these people call emergencies—they don't have any idea what a real emergency is. My whole outlook on life has changed and to be honest, it is spooky!

• • • • •

Our life has returned to normal in most ways. We are having a normal school year, which is important to my daughter. Her illness has left many scars and fears with all of us, including not knowing what is going to happen tomorrow, long-term effects of chemotherapy, financial destruction that we still have not recovered from, and more.

But I also have a deeper appreciation of life. I tend to look at life differently now and enjoy the little things: a smile, a hug, watching my child act normal and be with friends. A laugh, a cry—they each have a deeper meaning. I definitely take more time to be with my children and listen and understand them. My daughter and I have a much closer relationship. Our bond is a gift as she enters her pre-teens.

In some cases, cancer results in disabilities that affect the survivor's ability to live independently. Some survivors are never able to live on their own, while others return intermittently to live with their parents for financial or health reasons. These situations create a tremendous challenge for the family. Parents need to adapt to having an adult child as a temporary or permanent resident in their home, as well as make arrangements for care when they are no longer able to provide it.

I still live with my parents off and on, depending on my health. I lived on my own for 4 years as an undergraduate and for the first year of grad school. When I was diagnosed with breast cancer in February, I moved back home for the surgery and recovery. This year, I'm back at grad school Tuesday through Sunday and the other days I come home. Next semester I'll be back in school full time and living on my own again.

• • • • •

I am 25 and had astrocytoma when I was 10. I had chemotherapy, radiation, and surgery. They ended up removing some of my vertebrae to relieve the tension, and I was in a body cast and halo for 6 months. I'm now 4'6" and in a wheelchair. I live with my mother and stepfather because I still need a lot of help.

*Our daughter's math skills and judgment have been affected by cranial
radiation at a young age. She lived with us until her mid-20s but is now
independent. We do subsidize her rent so that she can live in a safe place,
because she gets a low salary from her job. After moving out she got into
serious credit card debt, so now we limit her to one card with a low credit
limit and check up on it to make sure it doesn't happen again.*

Adult survivors sometimes revisit their cancer experience by asking their
parents questions and soliciting their memories. These conversations may
help survivors gain an understanding of the trauma from their parents'
perspective. One method is to sit down together and compare recollections. Individual views of the same experience can be incredibly different.
Another method used to explore the past is to join an online discussion
group (listserv), chat room, or survivor support group.

*One nice thing about belonging to the listservs is that I print out some
of the postings and give them to my mom. She went through my cancer
20 years ago on her own and it was pretty traumatic. I think it helps her
to feel like she was not the only one who went through that and felt that
way. Plus, it helps us because we can discuss more things. I'm interested
in knowing what happened (I had cancer when I was 2) and how she felt.*

· · · · ·

*My parents didn't tell me I had neuroblastoma when I was an infant
until I was 12 years old. Even though I remembered a few experiences,
I really didn't have a clue what it meant. It wasn't until my own child
was very sick that I gained an appreciation of what my parents went
through. My parents divorced, and my own experiences as a mother
helped me develop a more mature attitude and understanding about my
parents' divorce. I have a lot more appreciation for what my mother went
through.*

Relationships with siblings

Childhood cancer touches all members of the family and can have especially long-lasting effects on siblings. The diagnosis, treatment, and aftermath
can all create an array of conflicting feelings in siblings. Not only are they
concerned about their brother or sister, but they usually resent the turmoil
the family has been thrown into. They feel jealous of the gifts and attention
showered on the sick child, yet feel guilty for having these emotions. Some
siblings feel that the child or teen with cancer continues to consume most
of the parents' attention long after treatment ends. In other families, siblings and the child with cancer form deeper and closer relationships.

My son had panic attacks in college. During therapy, he learned it was from sublimated worry and anger about his younger sister's cancer many years earlier. He's 30 and it still occasionally appears. He says he can't believe he's this age and he still falls apart when something goes wrong. He's had lots of help since then, but we didn't know anything was wrong before. We thought everything was taken care of—there were loving friends. But the truth is, he was farmed out at the time. And he did resent it. And I realize now that it must have felt like the epitome of desertion.

• • • • •

I have two older brothers. They were 13 and 11 when I was diagnosed. I haven't ever had the best of relationships with my brothers. There was lots of sibling rivalry and fights. I didn't notice any problems when I was sick, but my mother said my brothers were jealous of the attention that I was getting. When I went to the camp for kids with cancer, I didn't let my brother come, I took a friend. I thought of the camp as my time to get away. I didn't want him there with me. It's been 13 years and we've never talked about it.

The most common reactions of siblings to their brother or sister's cancer are concern, fear, jealousy, anger, guilt, fear of abandonment, sadness, and worry about their parents. Younger children may also feel that something they did caused their brother or sister's cancer. These feelings can cause academic and social problems or feelings of anxiety and depression.

I have two older brothers—one was in ninth grade and one in his first year of college when I was diagnosed. My youngest brother and I were only 18 months apart and were always really close. It was hard for him when I was going through treatments and he lost a lot of attention. They also were left to fend for themselves because my father was stationed far away when I was sick. I think my younger brother resented it, and this came out when we attended camp together. He realized there that his feelings were shared by other siblings and were valid. He never expressed his resentment at the time, though, because he was old enough to know what I was going through was pretty difficult. And sometimes I milked it. I'd poke at them and make comments because they weren't allowed to hit me.

Brothers and sisters within the same family can have markedly different reactions to their sibling's cancer treatment and survival, depending on their age, temperament, and social support. Family therapy can be very effective in exploring the various reactions of members of the family and working out ways to communicate well and support one another.

My youngest daughter was 9 when her 13-year-old sister had her bone marrow transplant. They had always been close and we worked to maintain that. She really looked up to her older sister and wanted to be like her. She wanted a central line and went so far as to tape an external line with an empty attached bag to her chest when she accompanied us to clinic. She showed her stress by biting the skin around her thumb and fingers until they bled. She had never done that before the cancer. It's improving now—after over 2 years—but she still does it when she's stressed.

My son, on the other hand, was in eighth grade and I was pretty much gone until he was a sophomore. It was difficult for him, but he doesn't talk about it. He thought being in the hospital was "boring" so he didn't visit very often. I really missed sharing a lot of his life—all of the successes such as wrestling when he went to state, won the tournament, and got a trophy. I missed it all—I can never go back and experience it, it's just gone. Over time, he chose to deal with our absence by spending less time at home and running with a new group of friends. He's made some bad choices and it's hard to know if it had anything to do with our disrupted life or if it's normal teenage experimentation. We are really concentrating on encouraging him—and my other kids too—because they have so much potential. While he's made some mistakes, he's done some really neat things too, so we're still hopeful. We're just trying to reclaim all our kids and it's been a real struggle.

Siblings also learn important lessons about compassion, sharing, and coping skills. Most realize that should they ever become as sick, the same attention would be paid to them and that all possible efforts would be made to help them survive. That can be a comfort when jealousy or feelings of neglect arise. Their empathy and compassion may grow through the crisis. Brothers and sisters of children with cancer sometimes feel that they benefited from the experience in many ways, such as increased:

- Knowledge about health and disease.
- Empathy for the sick or disabled.
- Sense of responsibility.
- Self-esteem.
- Maturity and coping ability.
- Family closeness.

Many of these siblings mature into adults interested in the helping professions such as medicine, social work, or teaching.

One experience in my life that was in no way comfortable for my family or myself and caused me a lot of confusion and grief was when my brother had leukemia. The Thanksgiving of my third-grade year, Preston became very ill and was diagnosed with cancer. Along with the disruption of this event, it also caused me to grow tremendously as a person.

When my brother had very little hair or was puffed out from certain drugs, I learned to respect people's differences and to stick up for them when they are made fun of. Also, when Preston was in the hospital I was taught to deal with the great amount of jealousy that I had. He received many gifts, cards, candy, flowers, games, and so many other material things that I envied. Most of all, he received all of the attention and care of my mother, father, relatives, and friends. This is what I was jealous of the most. As I look back now, I can't believe that I was that insensitive and self-centered to be mad at my brother at a time like that.

The thing that made this a graced period for me was the fact that it enabled me to be very close to my brother as we grew up. My brother and I are now good friends and are able to talk and share our experiences with each other. I don't think we would have this same relationship if he never had leukemia and I think that has been a very positive outcome. Another thing that has been a positive outcome of this event is the people I've been able to meet. Through all the support groups, camps, and events for children with cancer and their siblings, I have met some people with more courage and more heart than anyone could imagine. In no way am I saying that I'm glad my brother had cancer, but I will say I'm very glad with some of the outcomes of it.

Survivors themselves often have strong feelings about the effect their cancer had on family functioning and the long-range effects on siblings.

It was only over the course of years that I realized how guilty I felt about my brother. I know that the year I was ill was one of terrible disruption for my family, and my brother really seems to have suffered for it. I won't go into the nature of his emotional problems, but I realized that I held myself responsible—that I somehow felt that while my parents attended to my needs, they neglected my brother. Now I know this is not rational, but it feels so real.

I think these kinds of feelings are not uncommon in those touched by a life-threatening illness, but somehow surviving such an illness exacerbates and enhances them and sometimes traps us in them.

• • • • •

In a focus group for adult survivors of childhood cancer, we recently started talking about sibling guilt. It's been an enormous problem for me. My brother was 6 when I was diagnosed at 5. Even before I got sick, he was so smart and used to watch all of the science shows. He knew that I could die, and he lost a lot of attention when I was sick. He is still socially awkward (in his late 20s) and is still having problems sorting life out. We've never talked about it, but I think we should.

Relationships with friends

Cancer can slam into friendships like a hurricane. When treatment ends, you look around to assess the damage and see how many friendships are still intact. You may find that many remained firm through the storm, while others disappeared.

Losing friends

Unfortunately, childhood cancer occurs at a time when friendships normally change rapidly. When the diagnosis occurs in elementary school, friendships often depend on what classroom you are assigned to or who shares your lunch table. If you are gone for an extended period of time, the group may welcome you when you return, or the groups may have shifted so that you are now on the outside. When cancer strikes middle-school-aged children, friendships often dissolve. Social groups are forming, peer pressure is at an all-time high, and compassion is often a temporary casualty of puberty. In many cases, high-school-aged adolescents are more mature and understanding, and friendships remain strong throughout treatment. A high school football player describes how his friends rallied around him after diagnosis:

My friends were supportive from diagnosis and were very much a part of my coping. Being around them helped me feel normal. The ones who were exceptionally supportive, the ones who visited me in Rochester immediately after diagnosis and those who visited me often, I am still very close to, despite all the changes that take place in high school. Most of my friends were very curious and asked questions like: "What exactly is it?" "When are you cured?" "Can you do everything that you used to?" I think the more they knew, the more they felt comfortable talking about it with me; and I never had any problems talking about it with them if they had questions.

His mother adds her perspective:

On the Sunday after diagnosis, I was walking out of his room and looked up and there stood his friend, Brent, and his mother. I didn't know his mother very well, but was so surprised that they would drive over 200 miles to see Joel for just a few minutes. Later the same day, another

*friend and his parents appeared. Seeing those two guys made a big differ-
ence in how Joel felt in those early days. They gave him back a sense of
normalcy.*

*When Joel returned to school, his broader circle of friends was very sup-
portive. They asked him to come to football games. They brought homework from school. They'd come over and watch videos when he didn't feel
like going out. They shaved his head for him when he thought his hair
would fall out. (It didn't.) They treated him like a normal ninth grader.*

*His friends have stood by Joel throughout treatment. They have treated
him just as they would treat any other friend. There is one boy who told
Joel he didn't like to wrestle around with him because when he bumped
Joel's port, it felt "creepy." Joel's response: "Yeah, well, you should feel it
from my side." And then they went back to horsing around. Now that
treatment is over, he still has the same strong circle of friends around
him. They are now helping him to rediscover what it feels like to be 17
and not on treatment.*

*His experience with his friends has made him very sensitive to what it
takes to be a good friend. On a college application, he was asked to list
one book, song, movie, or play title that best describes him. His choice:
"You've Got a Friend" by Carole King.*

Friends disappear for many reasons—they can't think of what to say, or are
afraid they will cry or say the wrong thing. Or they simply grow unfamiliar
with the child who, in the midst of a rapidly changing social scene, misses
huge chunks of time with friends. The friends may even think they can
catch cancer. Many survivors have painful stories to tell of lost friendships.

*I had rhabdomyosarcoma when I was 12, right before junior high. I had
to grow up real fast. It was really tough because everyone was forming
their peer groups and I missed 105 days of school that year. Kids can be
pretty mean and nasty when you are losing your hair. I also didn't want
my friends to suffer with me so I pushed them away. When I went back
in eighth grade I had no friends. So I had to start all over again and it
was tricky.*

• • • • •

*People lose so many friends during treatment and even later when you
tell folks. You get so isolated. People have a tendency to avoid you. They
are afraid. I think they think, "Oh my God, that happened to my friend,
maybe it could happen to me." I think much of the avoidance is so they
won't have to think about it.*

I lost all my friends but one when I was diagnosed at 16 years old. She stuck with me through everything and is still my best friend. I lived in a small town and everybody knew my business. I never went to any proms and pretty much was left out of all high school activities.

Friendships depend a lot on how the child's school and teacher handle the cancer. It can be an unparalleled opportunity for the school to teach many vital lessons about friendship and compassion. Sadly, many schools miss the boat. My daughter's principal was horrified that I would dare suggest hospital personnel conduct a special assembly at the school. Few teachers knew why she wasn't in school. When she had good days and attended, some were shocked and horrified when she took off her hat. Some of her peers and their parents thought she had AIDS and they shunned her. I finally contacted the superintendent and he set the school straight.

I explained all this to my daughter and somehow we found humor in it. She persevered and triumphed. Yes, she lost some friends, but we both believe that would have happened anyway. Those who were meant to remain lifelong friends have remained so even 7 years later.

Survivors also lose friends to cancer, and this is very difficult for children and their parents. During treatment, children and teens become extremely close to others going through treatment for cancer. And some of these children and teens die.

One of my favorite songs from the musical Les Miserables is "Empty Chairs at Empty Tables," sung by Marius, slowly recovering from his wounds from the battle at the barricades. It is so clearly the lament of a survivor. I've grown to understand that song more and more as I've lost friends to cancer: my bunkmate who, at 12, insisted that she would grow up and become the doctor who cured cancer; my beloved "big sis" who died from complications of a bone marrow transplant for recurrent Hodgkin's in her early 30s; the spunky counselor-in-training who was my best friend as well as my trainee; the dear friend who dreamed of becoming a teacher and insisted on remaining in college even while undergoing treatment, treatment, and more treatment for recurrent Hodgkin's; and I don't even know where I'd begin about the younger children I've known.

One thing that I think is important to realize is how double-edged grief can be for us. For me, it's the obvious pain of losing a beloved companion and confidant...but there's also the part of me that fears I'm next, and the part that feels guilty for even thinking such a thing. One of the most difficult aspects, though, has been survivor guilt—a sense that somehow I don't deserve to be alive when so many wonderful people close to me have died. Marius' "Oh, my friends, my friends, forgive me/That I live and you are gone/There's a grief that can't be spoken/There's a pain goes on and on..." truly sums this up best. But I try to remember that it wasn't my decision, and that my friends would not want me to become despondent.

Near the close of the song, Marius bursts into, "Oh, my friends, my friends, don't ask me/What your sacrifice was for..." That's exactly my feeling, and exactly my reason to go on living and try to live well. What is the point of all the empty chairs at my table? What was the reason that I buried two maids of honor before my wedding? Why has half of the Sunflowers cabin—my girls, my counselors-in-training—died in the 5 years since that year of camp? I don't know.

Making new friends

Friendships in childhood are fluid; they depend on what class, school, neighborhood, church, or sports team you are involved with. Some survivors renegotiate or rekindle friendships and others make new friends during and after treatment.

When I got to high school I realized that people will always be the way that they are, and because I am blind, I will always need to overcome barriers. So I decided to take it on myself. I go out of my way to start conversations, and it's tough. But sometimes you just have to take chances and smile and say hi.

• • • • •

After my diagnosis of leukemia (ALL), I was tutored at home for my entire eighth grade year. My junior high went from seventh through ninth grade. One of the most difficult things about being on treatment was that all the people I hung out with and claimed as friends were too afraid to talk with me when I came back. They would walk past me in the hall and not even acknowledge me. Maybe they didn't recognize me. Before, I had long hair, a great figure, and was very athletic, and when I returned I was overweight and I only had a dusting of hair. Only one friend from school ever came to visit me in the hospital. When I went back in ninth grade, the teachers were incredibly supportive, but dealing with friends was very, very difficult. I just started hanging out with a new group of friends. By high school, there was nothing noticeably wrong, so I made lots of new friends.

I had bilateral retinoblastoma when I was 2½. They had to remove both eyes, so I'm totally blind. I am an athlete, and have been involved in several sports. Right now I'm into mountain biking. I use a tandem bike— I'm in the back (called the stoker) and have a pilot in the front. It's really a liberating experience and I find it to be a wonderful icebreaker. It's a great way to get out in the community and meet people with similar interests. It also promotes disability awareness and hopefully gets people involved. But whether you have a disability or not, athletics is rewarding to anyone who is involved.

Many parents of young children take an active role in encouraging new friendships. They can ask their child whom they like the most in their class at school and invite that child over to play or watch a movie. They can befriend parents of children with similar interests and invite the whole family over for dinner. Encouraging participation in school, music, church, or athletic activities exposes the child or teen survivor to new groups of peers.

My daughter was diagnosed with AML (acute myelogenous leukemia) in sixth grade, and the people in the school system were concerned but awkward about what to do. There was not much support from the faculty, and her peers followed the teachers' leads. We did a lot of things to try to keep her connected so that when she was well enough she could easily rejoin her group. We did a presentation with her class to help them understand and prepare them. We also filled up picture books with happy pictures of her daily life. For instance, we took pictures of the hospital school, the playroom, bingo games, her with her gifts. The hospital was an hour away so it was not easy for the kids to drop by to keep in touch. She missed all of sixth grade.

She was able to start seventh grade and play on the school softball team, and she made tryouts for the basketball team. She was accepted pretty much back into her group, but then she relapsed. The seventh grade was at the junior high and had a different faculty and principal, and they were great. The teachers all came to visit her. They encouraged the kids to write notes and set up a mini-mailbox in the office for the kids to drop their notes or cards in to be delivered. We were stunned to have so many visitors. She didn't get back to school until eighth grade. The aseptic necrosis in her legs made it impossible to play sports. The kids were really nice to her, but by now they had new social groups that didn't include her.

The kids included her after each episode of sickness. But by eighth grade they were a bit scared. She told me one day that she thought the kids were thinking she might die. She said, "Nobody likes me, I don't fit in, I'm not part of the group." But we encouraged her to do what she could—she participated in a scholastic bowl, speech teams, math teams, and a school play, managed the softball team, and had tutoring by teachers during their free periods. She's also a talented pianist. I think she's going to blossom this year in high school because there are a lot of musical opportunities.

Some survivors worry about making new friends because they don't want to cause their friends pain in the event the cancer returns.

You know, it's tricky starting new relationships when you have a health problem because you know it might happen again. I have a hereditary cancer and it could happen again. I don't think about it often, but it does lurk in the back of my mind. I really love my friends and don't want them to suffer. But I realize it's not fair to my friends to push them away. My friends are very important to me.

Some survivors blend back into their peer group after treatment, while others, even many years later, still feel different. Some survivors feel that they are rejected socially due to their cancer history, while others feel mature beyond their years because of what they have experienced. This can create differences in interests and value systems between survivors and their peers.

I'm in college now and I still feel older than everyone else. I've faced life and death, and I just don't relate to what they are interested in doing, like drinking and partying. They seem so immature and my mind frame is so different. I feel like the oldest woman on the planet.

• • • • •

It's been over 20 years since I had cancer. And the older I get, the more I realize what's really important in life. Believe me, I'll take the wrinkles to get the wisdom any day. So many of my friends just talk about decorating their homes, their haircuts, and the latest fashions. I feel like the cancer helped me evolve more. It made me less interested in the superficial and made it harder to relate to the petty stuff. Not to sound like I'm better than anyone else, but I just think there's a whole lot more to life—a life that is more meaningful, deeper, and different from what I imagined it would be before I had cancer.

• • • • •

I used to be very social and now I'm afraid of people. I thought after the chemotherapy everything would be normal again, but I found I still wanted to be by myself. I used to be into how I looked and what was cool. Now I know it's what's on the inside that counts.

I was diagnosed with ALL in 1972 when I was 15. I felt like I was fast-tracked into adulthood. My peers became adults and most of the kids I knew in the hospital died. I missed a lot of school and didn't develop normal peer relationships. I became more mature, more serious. I just didn't horse around anymore. I was different from my peers and couldn't make that up. I gained a lot, though. I gravitated toward serious, goal-oriented, genuine people in college. I had a normal social life and am happily married.

Late effects from cancer treatments can create additional barriers. Graft-versus-host disease skin problems, thin or absent hair, very short height, amputation, hearing loss, or poor social skills from neurological side effects all can impact the ability to make friends.

My daughter really likes people. But she has an apathy about relationships and interests that makes it hard to make and keep friends. She's only 4'7" so new people she meets automatically know that there is some health history. She was really shy and embarrassed about her height in high school, but she's matured now and is less bothered by it.

· · · · ·

In grade school I was kind of an outcast. I don't think people avoided me because of the cancer, rather I think I felt awkward and unsure about how to be accepted. I had a really wonderful friend in grade school. Every year the popular group would shun one of the girls. So we would make a clique of the unpopular girls—we pulled everyone in. I'm now 28 and we are still best friends. We recently talked about it, and I realize how much she helped me deal with the horrible things that went on in school. She knew I was fragile and she really looked out for me. It was very powerful for me to realize how much she helped me.

Cranial radiation at a young age or high-dose radiation to the brain at any age can affect a survivor's social skills. Parents can help their young children by role-playing social skills, enrolling them in social skills classes, and encouraging friendships with schoolmates. Peer support groups for teen and young adult survivors can provide a safe place to make friends, talk about feelings, and have fun.

My daughter had cranial radiation for her relapsed ALL. She has big social problems at school. The other kids don't know what to make of her. She says whatever she thinks, whether it hurts someone's feelings or not. We have always thought that it was because she lost so many years of her childhood being sick and primarily interacting with adults. But the more I learn about radiation, the more I think that may be the culprit.

• • • • •

My daughter was irradiated at age 4 and she really has trouble with games. The rules just change too fast for her to keep up with, so she's always left behind by the kids on the playground. Even though the kids like her and help her, she just can't figure it out. I think the social disabilities are worse than the academic disabilities. With academics, you can learn to compensate for the weak areas. But you can't memorize how to react to the world. Academic disabilities are accommodated in the schools—modified to the child's strengths and weaknesses. But social disabilities are judged by your peers. And they are tougher judges than adults.

Having other survivors as friends

You may find that you don't get the support and understanding you need from your friends who don't have cancer. Perhaps you need people who are willing to listen without judgment when you talk about your cancer. Or you may not like to talk about it at all. You may feel strongly that you need to live a healthy lifestyle to lessen the chances of late effects, and your friends may not respect your decision not to smoke or drink. For a variety of reasons, you may seek out or continue friendships made during treatment with other people who had childhood cancer. This shared experience can create deep and long-lasting bonds.

I was diagnosed with cancer when I was 16. Back then I was a cheerleader, very attractive, very popular. I guess you could say I was one of the cool kids. I was very busy and had lots of friends. I was also judgmental and snobby. What pointless stuff I was interested in. But after the diagnosis I became an outsider. All of my friends disappeared. I dropped out of school and was tutored during chemotherapy and when recuperating from my surgery. So I never really entered back into the high school scene. I just couldn't relate to them anymore. But I did become very, very close to five other teenagers on treatment for cancer. Four of us are in college and one's in high school. We all survived and are the best of friends. I talk to them all the time. Even our parents are close.

• • • • •

I've been involved in young adult support groups for years. I'm starting to have some mixed feelings. Just because of our shared experiences, they tend to be really nice and sensitive people. You only socialize with people you know, so if you use these groups as your only social outlet, it's not a good thing. I think you should use those groups to build skills, then move on. Or at least branch out and develop other friendships, too.

Dating

Close and intimate relationships are hard at times for everyone, whether or not they had cancer. Some survivors have a more difficult time starting relationships than others. Whether you are merely looking for some fun or searching for a partner for life, you may find that your cancer history is an impediment. If you missed months or years of middle school or high school, re-entering the dating world can be especially complicated if your appearance is altered by baldness, weight gain, or scars. People you are attracted to may avoid you due to phobias about cancer or because of peer pressure. You may not feel ready to date after enduring the physical pain and social isolation that usually accompany cancer treatment. Or you may just pick up where you left off pre-cancer.

I was treated for ALL from ages 12 to 14. Dating was a very big issue for me. I didn't really date until I'd been in college for a couple of years. In high school, when dances came around I always wondered who I would go with. I had lots of really good male friends, but no boyfriends. It seemed to never go past friendship and I was pretty traumatized by it. But my mother and I decided that they were intimidated because I did so well in athletics and schoolwork, and I had cancer. The combination was just too much.

· · · · ·

After completing my treatment for cancer, I fell for the first loser who came along. My hair was still short and he told me I was beautiful. I look back now and can find nothing attractive about him, but at the time he said what I wanted and needed to hear. He made me feel good. He had no job, no prospects, and no plans. Then I got pregnant and realized from his reaction after the twins were born that he was bad news. I kicked him out and it was the best decision I ever made. I decided after getting rid of the loser that I didn't want a family like the one I grew up in—alcoholism, smoking, abuse.

I met the man I eventually married shortly after that. He loved my babies and he loved me. He had grown up in a very stable, loving home and has been wonderful to us. He's a sweet man and a great dad. We've been married for 6 years and have four kids.

· · · · ·

I was treated for cancer during high school. Everybody knew about it, but it wasn't a big deal to them. It never posed a problem with dating other than I was mature beyond my years and attracted to interesting, genuine people. I just seemed to miss the party-and-be-crazy stage.

Body image and sexuality

Cancer can change not only your physical appearance, but how you view yourself. You may have an obvious difference (amputation) or a more private one (loss of a testicle). You may have scars that can be seen by anyone you meet (on your face) or only by loved ones (on your lower abdomen from a laparotomy). Even if you have no physical scars, you may have an altered sense of your own appearance. If you don't think you are attractive, it may be hard to convince yourself that someone you want to date will be attracted to you. On the other hand, many survivors and those who love them feel that the scars represent life and thus are beautiful.

> *Before I was sick I had long hair and I looked good. I based a lot of how I felt about myself on my looks and how people reacted to them. On chemo, I lost my hair, eyebrows, and lots of weight, especially in my face. I looked really horrible. I hid a lot. I wore wigs and penciled in eyebrows, but I still felt bad about my looks. People would stare, whisper, and point. I became very afraid of people. It's been years, and to this day I have a problem with people looking at me. I know there is nothing wrong with the way I look, but subconsciously I still think I look weird. I feel panicky if someone looks directly at me. I just can't get over the feeling.*

· · · · ·

> *I think there are lots of reasons some of us aren't comfortable with our scars and don't "wear them with pride" like the Nike® commercial. I don't disclose my cancer history to co-workers, so having scars can bring questions and difficult answers. Many of us want to "feel normal." We grow back the hair, we lose the "moony-face," we grow back the eyebrows, and we want to look like our old selves—like a regular face in the crowd. The scars stick around.*

> *I think we all go through different phases with our cancer—needing to talk about it, needing to not talk about it, being proud of our survival, wanting to forget it ever happened, etc. The scars are constant reminders of what we've been through. Sometimes that is a good thing; sometimes it's a reminder you don't want.*

Most studies of childhood cancer survivors show that overall emotional well-being is good. However, some areas can become problematic, including sexuality. Healthy adult sexual relationships have psychological, interpersonal, and physical parts, one or more of which can be affected by treatment for cancer.

> *I feel fine about the way I look now. It was hard being a guy and wearing a wig in high school. But as soon as I had a little hair, I stopped wearing the wig. That was in ninth grade and no one was dating then anyway. I was into academics and athletics. But when I started dating, everyone knew, but it wasn't a problem.*

People with histories of cancer can view the body as a source of health concerns rather than sexual pleasure.

> *My oncologist has children my age (late teens) and he treats me like one of his kids. If I tried to talk to him about sex he would probably fall off his chair and faint. He has never asked me a thing about it. My hormone levels are wacky and it affects my moods. My sex drive has completely disappeared; I don't know how my boyfriend puts up with me. I think I've been so poked and prodded that I just don't want to be touched anymore. I don't mind hugs, but don't want anyone near any of my lymph nodes. I'm embarrassed about all of my scars. All of this together makes it really hard to have a decent sex life.*

· · · · ·

> *For many, many years I had a terrible nightmare following treatment. I would dream that I was sound asleep in my bed at home and then I would hear the smallest noise and know that someone was breaking into my house. I would then wake up in terror and be unable to go back to sleep because the dream felt so real. I was always sure someone was indeed breaking into my house. I no longer have this dream, but it took some years of seeing a psychoanalyst to figure out what this dream was about and why it troubled me so much.*

> *I love my home and am very much a homebody. I like making my house nice, comfortable, and welcoming. I do with my home what I hope I do with myself: be warm, welcoming, and comfortable. So I came to understand that the house stood for myself. That in this dream I am the house and the house is me. In the dream something very bad and scary happens to the house/me. The house/me is broken into. I had my first surgical procedure when I was 10 years old, an appendectomy. My house was broken into. And at the time of the surgery I was very ill and very scared. Since that first surgery I have had seven more surgical procedures with general anesthesia and numerous invasive procedures. All of these came to constitute multiple experiences of having my body broken into.*

> *I think if it just ended there, I would have recovered very quickly from these nightmares and gone on about my business. But during my*

analysis, I discovered that I had in my mind a fear of being broken into sexually. That is a place that I didn't want to know very much about. I was scared of sex and scared of what men do to women sexually. Now, I am an educated woman (I had even been married before), and that seemed very silly—a silly notion and silly that I would find that some part of me was scared of sex. But the more I knew about it the more it began to make sense. And when I started knowing more about this fear from both perspectives, being broken into physically by medical procedures and sexually, the dream stopped and I stopped pushing away all of the eligible men who wanted to date me.

The final outcome was that even though I am considerably overweight, and not young, I married a wonderful man. And enjoy a wonderful sexual relationship with him.

Some young men and women have positive dating experiences during or after treatment that help them feel better about their appearance.

I started dating my first boyfriend when I was 16—a few months after I finished my treatment for Hodgkin's. I was still wearing a wig, and he talked me into taking it off. He told me he thought I was pretty without it. I felt ugly and bald until he said that. He liked to run his fingers through the little bit of hair that I had. It was the sexiest thing and it meant the world to me.

Although disability awareness is changing, there are still plenty of people who stare, make rude remarks, or just act uncomfortable around people with disabilities.

I had non-Hodgkin's lymphoma and have two fairly noticeable scars— one on my neck and one that's about 5 inches long on my upper arm. Whenever I wear sleeveless tops, I get asked about it. I either say "It's from surgery" or "It's from when I had cancer." What I say depends on what my relationship is with that person. For a long time, I felt uncomfortable about them and I covered them up. But it's been years now, so I'm not quite as bothered by it.

• • • • •

I developed a secondary breast cancer when I was in my late 20s and had a mastectomy. I wanted to have a reconstruction and implants, but the surgeon said it would be a 10-hour surgery and insurance wouldn't pay for it. I can't pay out of pocket for it, so I use a prosthesis. It really affects what I can wear. If I put on a sleeveless dress or one that is a tiny bit low in front, the prosthesis shows. I really hate it.

I am in a wheelchair and am small. People stare at me and some think I'm stupid. If I am in a store trying to buy stuff, they will ask my mom, "Oh, can she sign her name?" It bothers me that they talk to her and not me.

Survivors with hormonal problems should be evaluated by an endocrinologist or obstetrician/gynecologist with experience treating cancer survivors. Some sexual problems can be caused by hormonal imbalances (see Chapter 9, *Hormone-Producing Glands*) while others are rooted in psychological distress (e.g., fears of being touched). These are normal late effects from treatment for which help is available.

The healthcare provider at your follow-up clinic should discuss any sexual concerns you have. They can also suggest therapists who help individuals or couples understand and deal with sexual problems. The American Association of Sex Educators, Counselors, and Therapists (AASECT) can suggest accredited therapists in your area. Its website address is *www.aasect. org*. Another resource that contains a wealth of information about sexuality after cancer is Leslie Schover's book *Sexuality and Fertility After Cancer* (see Appendix B, *Resources*). The Lance Armstrong Foundation has information about female and male sexual late effects at *www.livestrong.org*; click on "learn about cancer," then "cancer support topics," and then "physical effects of cancer." For more information about this topic, see Chapter 14, *Kidneys, Bladder, and Genitals*.

Disclosure

No one else can decide the right time for you to disclose your cancer history. You might want to find out right away if someone you are interested in is cancer-phobic. On the other hand, you may wish to establish a relationship first so the person already cares for you and will be less likely to respond negatively. Some survivors feel strongly that quick honesty is the best policy, while others feel equally strongly that it's better to wait awhile. Only you can decide when the time is appropriate to share such an important part of your life.

I was beginning to feel like myself again 3 years after treatment for cancer when I went on my first date since diagnosis. I met my date at the beach and we went on a long bike ride. I had a great time and it sure seemed as though she had a great time too, until the word cancer came up. We were talking about what we had been doing recently and because I am not ashamed of having cancer, I told her, and wow, was she shocked. Her whole attitude changed and I have called her twice since and she has not called me back.

Of course I realize that she might not be calling me back because she simply didn't like me, but I can tell when a girl is interested in me and she was. I totally freaked her out by telling her I had cancer.

People are afraid of what they don't understand. I am still the same person I was, I have nothing to be ashamed of. Actually, I am very proud of myself for enduring the treatment, and other people should be proud of me too, but they are not. They are afraid of getting close to me because they are afraid I will get sick again. Even though I am 3½ years in remission and my prognosis is excellent, I can understand how people would feel that way—it is a possibility.

The best plan is to let a person get to know you really well before you spring the notion of the cancer on them. Hopefully by that time they will love you enough not to care. When I go on another date and some-one asks me how I got my scars, I'm going to answer, "A motorcycle accident!"

· · · · ·

In my freshman year of college, I met a man I just adored. He was a gor-geous, blond composer. I had a major crush. He was in the same choir I was and loved all of the same things I did. He was very interested in me and we started to date. In English class, the first assignment was writing an essay about a personal experience. I wrote about having had cancer. The teacher made us read them aloud. After hearing that, the fellow I had a crush on cooled it immediately. I went to my support group and just started to cry. The social worker suggested that I try to talk to him about it. So I was talking to him about things in general (no mention of cancer), and when I put my hand out to touch him on the arm he jerked back. I didn't think people did that kind of thing anymore. It still hurts to think about it.

· · · · ·

I met my fiancée at a camp for kids with cancer. We are both cancer survivors so there was never any issue about disclosure. We were both up-front from the very beginning and shared our stories.

If you have obvious scarring or a disability resulting from cancer treatment, you might not have a choice of when to share the information. Some sur-vivors enjoy educating the public about disabilities or differences. Others say there are days when they don't mind explaining, and days when they just wish strangers would keep their stares and personal questions to themselves.

Disclosure is not much of an issue for me. I either use a cane or a guide dog to get around, so it's pretty obvious I'm blind. Although my eye

*prostheses look natural, one eye droops a little bit from the radiation.
Little kids do ask me what happened to my eye. I'm really open about
my cancer history, which helps make other people comfortable with it
too. When I had the rhabdomyosarcoma, they removed part of my jaw
and a muscle there. However, I have long curly hair and I have it cut in
such a way that it covers it up. Now if I pull it back, it bothers my mom,
but other people tell me it's not that noticeable.*

· · · · ·

*I had a brain tumor and am in a wheelchair. Kids stare at me a lot.
Adults assume I was in a car accident because of the wheelchair and my
bent leg. If anyone asks me why I am in the wheelchair I say, "Oh, I had
a disease, so I can't walk." Sometimes I tell the whole story depending on
how I feel.*

· · · · ·

*I had a leg amputated when I was young and use crutches. Sometimes
I feel like I'm on display. I don't mind using the crutches, but I wish I
didn't need them. Other times, I don't mind talking about it. It's pretty
obvious that something is different—I only have one leg! It's often a conversation opener. They ask what happened and I say, "Oh, I had cancer
when I was a kid." That's how I've started conversations with most of the
women I've dated. Everyone knows someone with cancer—a mother, a
cousin, a neighbor. So we instantly have something in common. I really
have no choice about disclosure.*

Disclosure may be especially problematic for survivors at risk for fertility
problems. Having cancer as well as losing the ability to have children can
be a crushing blow. It can also undermine relationships if having biological children (rather than adopting) is an important life goal of the partner.
Some survivors choose not to get fertility tests to avoid the necessity of
dealing with the issue before marriage. Others do not disclose the possibility of infertility due to fear of rejection.

*I'm very short and young-looking as a result of my cancer treatment.
As a man, my appearance is a real impediment to having relationships.
I really would like to get married. There is also the possibility I may be
infertile, but I don't want to be tested. I just don't want to deal with it
prior to a commitment; I'd rather figure it out together.*

When and how to disclose your cancer history to friends or partners is a
purely personal choice. Most survivors opt for sizing up the person and
deciding on a case-by-case basis. Often, survivors adopt the concentric circle method of sharing information. Those in the innermost circle know the

entire history, those a bit farther out are given a little information or only what they need to know, and those on the outer perimeter know nothing. Some survivors find it helpful to practice what they will say when disclosing their cancer history.

> I was treated for osteosarcoma during my dating prime—ages 16 to 18. I never dated. I rationalized it by thinking I didn't want to put anyone in the position of having to deal with my cancer. The truth was that I felt too ugly to date and my self-esteem was very low. My first year in college I decided not to tell anyone. Since I have a big scar on my leg, I made up various stories to explain. I tried to make the stories fun...I was attacked by a shark, fell off a Ferris wheel, was in a motorcycle accident. I thought if I told them the truth, they would desert me like all of my high school friends had. I didn't want to go through 4 years of college alone.
>
> By my second year, I felt comfortable enough to tell the truth, but I downplayed it. For instance, if someone looked shocked and said, "I'm so sorry," I'd say, "Oh, it happened a long time ago. Don't worry about it." Then I'd change the subject. I wanted people to know, but not to dwell on it or feel sorry for me.

Some survivors just pick up their lives where they left off. They find that their cancer history makes no difference in their social lives.

> Talking about cancer isn't a big issue for me. I had ALL and everybody knows it. Other than the fact that the experience changed me and made me who I am today, there are no outward signs. At a certain point in relationships I make a point to let the person know, because it was a huge part of my life. My life is normal and good.

Disclosure of cancer history to potential employers or coworkers is a completely different matter, which is covered in Chapter 4, *Navigating the System*.

Communication

Communication about cancer history is very important for those who live with the memories and late effects of their treatment. Sometimes survivors have one or two close friends from the hospital with whom they continue to share their thoughts and feelings about the past and their hopes and worries about the future. Joining a support group for survivors is a way to connect with others who have lived through similar experiences. These groups are a great resource for talking over practical matters with people who have traveled the same path. If there is no peer support at your hospital or follow-up clinic, ask a social worker or nurse to connect you with someone in similar circumstances. You could also train to become a counselor at the closest camp for children with cancer. Most of the young adults who are counselors at the camps share a history of cancer, and many form lifelong friendships there.

> *My fiancé and I both had cancer. We deal with it very differently. He doesn't get worked up about it—when it's over, it's over. But the nice thing is that he understands that I deal with it differently. I have to remind him about how upset I get around diagnosis and anniversaries. I had to learn how to tell him what I need. It took a while to get used to that. But we really think alike on most things, and respect our differences on the others.*

The Internet is a way to contact those who have lived through cancer. There are numerous support groups and websites where survivors can connect, chat, and share stories and advice. The Internet is a great leveler—it doesn't matter what you look like or whether or not you have any disabilities—you are valued for the thoughts, words, and ideas you choose to share. Addresses of some of these sites are listed in Appendix B, *Resources*.

> *I am a member of several Internet support groups. I believe in facing the future squarely, even though it is scary sometimes. I really like to help people and share stories. It's my way of giving back.*

· · · · ·

> *I had bilateral retinoblastoma when I was 2 and am blind. When I first got access to the Web my senior year in college, I started looking around for information on retinoblastoma and only found clinical and treatment facts. Nothing on psychosocial or emotional issues. From firsthand experience I knew about some long-term effects and realized that people really need to know these things. I didn't know other survivors, so I started an Internet discussion group with the help of Gilles Frydman, the founder of the Association of Cancer Online Resources, Inc. (ACOR: www.acor.org). We started with very few people, most of us in our 20s, 30s and 40s. It was neat when it branched out to include parents of newly diagnosed kids. It's gone global now.*

Marriage/life partnerships

Marriage (or a lifetime commitment) is one of life's major events. But for survivors of childhood cancer, making a life-long commitment may take on even greater meaning. A lingering fear of recurrence makes some survivors hesitant to link their future to another. Coming to terms with uncertainty, however, allows you to acknowledge you have a future that includes love and companionship.

> *I had cancer when I was a young teen. The only effect it had on my dating was that it made me value thoughtful, caring people. Not a bad thing! I had normal relationships through college and am happily married now. My wife and I have three beautiful, healthy kids.*

Some young adults rush into relationships while they are feeling vulnerable and uncertain of who they are or what they want.

> *I was very dependent on my family after my diagnosis of Wilms tumor at age 18. I married right out of college and was totally dependent on my husband. He handled all the money, made all the decisions, and pretty much ran my life.*

· · · · ·

> *When I had cancer at age 15, over 30 years ago, my parents didn't know if I would survive. As a result, I had no rules or guidance through my teen years. I went quickly into a bad marriage and then divorced. Several years later I married my wonderful husband who has been the best thing that ever happened in my life.*

Others feel that having cancer gave them a maturity that helped them find a partner who shares their values.

> *Hanging around adults for several years during treatment matured me beyond my years. After cancer, I was serious about big decisions. I still knew how to have fun, but I was more thoughtful, more discerning. I married a wonderful woman 20 years ago, and we have three beautiful kids. I'd be having a different life if not for cancer.*

· · · · ·

> *My husband has been with me through a lot in the 22 years since I had cancer. I have several late effects that have changed our lives. But I believe in following your dreams. We just took a different attitude and we enjoy what we can do together. The things I can't do with him, I just adapt. My heart is in the mountains. We have taken many hikes through the years. When my husband decided to climb Mt. Whitney, I wanted to go. It was the ultimate hike, but due to my chronic fatigue, I had to miss out. I trained with him on the local hills. When he climbed Mt. Whitney, a little bit of me went along. I accept the restrictions in my life and enjoy very much what I can do. We both have wonderful senses of humor and that has helped us through the years.*

Fertility

A big concern of some childhood cancer survivors is whether they will be able to have healthy children. Evidence indicates that cancer survivors are not at greater risk of having children with disabilities or cancer when compared with those who never had cancer (see the "Health of offspring" section later in this chapter). The vast majority of survivors remain fertile, and many have one or more healthy children. In some cases, however, the treatment used to save lives takes away the ability to create new life. This is an especially poignant and difficult loss.

> I am lucky to not have many late effects from my bone marrow transplant. Many of my peers whom I grew up with at the hospital have serious side effects. I have been truly blessed that I lead a very healthy life. I do have a couple of side effects that might play a larger role in my life as I get older, but as of right now they are pretty insignificant. I have cataracts in both eyes, and a mild heart problem caused by one of the drugs I received taking chemotherapy. The other side effect is due to damage to my endocrine system. I don't think I will be able to have my own children, and as I get older, I am finding that difficult to deal with, as I absolutely love kids. But there are always options. If medical advancements do not provide me a way to have my own children when I am ready to have them, then I would definitely adopt.

· · · · ·

> When the doctors told me that I probably was infertile, it was the most devastating part of the whole experience. By the time they told me about sperm banking it was too late. My urologist looked at the results and said, "No way, buddy." When I was dating, I told my future wife that I was told I'd be infertile. But in the back of my mind, I always had hope. My wife stayed on the pill until we thought we were ready to be parents. The first month she went off, she got pregnant. We have an 18-month-old boy, and my wife is pregnant again. It's wonderful. He's a miracle.

Those most likely to be infertile or have impaired fertility are:

- Survivors who had high doses of alkylators—cyclophosphamide, carmustine (BCNU), lomustine (CCNU), busulfan, melphalan, ifosfamide—and/or total body radiation.
- Male children and teens who had direct radiation to their testes.
- Female children and teens who had direct radiation to their ovaries.

Children treated before puberty tend to have fewer fertility problems than those treated after puberty, and girls usually are less affected by treatment than boys. For more information about the effects of radiation and chemotherapy on fertility, see Chapter 9, *Hormone-Producing Glands*.

In addition to the treatments listed above, many other factors affect the nature and degree of fertility. These include the type of cancer, its location, the treatment, gender of the survivor, and age at diagnosis. Physical and psychological late effects also impact the desire and ability to have children.

> *I had Hodgkin's 15 years ago and again 2 years ago. I used a sperm bank because my wife and I really want children. It's funny how the pain is so temporary, but loss stays. Even the memory of pain is gone, but losing an ability is forever. The hardest thing is loss. And the worst loss is infertility. We are running out of vials and none of the inseminations have worked. For me, this is the hardest part of having cancer.*

Fertility is affected if female survivors have an early menopause. Normally, fertility tends to decrease when women are in their mid-30s. In some women treated for cancer, this decrease in fertility can occur much earlier. Those most at risk for early menopause are:

- Adolescent girls treated after puberty.
- Female children or teens treated with both cyclophosphamide or other ovarian toxic drugs (ifosfamide, BCNU, or the combinations of medicines called MOPP and COPP) and radiation below the diaphragm.
- Girls who had an early puberty due to cranial radiation.

If you are at risk for early menopause, talk with your healthcare provider about family planning. You may be fertile for fewer years because of your treatments. If your periods become irregular or stop completely, see your gynecologist. Fertility can decline even with regular periods, so survivors at risk of early menopause should not rely on their periods as evidence of fertility—they need to have hormone levels monitored by their healthcare provider. Survivors who experience early menopause should get routine medical care to check for osteoporosis (thinning bones) and heart disease. These medical issues are covered in Chapter 9, *Hormone-Producing Glands*, and psychological issues are discussed in Chapter 2, *Emotions*.

> *I had ABVD (combination of four chemotherapy drugs) to treat my Hodgkin's. I'm glad because we really want children, and MOPP has an increased rate of fertility problems. I don't think I'll have any fertility problems. We've done all the tests and I seem to be fine. During treatment, of course, my periods stopped. But I have them now like clockwork.*

There may be factors other than physical problems that affect childbearing. Some women worry that pregnancy may be risky because of their treatment for cancer—a true medical concern for those who had certain treatments, such as pelvic radiation. Others fear they may pass on cancer to their children, a fear that is, in most cases, unfounded. Yet other survivors are concerned about relapse or secondary cancers and may hesitate to bring a child into the world whom they might not be able to parent into adulthood.

I was told when I was about 15 years old that the retinoblastoma I had as a child was possibly genetic. No one could say for sure. That was a blow at that age, because even then, I was babysitting a lot and imagined having my own little ones someday. I had several years to let this news sink in before I met the man I married. He was aware of my medical history, and it was okay with him if we adopted. Although on the surface, all seemed to be settled, the decision became very real and not so logical when the time came to decide on some permanent form of birth control. It made no sense for him to have a vasectomy, since he was healthy. What if I died young or we divorced? He should still be able to father his own children. So logic and common sense said I should have a tubal ligation. This was in 1970, and although my head said this was right, my heart and emotions made it difficult. What if a cure was found while I was still of childbearing age?

Logic won out when I considered how sad I would feel if my children developed retinoblastoma in both eyes. The agonizing over my decision was also not something I would want my children to go through. It just made more sense to stop the spread of this disease. My older sister, who did not have RB, was unable to have children due to a medical problem that was unrelated. Once we knew more about the heredity factor, she admitted relief that she had adopted, because she was afraid that perhaps she carried the gene, too.

This is not an easy decision to make, and no one can make it but the survivor. If I had my own children, they would be at an age to parent also, and I am glad I don't have to watch them make that decision. My adopted daughter had a baby boy 2 years ago, and it was a relief to know neither she nor I had to worry about little Devin.

Some survivors who are told they are infertile from their treatments are surprised to find out that they or their partners are unexpectedly pregnant. Even if it is likely that you are infertile from treatment, it is best to use birth control if you do not desire children.

I was diagnosed with non-Hodgkin's lymphoma stage IV when I was 16. It had already metastasized to my lungs, bones, and spine. The tumor in my spine paralyzed me from the waist down and I had lots of radiation to my lumbar spine to help me regain my mobility. The doctors told my mother that my ovaries probably got so much radiation that I would never have children. Well, I didn't believe them so I started using birth control pills when I was 18. Even using birth control pills I got pregnant—with twins. Since then I've had three more children.

· · · · ·

I had ALL 25 years ago. My wife and I have had no problems conceiving. As a matter of fact, we have three children, each 19 months apart. We're very fertile. I had a vasectomy because three was all we wanted.

Some adult survivors were never told or do not recall hearing that infertility was a potential consequence of treatment for their cancer. Prior to the early 1970s, many parents were advised not to discuss the cancer with their children. Young children knew they were sick, and when treatment was complete, the family acted as if the cancer had never invaded their lives. Many young adults do not learn that their ability to have children may have been compromised or destroyed until they have spent several emotional and expensive years trying. Learning the truth can unleash overwhelming feelings of anger and devastation. Survivors who were told of their probable infertility have varying feelings, and these may shift over time. Counseling from an expert in grief and loss can be of immense help to those struggling with these strong feelings.

About the issues of fertility—life and living is better. In 1972 at the age of 21, because of treatment, I lost my capacity to have children. I thought I would never recover, but life is funny and I did. I found myself working with children in all sorts of ways that I had never imagined. And I can say that although at times it has been hard, my life has been incredibly rich even without children.

I have found in strange ways children do come to you. I was a children's librarian, I love my nieces and nephews, and I enjoy the children of my friends. But I did have to go through a lot of therapy before I properly grieved my infertility.

In terms of dating and finding men—I found that my infertility was a funny way of weeding out the chaff from the keepers. The good and wonderful men in my life have never found my infertility a problem, including my wonderful and loving husband. Not having children is something we have mourned together. We have a rich life nevertheless.

· · · · ·

I was told when I was treated for Hodgkin's in 1977 that I would be sterile. It was hard because I'd always wanted twin girls. The whole bubble burst—your health and looks go, and you can never have children. It was like every door started slamming closed one at a time. I thought I'd adopt. When I was in my early 20s, my husband and I went to three preliminary meetings. Then a friend asked what was our hurry, and that made sense so we decided to wait. After that we realized we liked our freedom. I also had problems with my immune system so I've been sick a lot, plus I have chronic fatigue, so it would have been really hard to have kids. I couldn't have children, but I've always loved cats. I filled the void of being childless by raising a cat. Whiskers was with me for nearly 20 years. She was my constant companion and my strength throughout my illnesses. I have no regrets. I have loved my life.

· · · · ·

Sadness, like anger, is one of those emotions in life that has its appropriate place. We can't protect ourselves from sadness, nor should we want to. Sadness that sweeps over us from time to time allows us to savor our joys and thrills.

I think that surviving a life-threatening illness sometimes makes us a little more susceptible to sadness because it places us on a life journey where we will be altered in ways that may not suit us. From time to time, even though it is 28 years later, I am caught up in a tremendous sadness at not having children. It is a deep and abiding grief that washes over me at odd and unexpected moments. But it does wash over me and then pass. And I am able to go on and savor the joys of my life.

Support and empathy from family and friends may not occur if you are infertile. Leslie Schover, in *Sexuality and Fertility After Cancer*, writes:

The most profound loss is giving up the dream of having one's own, genetic child. Cancer survivors are often told by physicians, family, and well-meaning friends that they should be glad to be alive. Their pain at being infertile is dismissed as ingratitude. But many people see having a child as a very concrete way of defeating death and leaving a part of oneself for the future. Many men and women grow up assuming they will be parents one day. For a couple, that longed-for child was to be the blending of their individual strengths and the product of their love. Mental health professionals who treat infertile couples often point out that it is difficult for them to grieve adequately or to get true understanding and support from family and friends because what has been lost is potential, rather than an actual child. The loss is no less real, however.

In order to make informed decisions about childbearing, you need to ask questions and get thorough, understandable answers. Start off by asking yourself the following questions, and then consult a medical professional at a comprehensive follow-up clinic to get an honest evaluation of your individual situation.

- Am I in a stable relationship and do we both want children? Not having children is a choice made by many couples, with or without a cancer history.

- Am I experiencing any anxiety about the health of my future children? The next section discusses health of offspring, and for the vast majority of survivors, the news is very encouraging.

- Am I worried about my ability to physically carry a child? Pregnancy places additional stresses on the heart and lungs. If you received anthracycline drugs (doxorubicin, daunorubicin, idarubicin, or mitoxantrone) or lung, heart, or uterine radiation, you may have a higher risk for pregnancy complications. Prior to pregnancy, obtain expert advice about your actual risks so you can make an informed decision. If you do have any increased risk, get obstetrical care from a specialist in high-risk pregnancies during your pregnancy.

- If I wait to try to get pregnant, will I have problems conceiving? Much is known about risks to fertility from various treatments. Opinions from your caregivers will be about risks to groups of survivors, not you as an individual. Fertility is a complicated matter, and your healthcare provider will consider your type of cancer, age at diagnosis, your gender, and your treatment. Keep in mind that you are getting an educated opinion (or two), but not having your future told. The honest answer is that knowledgeable healthcare providers can give you their best guess, but no one can accurately predict your future.

- If I am infertile, what technologies are available to help me become pregnant? Donor sperm, donor eggs, in vitro fertilization, and surrogate mothers are methods of reproduction for infertile survivors. To find out about the most up-to-date techniques available, contact Fertile Hope at *www.fertilehope.org* or RESOLVE at *www.resolve.org*.

- What are the costs of the various options—adoption, infertility treatments— and how will they be financed?

- Would we rather adopt a baby, go through infertility treatments, or choose not to have children? Spend time talking over your priorities before making these important decisions. Consulting a mental health professional with experience helping couples cope with infertility may help you clarify your feelings and sort out your options. Infertility clinics in your area or your oncologist can provide the names of skilled therapists.

Explore whether there are local support groups for infertile couples in your area. Sharing experiences and talking over your situation with others can yield understanding and empathy you may not get from family or friends.

Health of offspring

Cancer survivors often worry about the health of their future children. They are afraid that a child conceived after surgery, radiation, or chemotherapy might be born with serious or life-threatening health problems. They also sometimes wonder if they could pass on their cancer genetically to their children.

> *Because I had bilateral retinoblastoma, I have a high chance of passing it on to any offspring. A doctor told my mother when I was in my early 20s that the disease could be passed on, so my wife and I chose not to have any kids.*

The results of studies looking at the rate of birth defects in children born to childhood cancer survivors are very encouraging. In general, children born to survivors are just as healthy as those born to people who never had cancer. Doctors caring for survivors encourage them to have children if they desire them, and except in certain circumstances, no special tests are recommended. However, close monitoring is necessary for certain risk groups, such as those who had pelvic radiation or received drugs that can damage the heart.

An article published in the *New England Journal of Medicine* in 1998 described the results of the largest study done to date on the health of the children of survivors of childhood cancer. Researchers in Denmark, Finland, Iceland, Norway, and Sweden examined their national databases to assess the risk of cancer in offspring of 14,652 cancer survivors who had produced 5,847 offspring. Other than survivors of retinoblastoma and other hereditary cancer syndromes (e.g., Li-Fraumeni syndrome, von Hippel-Lindau disease), offspring of cancer survivors were just as healthy as the children of their healthy siblings.[1] More recently, a study of 4,699 children of 1,128 male and 1,627 female childhood cancer survivors provided strong evidence that the children of cancer survivors are not at significantly increased risk for congenital abnormalities resulting from their parents' cancer treatments.[2]

> *I had leukemia 20 years ago. I have three beautiful children. All healthy, all smart. What a blessing.*

Many evenings I go into the bedroom of my 18-month-old son to just look at him. He is so perfect, such a miracle. I hope that I will always be able to protect him from harm.

This encouraging news concerns survivors treated in the 1970s and 1980s. Results about the effects of newer protocols will unfold over the next 2 decades, as those survivors reach adulthood, marry or enter committed relationships, and have children.

Physical changes in the bodies of some female Wilms tumor survivors can cause health problems in offspring. Women who had abdominal or pelvic radiation may have a uterus that does not expand well during pregnancy. This can cause spontaneous abortion (miscarriage), low-birthweight infants, and a higher rate of babies who die in the uterus or soon after birth. Any pregnant survivor with a history of radiation that included the uterus should be followed by an expert in high-risk pregnancies.

I had Wilms tumor when I was 2 years old. I have had three sons and all were around 7 pounds and full term. I do have one badly damaged fallopian tube from the radiation, but it didn't seem to affect my fertility. The only problem I've had is that the slight scoliosis (curvature of the spine) from the radiation makes epidurals during labor difficult.

• • • • •

When I was treated for Wilms tumor with flank radiation and chemotherapy as a teenager, I stopped having periods. When I was finished, I had a complete endocrinology workup and was told my chances for having children were between slim and none. They told me if I ever wanted children they could try some fertility drugs. Since I was planning on getting married, I asked about birth control and was told none was necessary. So I got married and within a month started a new job doing public relations for a regional hospital, which required mandatory blood testing. The very first day on the job they called me to make sure I knew that the pregnancy test was positive! I was shocked, but absolutely thrilled because all my life I'd wanted children, and yet I had so much fear that I never would. I had my first healthy son when I was 22 and my next healthy son 4 years later.

Pregnancy is a stress on the heart, so if you were treated with drugs that can weaken the heart (see Chapter 12, *Heart and Blood Vessels*), you should have your heart evaluated prior to pregnancy and be cared for by a specialist who can monitor your heart during pregnancy and labor.

Very few types of cancer can be passed from parent to child genetically. Familial retinoblastoma, Li-Fraumeni syndrome (clusters of different cancers such as breast cancer, leukemia, brain tumors, and sarcomas in a family), and rare cases of Wilms tumor may be caused by genetic mutations.

> I had retinoblastoma in one eye 30 years ago. They thought it was the non-hereditary form because it was one tumor in just one eye. The eye was removed, and I had no chemotherapy or radiation.

> Ten years ago, my newborn daughter was diagnosed with retinoblastoma in both eyes. She had one eye removed and the remaining eye was radiated with 2200 cGy (centigray). Two years later the tumors returned in her remaining eye. The tumors regrew only 3 weeks after chemotherapy ended, so she had more chemotherapy. When that course had to be cut short due to side effects, they decided to remove the remaining eye.

> I was 6 months pregnant when my daughter's retinoblastoma returned. The doctors knew that there was a chance that the child I was carrying could inherit the disease, since both my daughter and I had it. After my son was born, he was checked over carefully, and the cord blood was sent away for DNA testing. The results came back and showed that he had not inherited the disease. He's fine, but still goes every year for a checkup.

If you are one of the survivors whose family history puts you at higher risk for having a child with health problems, you might want to consider genetic counseling and possibly genetic testing. Prior to the testing, take steps to protect the confidentiality of the information. One way to do this is to learn about the Genetic Information Nondiscrimination Act (GINA), a federal law passed in 2008 to limit disclosure of genetic information without your permission. Consumer factsheets about GINA are available at *www.ginahelp. org* and *www.genome.gov/10002328*.

> I had non-Hodgkin's lymphoma when I was 16. When I was 21 my third child Danielle was born. On her first birthday, she was diagnosed with neuroblastoma. The doctor, who had treated me, had big tears in his eyes when he told us. Two years later, she died. We've had a lot of cancer in my family, and I've since been treated for breast cancer (at age 27) so we just may have cancer genes running in the family.

State-of-the-art genetic counseling is a multi-step process, with several sessions and chances to change your mind about testing. It also includes follow-up to thoroughly explain the report and what it means. A good genetic counselor can help explain the nature of the risks (if any) your genetic profile could cause an unborn child. Your test results and counseling sessions should be confidential. Genetic testing is a rapidly evolving field. To learn more about genetic testing for cancer, you can view the National Cancer Institute slide program, "Gene Testing" at *http://cancer.gov/cancertopics/understandingcancer/genetesting.* Make sure you go to a well-respected genetic counseling program. You can get a referral from your doctor, your nurse practitioner, or the National Society of Genetic Counselors (go to *www.nsgc.org* and click on "Find a Genetic Counselor"). Various resources related to genetics are available at *www.geneticalliance.org.*

Adoption

Whether to adopt children is an intensely personal decision. If you wish to adopt an infant, you may find that it is a difficult and time-consuming process. If you are open to adopting a toddler or older child, or a child of mixed race background, the waiting time is almost always shorter. Many of these older children are healthy and well adjusted, although others have medical needs, disabilities, or emotional issues. When applying to adopt, you may face barriers from agencies based on your health history. Nevertheless, many adoptive parents describe the process as worth every second once they fold their new infant or child into their family.

Domestic or international adoptions can be arranged through public or private licensed adoption agencies. Title III of the Americans with Disabilities Act prohibits agencies from discriminating against cancer survivors based solely on their cancer history. They must consider applicants on an individual basis. You can also arrange adoptions privately through an attorney.

During the adoption process, a home study is done by the agency involved. This study will require a medical exam by the prospective parents' physicians. Make sure your doctor explains your medical history in an honest yet positive way and stresses the length of time you have been off treatment and your current health status.

Choose your agency or attorney carefully to ensure that your emotional and medical situation is clearly understood. Try to put together a team that works well together to give you the best chance to adopt.

Chapter 4

Navigating the System

The best prescription is knowledge.
—C. Everett Koop, M.D.

EVEN IN the 21st century, a cancer history can still create challenges for survivors. Knowledge, networking, and advocacy are necessary to overcome barriers to obtaining an appropriate education, insurance, and a job.

It helps to have a map for the cancer survivorship journey. This chapter offers basic information to help guide you on your journey. It covers education from elementary school through vocational training or college. It outlines your legal rights and gives specific suggestions about how to understand and use the system to get the most appropriate education for yourself (or your child). It then discusses how to obtain comprehensive and affordable life and health insurance; how to obtain free or low-cost medications; how to handle job interviews and strategies for avoiding discrimination; and ways to enter the armed services. Finally, individual and group advocacy are discussed.

Education

Childhood cancer and its treatment can leave survivors with unique educational needs. Treatments that sometimes affect school performance are brain radiation, brain surgery, intrathecal methotrexate, and high-dose systemic methotrexate. Chapter 8, *Brain and Nerves*, covers these possible late effects in detail. In addition to these treatments, learning potential can be impacted by numerous or lengthy hospitalizations, persistent fatigue, hearing or vision loss, fine or gross motor impairments, and social difficulties.

> *I get help from the Lighthouse, which helps people with vision problems or blindness. I'm a rare case for them—hard to classify. I have severe vision cuts, but my remaining vision is quite good. I'm starting high school next week and feel a little odd entering a mainstream school because I have trouble navigating, although the academics are manageable.*

Comprehensive follow-up clinics have skilled personnel who help families work with school systems to get the best possible education for their children. But many individuals and families do not have access to these resources and must navigate the special education system on their own. You have many legal rights, and knowing what they are can help you advocate for yourself or your child.

Legal rights

The Individuals with Disabilities Education Act (IDEA) requires every public school to provide a free and appropriate education in the least restrictive environment to all disabled individuals between the ages of 3 and 21. That means providing, without charge, special education programs, speech therapy, occupational therapy, physical therapy, psychiatric services, assistive communication techniques and technology, and other interventions as needed to help children learn. This law has been extended and modified by the Individuals with Disabilities in Education Improvement Act of 2004 and updated regulations published in 2006, 2008, and 2011 (see *http://idea. ed.gov/explore/home*). The major provisions of these laws are the following:

- All children, regardless of disability, are entitled to a free and appropriate public education and necessary related services. Schools are required to provide an individually designed instructional program for every eligible child, including early intervention programs for at-risk toddlers.

- Children will receive fair testing to determine if they need special education services.

- Parents of a child with disabilities participate in the planning and decision-making for their child's special education.

- Children with disabilities will be educated in the least restrictive environment possible, usually with children who are not disabled.

- The decisions of the school system can be challenged by parents, with disputes resolved by an impartial third party.

- Planning for transition to postsecondary schooling, work, or independent living must start by the time the student turns 16, or younger if appropriate.

- Parents have the right to withdraw consent for special education and related services, but they must do so in writing.

These laws cover survivors of cancer whose medical problems affect their educational performance, and eligibility is usually obtained using the categories known as "other health impaired," "traumatically brain injured," or "learning disabled." Special education services are also available if the child's medical condition limits energy, alertness, or strength. Many survivors do not need special help in school, but those who do have a legal right to it.

Children on and off treatment may also be eligible for services and accommodations under Section 504 of the federal Rehabilitation Act. This law applies when the child does not meet the eligibility requirements for specially designed instruction but still needs accommodations (provided through a "504 Plan") to perform successfully in school. For example, special accommodations to address health needs can include a water bottle on the desk, reduced homework during periods of illness, waiving regular attendance/ tardy policies and procedures, or allowing additional time to get to class. Another example is that a child off therapy with cognitive impairments that do not meet the IDEA requirements might need to have accommodations that eliminate timed tests or provide more time to finish written assignments.

> My 12-year-old daughter is in seventh grade. She had a BMT (bone marrow transplant) 5 years ago for AML (acute myelogenous leukemia). She doesn't have any learning disabilities, but does have a 504 plan.
>
> The first week of school, we had a meeting with all of her teachers, the school counselor, the nurse, and the dean. She got a waiver for the 10-day absence policy. Otherwise, if she was absent over 10 days, she automatically fails her courses. She gets to carry a water bottle at school. She sometimes needs to lie down to breathe (she has scarred lungs). I go pick up her books from her locker so she doesn't have to carry them home. She gets to leave class after everyone else does to avoid the rush and is expected to be late to the next class. It's worked really well.
>
> I didn't expect much support from the teachers, but they have been wonderful. Her history teacher has offered to bring her homework by the house when she is sick and pick up the completed homework for all of her classes. She hand-carries it to all of JaNette's teachers.

The Canadian special education process is very similar to that used in the United States. Provincial guidelines are set down by the national Ministry of Education and governed by the Education Act, but most decisions are made at the regional, district, or school level. Evaluations are done by a team that may include a school district psychologist, a behavior specialist, a special education teacher, other school or district personnel, and in some cases a parent, although the latter is not required by law as it is in the United States.

In Canada, children between the ages of 6 and 22 may qualify for special education assistance under the Designated Disabled Program (DDP), the

Special Needs Program (SNP), or the Targeted Behavior Program (TBP), depending on the evaluation.

A full range of placement options is available for Canadian students, from home-based instruction to full inclusion. Students from rural or poorly served areas may receive funding to attend a day program outside their home area.

Referral for services

The steps necessary to obtain services in the United States are referral, evaluation, eligibility, development of an individualized education program (IEP), annual review, and triennial assessment.

Parents or teachers can make a referral by writing the school principal to request special education testing. Some school districts automatically set up an IEP for any child who had cranial radiation during cancer therapy, while other school districts are extremely reluctant even to evaluate struggling children for possible learning disabilities. Therefore, it is best for the parent or physician to send a written request to the principal, stating that the child is "health impaired" due to treatment for cancer, listing the child's problems, and requesting assessments and an IEP meeting.

> My son had problems as soon as he entered kindergarten while on treatment. He couldn't hold a pencil, and he developed difficulties with math and reading. By second grade, I was asking the school for extra help, and they tested him. They did an IEP and gave him special attention in small remedial groups. The school system also provided weekly physical therapy, which really helped him.

· · · · ·

> Initially, the school was reluctant to test Gina because they thought she was too young (6 years old). But she had been getting occupational therapy at the hospital for 2 years, and I wanted the school to take over. I brought in articles from Candlelighters Childhood Cancer Foundation [now called the American Childhood Cancer Organization] and spoke to the teacher, principal, nurse, and counselor. Gina had a dynamite teacher who really listened, and she helped get permission to have Gina tested. Her tests showed her to be very strong in some areas and very weak in others.

> Together, we developed an IEP, which we have updated every spring. Originally, she received weekly occupational therapy and daily help from the special education teacher. She's now in fourth grade and is doing so well that she no longer needs occupational therapy, and she

only gets extra help during study hall. They even recommended her for the student council, which has been a tremendous boost for her self-confidence.

Once the referral is made, an evaluation is necessary to find out if the school district agrees that the child needs additional help, and if so, what types of help would be most beneficial. Usually a multidisciplinary team—consisting of the teacher, district psychologist, speech and language therapist, and resource specialist—meet to administer and evaluate the testing. Your written consent is required prior to your child's evaluation, and you have the right to obtain an independent evaluation if you believe the school's testing is biased or flawed in any way. However, you may be responsible for this cost. The evaluation usually includes a review of educational, medical, social, and psychological status.

Survivors of childhood cancer at risk for learning difficulties require neuropsychological testing, which is best administered by psychologists experienced in testing pediatric patients. Most large children's hospitals have such personnel, but it sometimes takes very assertive parents to get the school system to use these experts. If you pay for the neuropsychological evaluation, you choose how much of the information to share with the school. You can cover portions that you wish to remain confidential and copy the rest to give to the team.

> *The psychologist who did my son's neuropsych report did a thorough job and wrote an excellent report. Unfortunately, she included paragraphs on family functioning and sections on my son's psychological history. Since I wasn't asking the school system to provide counseling, I didn't want them to have access to that information. I didn't want that to travel with my son throughout his elementary and high school career. We need the labels to get the services, but I also want to protect his privacy as much as possible. So, I only gave the school the parts of the report that I wanted them to have.*

After the evaluation, a conference is held to discuss the results and reach conclusions about what actions will be necessary in the future. Parents should attend this meeting and can bring a doctor, therapist, educational liaison, professional advocate, or friend with them. Make sure that in all written correspondence with the school, you clearly express your desire to be present at all meetings and discussions concerning your child's special education needs. You know your child best and have the right to be there. The school can still have the meeting if you choose not to attend or if you do not show up.

I had cranial radiation in 1976 when I was 5. My learning disabilities were identified when I was in third grade. I had problems copying from the board, so the teacher would let me use her notes. But I still had to copy them because it was part of the assignment. It was hard because I get letters transposed and skip words. But this made less and less difference as I went through high school and college, because copying wasn't important anymore. I now use spell check and grammar check and don't have as many problems in that arena.

Individualized education program

The IEP describes the special education program and any other related services specifically designed to meet the individual needs of a child with learning differences. It is developed collaboratively between parents and educators to determine what the student will be taught, and how and when the school will teach it. Students with disabilities need to learn the same things as other students: reading, writing, mathematics, science, history, and other preparation for college or vocational training. The difference is that, with an IEP in place, specialized services—such as small classes, home schooling, speech therapy, physical therapy, counseling, and instruction by special education teachers—are stipulated. These services are available to children with subtle learning difficulties, not just those with severe late effects. Parents must monitor the situation to make sure stipulated services are actually provided.

> *Chris gets help in school from physical and occupational therapists. He gets special education for math and reading, and he works with the occupational therapist on the computer and special projects. He also has an adaptive physical education coach twice a week and does regular phys ed with his class the rest of the time. He uses an auditory trainer— a hearing aid with a receiver that is connected to a piece the teacher wears. It directs the teacher's voice to his ear. He uses a hearing aid in the other ear. His comprehension level is now so much higher. Our IEP has worked very well.*

The IEP includes:

- Parental concerns, medical history, and information about the disability.

- A statement of present levels of academic achievement, social, behavioral, and physical functioning, academic performance, and learning style.

- Annual goals, objectives, benchmarks, and methods of evaluation.

- Services that will be provided and any program modifications or supports for school personnel that will be provided.

- The projected date when services/modifications will begin, and their frequency, location, and duration.

- Plans for standardized testing and graduation requirements.

- A description of the least restrictive setting in which the above goals and objectives can be met.

- Any individual accommodations needed for state and district-wide assessments.

- A statement of parental rights and responsibilities.

At least once a year, and more frequently if requested by a parent or teacher, a meeting is held (which your child can attend) to review the progress toward meeting the short- and long-term goals and objectives of the IEP. Some states have limits on the number of IEP meetings per year.

Someone from the school system is appointed to carry out and monitor each part of the IEP. However, the parent needs to know what it contains and work with the school if included services aren't being performed. A written copy of the plan is given to the family. It is best to create a positive relationship with the school so you are able to work together to promote your child's well-being. If, for whatever reason, communication deteriorates and you feel your child's IEP is inadequate or not being followed, there are several facts you need to know:

- Changes to the IEP cannot be made without parental consent.

- If parents disagree with the school about the content of the IEP, they can either withdraw consent and request (in writing) a meeting to draft a new IEP, or they can consent only to portions of the IEP with which they agree.

- Parents can request to have the disagreement settled by an independent mediator and hearing officer.

- Parents can hire a special education advocate—a person with special training and expertise whose profession is helping families get appropriate special education services for their child. The advocate will attend all meetings and give advice about legally mandated services and how to obtain them.

IEPs in Canada are almost identical to those used in the United States. In Canada, the IEP is updated yearly, or more frequently if needed. A formal review is required every 3 years. In Canada, if disputes arise between the school or district and the parents, the School Division Decision Review process is available to resolve them. The concept known as due process in the United States is usually referred to as fundamental justice in Canada.

My daughter's bilateral retinoblastoma was treated with surgery (both eyes removed), chemotherapy, and radiation. Paige goes to the public school where she has a half day with a special teacher for the blind and a half day in the regular class with a teacher's aide. She was having some problems in school for a couple of years, but it was hard to tell if it was because she couldn't see or was a late effect from the radiation. So we did neuropsych testing and found the problem areas: language processing and attention. This year we started her on a very low dose of Ritalin® to help her focus.

Since then, she's improved her reading from a 2.3 grade level to a 4.3 (she's in fourth grade)—two full grades in a year. I just came back from the school, where she received the Most Improved Student award.

Although some disabilities are physical and visible, others (such as educational and social competence) may not be as obvious. To help children and teens reach their true potential, changes in intellectual functioning and social skills must be diagnosed early and addressed.

One type of late effect that I don't see much about is limited social skills and deficits in emotional/social development. My daughter Sophie was diagnosed with standard risk ALL at 14 months old—so very young. Now at 7 years old, she struggles socially, is very impulsive and often angry at other kids, and has some anxiety (around the social skills I think). I believe that the methotrexate affected her brain development and this in turn affected her processing abilities, which are at play when she is trying to deal with social situations.

Recently Sophie had another thorough evaluation (four parts) by multiple professionals (developmental pediatrician, psychiatrist, psychologist, and speech-language pathologist). They diagnosed Sophie with low to average processing speed and indicated that she has executive function problems—when something is new/harder/changes, she processes slowly and can't figure out how to react. Then she gets frustrated and impulsively acts out. In addition, they told me that Sophie fits the criteria for ADHD and has a lot of anxiety. It has been very hard. I thought (naively) that post treatment things would get easier, but there is no prescription for what is going on now. I have had to push for every bit of help that she is getting (e.g., assessments, support in her after school care program, play therapy, IEP at school). While I believe that the chemotherapy caused a large portion of these challenges, I find that many healthcare providers and teachers do not know about this or understand.

For more information about IEPs, visit *http://nichcy.org/schoolage/iep/iepcontents*. In addition, parents and teachers can obtain a free copy of the book *Educating the Child with Cancer, 2nd ed.* from the American Childhood Cancer Foundation *(https://acco.org/Information/Resources/Books.aspx)*.

Individualized transition plans

Special education students also have a right to be prepared for graduation, higher education, and work—in ways that fit their needs. For some survivors, extra support will be needed to make the transition from high school to adulthood go smoothly. Under IDEA 2004, when a student with an IEP turns 16, the annual IEP meeting must include discussion about transition service needs, and the child must be invited to attend. In Canada, IEPs must include a transition plan for students ages 14 years or older. The statement of transition goals and services must be written into the IEP.

Transition plans should include the following:

- Desired post-school outcomes

- Necessary documents and support services

- List of transition resource team members

- Career preparation activities

- Transition services for instruction, community experiences, employment, post-school living, and daily living skills

- Vocational evaluation

- Summary of agency responsibilities

- Summary of designated instruction and services for transition

- A statement about the rights that will transfer to the child when she reaches the age of majority, beginning at least 1 year before that date

Obtaining a high school diploma usually requires passing a certain number of specified courses. Students sometimes need to have changes in the graduation requirements—for example, a deaf student faced with a foreign language requirement might ask that the requirement be waived or that fluency in sign language be allowed to substitute for foreign language proficiency.

> *I tell kids who are having a hard time in high school that the world opens up in college. It's such a bigger pool of people. I also think your peers are more mature. You won't be that kid who had cancer anymore. My learning disabilities were not such a big deal in college. No one knew about them; I had the tools I needed to work around them. The doors really open up in college.*

Some students will need extra coursework to make it through high school, such as special instruction in keyboarding or study skills. These abilities will also help with higher education or future employment.

Some students will not be able to earn a regular diploma. A special form of graduation called an IEP diploma is also available. If a student earns an IEP diploma, that means he has completed all of the objectives set out in his IEP for graduation. Passing a series of five tests called the general educational development (GED) tests may be an option for other students. In the United States, many states have implemented high school exit exams that must be passed to graduate. In some states, exemptions are available for students with an IEP or 504 Plan.

Students planning to attend trade school, a 2-year community college program, or a 4-year (or longer) college program need information far in advance about which high school courses will be required for admission. This is especially important for those students with disabilities who carry a lighter course load, as they may need to make up some credits in summer school or via correspondence or online courses.

Transition programs should address the move from high school to trade school, community college, or a 4-year college program. Students are eligible for publicly funded education and/or services until age 22, if needed.

Vocational training

Preparing for the world of work means gaining appropriate skills, such as typing, filing, driving, filling out forms, and using tools. These skills may be gained in school-based vocational-technical classes, in classes taken at a community college or vocational school while the student is still in high school, in a union- or employer-sponsored apprenticeship program, in an internship, or on the job. Vocational planning is mandatory for special education students in the United States by age 16 as part of an Individualized Transition Plan, but it should begin much earlier.

Transition-to-work services may include moving into the public vocational rehabilitation system, which trains and places adults with disabilities into jobs. However, in many states, the vocational rehabilitation system is severely overloaded, with waiting times for placement ranging from 3 months to as much as 3 years. Typical opportunities range from "sheltered workshop" jobs (e.g., sorting recyclables, light assembly work) under direct supervision to supported placement in the community as grocery clerks, office helpers, factory workers, and the like. Often the survivor works with a job coach, a person who helps her learn work skills and how to handle workplace stresses. In some cases, the job coach goes to work with the person for a while.

School districts may sponsor their own supported work opportunities, such as learning how to run an espresso coffee cart or working in a student-run horticultural business. Many schools have vocational programs that give students a chance to have a mentor in their chosen field, and that may include actual work experience with local employers.

Some public and private agencies may also be able to help with job training and placement, such as the state employment department, the Opportunities Industrialization Commission (OIC), and the Private Industry Council (PIC). Goodwill Industries operates a job placement service in many larger cities, as well.

The Texas Commission for the Blind helps people who are in school or looking for work assistance. The state pays tuition for public college, and they pay for a portion of your book costs. It's a free education. They will provide you with any necessary equipment to do your job. Whenever I'm transitioning into school or to a new job, they open my case and provide some services.

Students with disabilities should receive appropriate vocational counseling, including aptitude testing, discussion of their interests and abilities, and information about work possibilities. Parents need to ensure that students with the potential to do higher level work are not shunted into jobs that will leave them financially vulnerable and possibly unhappy as adults.

Every state has a vocational rehabilitation agency that provides services to individuals in the state where they live. The federal Rehabilitation Act requires states to provide the following minimum services:

• Evaluation of potential for rehabilitation

• Counseling

• Placement services

• Physical accommodations (the state does not have to provide equipment but does have to help determine what equipment is needed)

Some states have vocational rehabilitation scholarship money that provides an amount comparable to tuition at a state university that can be used for vocational training. They also provide information about private vocational rehabilitation programs within the state. The Rehabilitation Act requires that state vocational rehabilitation agencies work with schools to provide transition from high school to the workplace for youth with disabilities. For information about accommodations on the job, you can contact the Job Accommodation Network at (800) 526-7234 or *http://askjan.org*.

The U.S. Department of Education website lists the locations of all state vocational rehabilitation agencies. If you think your state is denying you or your child appropriate rehabilitation services, you can file a complaint with the U.S. Department of Education, Rehabilitation Services Administration, Office of the Commissioner, Office of Special Education and Rehabilitation Services, 400 Maryland Avenue SW, Washington, DC 20202, (202) 245-7488.

Extremely disabled survivors

Some survivors, primarily those who had brain tumors, can suffer devastating late effects that leave them unable to work or live independently. Families dealing with this situation face a difficult future, one that is not often discussed. In some cases, nothing can be done to improve the survivors' functioning, and families may feel isolated and desperate. They must cope with complex medical, social, and psychological issues because so many body systems can be affected by tumor location, extent of surgery, and cancer treatment to the brain. They must seek out professionals to meet all of the survivors' needs and are often frustrated by the many gaps in services. This can be a relentless and exhausting job.

In some communities, parents can find resources that address their needs, while in other locations they are on their own. One method of support is finding respite care, which allows parents or guardians to have a break from caring for their child. This can be arranged through local social services, regional programs for the developmentally disabled, or privately. Some families network and take turns taking small groups of survivors on outings.

> *The local American Cancer Society sponsors events five times a year here. They go bowling, dancing, out to eat. But that's just not enough to sustain the survivors who can't work, or to give their parents a break. I really think we need to focus on trying to help families network and support one another.*

One way for caregivers to get respite time is to try to link the disabled survivor with a part-time job or a volunteer position that matches an area of interest. Some examples are walking dogs in the neighborhood, working with animals at farms or shops, or helping at a daycare center. These jobs allow the survivor to earn money and improve self-esteem, as well as provide a connection to the community.

Parents can check into local head injury groups to see if they have organized outings or know about local resource organizations that might help. Some comprehensive follow-up clinics provide monthly activities for adult disabled survivors. In some areas, social groups have been established to provide a social community for disabled survivors.

One of my best friends is a medulloblastoma survivor. We were very concerned about the number of survivors from the 1960s and 1970s in our area whose social skills had been wiped out by treatment. Many of them live with their parents, are unable to work, and have no life to speak of. So we started a group, and 14 of us met and talked all weekend. Most of them didn't even know that the others existed. We now meet regularly, plan activities, hold conferences, and help each other out. Many of the most disabled have really blossomed.

Parents may also need help to ensure that a plan (such as a limited conservatorship) is in place to care for their adult child if they are no longer able to do so. Making arrangements prior to illness or old age with the help of an attorney who specializes in estates and trusts can ease parents' minds about this most crucial transition.

College for disabled survivors

Most survivors have no cognitive difficulties and continue their education through the level they would have reached if cancer had not been part of their lives. However, survivors with cognitive late effects may need some help applying for and attending college. They need to carefully evaluate colleges and apply to those that will best address their special needs.

When visiting colleges, consider any special needs you have and talk to admissions personnel or staff members in the disabled student services office (every college and university has such an office) about any additional help you may require. Survivors with disabilities that affect mobility may need to pre-plan class times to allow for crossing campus to get to classes. Some colleges offer learning-disabled students special studies majors (designed around the student's strengths), special help (e.g., untimed tests, tutoring, notetakers), a lighter class load, or waivers from course requirements. See Appendix B, *Resources,* for books about colleges for learning-disabled students, and visit the Learning Disabilities Association of America's website at *www.ldanatl.org.*

My daughter is a senior in college at a state university. She has quite a few challenges as a result of the cranial radiation she had when she was 3 years old. However, through a combination of some years in private schools (for the small class size and individual attention) and special education services in public schools, she has many ways to use her strengths to work around her weaknesses. When she applied to the university, she called the Office for Disability Services (ODS) to find out what she needed to do to get accommodations. She brought in her neuropsych reports, filled in the forms, and met with a counselor (her sister went with her to take notes, and we are glad she did because the counselor talked really fast which is a problem for survivors who process slowly). But, she qualified for 100% extended time and she takes all of her tests in the ODS office. The process works really well.

It's against the law to deny admission to students based on disabilities; of course, other admissions criteria generally must be met. Public universities and community colleges may waive some admissions criteria for disabled students on a case-by-case basis if the students can show they are capable of college-level work. For example, if a student's poor hand/eye coordination made getting a high score on the SAT® or ACT® exam difficult, but the student will have a classroom aide available at college to make up for this problem in class, he might be admitted despite the low score. Standardized test requirements might also be set aside if high school grades or the student's work portfolio look good.

Taking untimed tests makes a world of difference for people like me because the timing is everything. I took the SATs timed and could only complete half the items. I used to keep close track of the time, and when I only had 15 minutes left, I'd randomly fill in the rest of the circles. I took the GREs for graduate school untimed and it was great. When I took my licensing exam for social work, I also took it untimed and did well. Being able to relax makes all the difference. I wish I'd known earlier that untimed tests were an option.

Schools that normally require all freshmen to live on campus may waive this requirement for a student with special needs. If living at home is not an option, a group home or supervised apartment near campus might be. Before your child leaves for college in another city, make sure you have secured safe and appropriate housing, found competent local professionals to provide ongoing care, and rehearsed daily life activities such as grocery shopping and visiting the laundromat. You'll also want to work out a crisis plan with your child, just in case a problem arises. She needs to know whom to call and where to go in case of an emergency.

Paying for college

Paying for college is difficult for many families. For most students, with or without disabilities, the best place to start is at the financial aid office at the colleges being considered. A discussion with the high school guidance counselor may also yield information about scholarships. A frequently updated list of scholarships for survivors can be found at *www.ped-onc.org/scholarships*.

The following organizations provide information about ways to pay for college:

- Federal student aid programs (*http://federalstudentaid.ed.gov*) provide various types of student loans.

- FastWeb (*www.fastweb.com*) is an Internet site that matches individual students with eligibility requirements for more than 1.3 million scholarships. It also contains a college directory of more than 4,000 schools, with information about admissions, financial aid, and other topics.

- HEATH Resource Center (*www.heath.gwu.edu*) is a national clearinghouse for post-secondary education for individuals with disabilities.

- The American Cancer Society at (800) ACS-2345 can connect you with its state affiliates, some of which sponsor scholarships for survivors, or you can check the website at *www.cancer.org* (search for "college scholarships").

> *If you can't find scholarships, you could help start a scholarship fund through your child's cancer treatment institution. My daughter's treatment hospital has just such a fund—and gave out 17 or so scholarships last year.*

• • • • •

> *In my searching last year for cancer-related scholarships, I found no "universal" scholarships, that is, ones that any survivor could apply for. There are scholarships available through individual high schools and universities that look for individuals who have "overcome adversity." Tell the high school counselor that you're interested in these kinds of scholarships. There is also a trend at some private schools to have a single scholarship application that the scholarship committee then uses to distribute scholarship funds. These often require an essay. The essay is a good place to write about cancer survivorship issues.*

Many scholarships are given for unique endeavors or obstacles overcome. You may wish to take advantage of these opportunities to share with the college of your choice the values and perspectives you gained from facing and overcoming cancer.

Insurance

Survivors of childhood cancer frequently encounter discrimination when they try to obtain adequate insurance. Some survivors are unable to get insurance and others pay increased premiums because of their cancer history. Securing insurance coverage requires research and persistence.

Life insurance

Buying life insurance is not one of life's pleasures, especially for survivors of cancer. Many companies have strict medical requirements that sometimes exclude survivors, no matter how long they have been cured.

Before shopping for life insurance, consider first whether or not you need it. Three reasons for having life insurance are:

- To replace wages if the family wage earner dies.
- To support an aged parent if the family wage earner dies.
- To provide burial expenses for a child.

You probably don't need life insurance if:

- You have no dependents (e.g., spouse, children, elderly relatives who require financial support).
- You are married, have no children, and your spouse will not suffer financial hardship if you die.

> I never took out life insurance because I always felt invincible. I just didn't think anything would ever happen to me. Plus, I don't have any dependents, so there is no real need to have life insurance.

The easiest way to get life insurance if you have a cancer history is during open enrollment at your place of employment. Most companies have a period in which you can sign up and not have to provide your medical history.

> In my many jobs, I never forget to enroll in the first 30 days after I'm hired. The new-hire conditions I've read state that the insurance company can come back and demand that you be medically qualified if you miss this first 30 days. I know the experts say insuring your children is a bad risk, but as we all know, children do get sick and they do die.

The experts will say, if the unlikely happens and your child dies, you can dip into savings for their funeral. Hey, like any of us have savings after all we've been through? In my employer's case, each of my children is insured for $20,000, which is pretty generous since it's usually only $5,000. It only costs me 80 cents a pay period. May I never use it, and may it be money down the drain.

There are several ways to obtain life insurance:

- You or your spouse/partner can work for a large corporation, organization, or government agency that has group plans. The plans do not make individual evaluations of employees or their dependents. They may provide good coverage at reasonable rates and often have no waiting period for pre-existing conditions.

- You can get estimates from several companies by hiring an independent agent (who does not work for a specific company) to act as your broker. Your state insurance department can provide you with a list of all the licensed insurance brokers in your area. The broker can check with many companies to find the best policy for your particular needs.

- You can purchase a graded policy that will give back your premium and a percentage of the face value of your plan if you die within a certain number of years (called a "waiting period"). After the waiting period has passed, you will have full benefits.

When applying for life insurance, the company usually first asks you to fill out a health questionnaire. You should answer all questions truthfully, but be sure to only answer the questions asked. For instance, if it asks if you have cancer, you can truthfully answer "no" if you are cured. However, if it asks if you have ever had cancer, you need to answer "yes."

I recently bought a very cheap (pennies a month) policy on all my kids. The only statement I had to sign asked, "Has the insured sought treatment for cancer in the last 5 years?" So I thought, "Okay, the BMT was 6 years ago and she was effectively off treatment 1 year past that. That's 5 years." So I marked "NO" on the form.

One long-term survivor says he has never told the truth on his applications for both life and health insurance:

I have never had any insurance problems about the cancer I had 25 years ago because I lie. I just don't share that information. I suppose they could find out because I always tell my current doctor about my history. So if they requested the records they could conceivably find out.

In the above case, if the insurance company learned about his history, he or his family could lose some or all of their benefits. A parent of a survivor who is also a lawyer cautions:

> After the initial application process, the company may require a physical or medical history from your doctor. Again, only answer the specific questions asked, and don't volunteer any information. After reviewing all of the facts, the company will decide whether it will insure you and, if so, how much coverage they will provide.

> • • • • •

> I had cancer as a child 42 years ago. I can get life insurance, but it is restricted. I can stretch it to $15,000 or $20,000, but they won't give me more.

> • • • • •

> I was able to get term insurance for a good rate. I told my insurance agent about my ALL (acute lymphoblastic leukemia) history, gave him a glowing letter from my doctor about my health, the recent excellent results from my physical, and some technical literature of ALL cure rates. My term policy is for a million dollars, plus I got $150,000 through work with no questions asked. The bigger the employee base, the more diluted the effect of one person. They just want you to be honest with them. The more money they make, the less they care about whether you had cancer.

It makes sense to get as much life insurance as you can if a low-cost opportunity arises.

> When I started to work for the university and had the chance to pick up extra life insurance (they pay for the equivalent of my salary's worth), I maxed it. Quadruple my salary and no health questions. I felt like it would be well worth it just in case. This way, when we start a family, I will already have it. Of course, this is (hopefully) going to be a complete waste of money.

Health insurance

As survivors mature, seek employment, and move away from home, many have encountered barriers to obtaining health insurance, such as rejection of application based on cancer history, policy reductions, policy cancellation, pre-existing condition exclusions, increased premiums, or extended waiting periods. Recent U.S. healthcare reform legislation, the Patient Protection and Affordable Care Act (ACA) of 2010 and its companion amendments, has the potential to relieve many of these problems for survivors.[1] Several key provisions of the law will phase in over several years, but that may be affected by court challenges and legislative actions. You can find up-to-date information about the current status and features of the law at *www. healthcare.gov*.

The ACA offers the following provisions that are relevant to childhood cancer survivors:

- Young adults are allowed to stay on their parents' insurance plan until they turn 26 years old. One exception (until 2014) is that "grandfathered" group plans do not have to offer coverage for a young adult up to age 26 if the young adult is eligible for group coverage outside the parents' plan.

- Certain preventive services are covered, including services that are important aspects of survivorship care.

- If you are unemployed with limited income—up to about $15,000 per year for a single person—you may be eligible for health coverage through Medicaid (starting in 2014.)

- If an employer doesn't offer health insurance, you will be able to buy it through an Affordable Insurance Exchange, which will offer a choice of health plans (starting in 2014.)

- You may get tax credits to help pay for insurance if your income is less than about $43,000 for a single individual and your job doesn't offer affordable coverage (starting in 2014.)

- Health plans can't limit or deny coverage for a child younger than age 19 simply because the child has a pre-existing condition. This protection will be extended to people of all ages (starting in 2014).

- The Pre-Existing Condition Insurance Plan (PCIP) makes health coverage available if you have been denied health insurance because of a pre-existing condition, and you've been uninsured for at least 6 months.

If the ACA is changed or struck down by the Supreme Court or congressional actions, health history will again be an issue if you have to apply for health insurance. The following information about pre-ACA health insurance options will apply in that case.

Some companies consider a 5-year remission acceptable, while others exclude all cancer survivors from their life or health insurance policies. Most companies evaluate risk based on the type, grade, and stage of cancer you had, and how long you have been in remission. If you had a policy prior to diagnosis, it cannot be canceled because of your cancer as long as you pay your premiums.

The three main types of health insurance in the United States are group policies, individual policies, and public health insurance programs. Group and individual policies are either traditional indemnity policies or some variation of managed care. Publicly funded health insurance options include Medicaid, Medicare, state programs for low-income residents or residents with disabilities, county health programs, or state high-risk insurance pools.

> *I try to convince my teenaged son that he has to do well in school. He's had two cancers, and he will always need good health coverage. I want him to think about the future, do well, and go to college. Our insurance will cover him as long as he's in college. Not having any insurance will never be an option for him. It stinks that he has to think about this at 16, but it's just a fact of life.*

• • • • •

> *My son was treated at Group Health® until he finished college and went to work for a large investment brokerage house. He signed up for their group coverage and his cancer history didn't make a difference. I kept him on our policy for a couple of years just in case there was a problem with his insurance. But it's been fine.*

Group policies

The easiest way to get insurance is for you or your spouse/partner to work for a large corporation or government agency that provides a group health insurance policy. The larger the pool of employees, the less likely you are to be rejected for health coverage. In many cases, you will not be required to answer any questions about your health.

> *You really are doing well to have a big, expensive comprehensive policy with a huge lifetime limit. If you have to take a high deductible to make it affordable, do it. I always figured that I could borrow a few hundred to a couple thousand from Dad to pay the deductible if things got tough, but asking him for $100,000 to pay for something that our policy didn't cover at all would be out of the question.*

• • • • •

> *I've always worked either for a university or a hospital. I've never once been asked a question about my health. It doesn't matter if you are a janitor or a doctor, you get the same coverage, no questions asked.*

• • • • •

> *I stayed on my parents' insurance during college. The 2 years after college I had no health insurance. It was scary. I left that job and went to*

work for a huge organization so that I could be accepted into the group policy with no physical.

If you do not work for an employer with hundreds or thousands of employees, you may be eligible for group policies through other organizations such as labor unions, fraternal organizations, professional or business organizations, student associations, church groups, or other special interest groups. If their risk pool is large, they may be willing to provide you with adequate coverage if you are a member of the group. The *Encyclopedia of Associations*, available in the reference section of most public libraries, includes information about which groups offer insurance coverage.

Individual policies

If you explore all of the groups you are affiliated with and cannot get group coverage, check out individual policies. But be forewarned that individual health insurance policies can be exorbitantly expensive. An insurance broker may be able to help you find all of the options available to you. You might also consider whether:

- Your parents can extend their policy to cover you if you are "disabled or handicapped." Regardless of your abilities, your cancer history may qualify you as disabled.

- Your parents' policy will allow you to obtain a policy with the same company when you are no longer eligible for coverage on their policy.

- Your state might have a catastrophic insurance pool. Your state's Department of Insurance or Insurance Commissioner's office can tell you whether this is an option.

- You can get coverage through your spouse's/partner's employment.

    You need to go out and get a good job not just to make a living and support yourself, but to get your health insurance. I went without health insurance for awhile, which was scary, so I was just ecstatic when I got it. It was expensive, but I didn't care because I had it. Then I went to work for a big consulting firm dealing mostly with the healthcare industry and I got better health insurance. When I got married, I got an even better plan because my wife works for an even bigger company.

If you cannot obtain group or individual insurance, it's time to evaluate government programs.

Government healthcare plans in the United States

The U.S. government does supply low-cost health insurance to some citizens through the Medicare and Medicaid programs. It also has healthcare plans for those in current military service and, through the U.S. Department of Veterans Affairs, for former military personnel. In addition, some states have healthcare plans.

- **Medicaid.** Medicaid is a joint federal/state insurance program that covers approximately 36 million individuals, including children, the aged, blind, and/or disabled, and people who are eligible to receive federally assisted income maintenance payments like Supplemental Security Income (SSI). The federal government administers the program through the Department of Health and Human Services. Each state has an agency that administers Medicaid in that state (sometimes called the Department of Social Services or the Department of Public Welfare).

  Medicaid may pay for doctor and hospital bills, prescription medications, physical, occupational, or speech therapy, and home aides. Search online for the Medicaid office in your area or call your local or county social services department.

  In most states, disabled adults and children who qualify for SSI also qualify for healthcare coverage through the federal Medicaid plan. SSI is available to severely disabled children of low-income families or severely disabled adults who can demonstrate an inability to work. If married, the disabled adult and spouse must meet stringent income and asset limits. Survivors over age 18 years are evaluated based on their own income, not their parents' income.

  Too much family income, may not always bar a disabled child from qualifying for SSI and Medicaid. In some cases, family income will reduce the amount of SSI received to as low as $1 per month, but the beneficiary will get full medical coverage. Individual state rules also affect eligibility.

- **Medicare.** Medicare is federal health insurance funded through the Social Security program. You qualify for Medicare if you meet any one of the following criteria:

  - Sixty-five years or older and entitled to Social Security, Widow's, or Railroad Retirement benefits

  - Totally disabled and collecting Social Security benefits for at least 24 months

  - Legally blind

  - On renal dialysis, regardless of age

Only survivors who had Title II benefits as a child (a "Childhood Disability Beneficiary") are eligible for Medicare, and marriage terminates that benefit until the survivor becomes eligible by reaching age 65.

Medicare Part A covers hospital bills and charges from other healthcare facilities if eligibility requirements are met. Medicare Part B covers medical expenses, medical equipment, and some other supplies. Part B has a yearly deductible, and the premium is deducted from your Social Security check.

Participating physicians accept the Medicare fee schedule. Medicare then pays 80 percent of the charges and you pay 20 percent. If you see a non-participating physician, you are responsible for the entire charge.

- **Comprehensive Health Insurance Plans.** The majority of states offer high-risk individuals, such as survivors, access to comprehensive health insurance plans (CHIPs). CHIPs, also called "high-risk pools," are a means for individuals to obtain insurance regardless of their physical condition or medical history. For more information about CHIPs, call your state insurance commissioner or department.

If you have specific problems getting appropriate medical benefits under Medicaid, state health plans, or other public healthcare plans, a social worker at your treating hospital or survivorship program may be able to help. If your problems are of a legal nature, such as outright refusal of services or discrimination, talk to a disability attorney, call your state bar association and ask for its pro bono (free) legal help referral service, or contact the National Disability Rights Network in Washington, DC, (202) 408-9514 (*www.napas.org*).

Legal protection

Before the ACA, although neither states nor the federal government mandated a legal right to insurance, there were some legal remedies to insurance discrimination.

- **COBRA.** The Comprehensive Omnibus Budget Reconciliation Act (COBRA) is a federal law that requires public and private companies employing more than 20 workers to provide continuation of group coverage for 18 months to employees if they quit, are fired, or work reduced hours. Coverage must extend to surviving, divorced, or separated spouses, and to dependent children. You must pay for your continued coverage, but it must not exceed by more than 2 percent the rate set for your former co-workers. By allowing you to purchase continued coverage, you have time to seek other long-term coverage.

Some states require COBRA benefits from employers with fewer than 20 employees. Check with your State Insurance Department to see if your state has a "mini-COBRA" law.

If you are leaving a job that provides you with health insurance for one that does not, pursue a COBRA plan. These plans allow you to continue your coverage after leaving employment. You will pay the full rate, including the contribution previously made by your employer, but it will still be less than what you'd pay as an individual customer. Maintaining continuous health insurance coverage is critical to prevent being locked out of healthcare due to pre-existing conditions.

Insurance is a big worry for me. We have insurance, but it is always a big problem if my husband wants to change jobs, or we start a new company, or whatever. Right now, we have our own company, but we only have two employees on the insurance, and one is leaving, so that disqualifies our group! I haven't figured out yet what to do.

- **ERISA.** The Employee Retirement and Income Security Act (ERISA) is a federal law that prohibits employers from discriminating against an employee for the purpose of preventing the employee from collecting benefits under an employee benefit plan. For example, an employer may violate ERISA by firing a cancer survivor to exclude him from a group health plan. ERISA also prohibits employers from encouraging a person with a cancer history to retire as a "disabled" employee. ERISA does not apply to job discrimination (e.g., denial of new job due to cancer history), discrimination that does not affect benefits, and employees whose compensation does not include benefits.

- **Health Insurance Portability and Accountability Act of 1996** (HIPAA, also known as the "Kennedy-Kassebaum law"). This law allows individuals to change to a new job without losing coverage if they have been insured for at least 12 months. It also prevents group health plans from denying coverage based on medical history, genetic information, or claims history, although insurers can still exclude those with specific diseases or conditions. It also increases portability if you change from a group to an individual plan.

I really think the HIPAA law has helped us (cancer families) a lot. Before then, no insurer could really afford to write a good policy that would be free of pre-existing condition hassles, because then everyone with pre-existing conditions would switch over to them at once. It would be like putting a big "KICK ME" sign on the insurer: "If you're expensive, come to us!" They'd have to raise rates to compensate for the higher claims, and the "good" risks would bail out for cheaper competitors.

With HIPAA, all insurers are forced to take the bad risks. And they did all raise their rates to compensate. But no one insurer got hammered with all the bad risks and high rates, because they all had to adapt at the same time.

It's not perfect. If you are stuck without insurance at all at diagnosis, you've got a whole year of exclusion ahead of you. But it really does work pretty nicely for families that can keep at least one steady full-time job with benefits going at all times, even if that job changes.

ERISA, COBRA, and parts of HIPAA are enforced by the Pension and Welfare Benefits Administration of the U.S. Department of Labor, (866) 487-2365 or 866-4-USA-DOL (*www.dol.gov/ebsa*).

To obtain more detailed information about insurance issues:

• Read the 2004 edition of *A Cancer Survivor's Almanac: Charting Your Journey*, edited by Barbara Hoffman, J.D.

• Get the booklet *What Cancer Survivors Need to Know about Health Insurance* from the National Coalition for Cancer Survivorship.

• Consult the Cancer Legal Resource Center (CLRC). The CLRC provides free information and resources about cancer-related legal issues to cancer survivors, caregivers, healthcare professionals, employers, and others coping with cancer. Contact the national office at (866) 843-2572 or *www.disabilityrightslegalcenter.org/about/cancerlegalresource.cfm*.

More information about these books and organizations is available in Appendix B, *Resources*.

Canadian health insurance

The Canada Health Act ensures coverage for all Canadian citizens and noncitizens who require medically necessary (as defined by provincial and territorial health insurance plans) hospital and doctors' services. Healthcare regulations are the same nationwide, although providers can be hard to find in less-populated provinces. A wide variety of specialists is available through the Canadian health system. Many of the best are affiliated with university hospitals. Some services not covered under the Canada Health Act (e.g., drugs prescribed outside hospitals, ambulance costs, and hearing, vision, dental care) may be funded by supplementary benefits from provinces and territories, by an employer-based group insurance, or by purchasing private insurance. More information about Canadian healthcare coverage is available at *www.hc-sc.gc.ca/index-eng.php*.

I'm Canadian so I have insurance through the province. I have a plan so I can't be denied medical care. Some things are excluded, like cosmetic surgery. The insurance is paid for through my wages. If you want extras like a semi-private room or dental care, your employer would have to have an additional plan. Through my work I have 100 percent of my prescriptions covered, prosthetics, semi-private room, and out-of-province medical care. My boss actually complained about premiums going up because of me, but I just said, "Sorry, it wasn't like I could help it."

Free or low-cost medicine programs

Survivors often need expensive medications, and they sometimes cannot afford them. Most major drug companies have patient-assistance programs, and you can apply to obtain free or low-cost prescription drugs. Although each company has its own criteria for qualification, in general, you must:

- Be a U.S. citizen or legal resident.
- Have a prescription for the medication you are applying to get.
- Have no prescription drug coverage for the medication.
- Meet income requirements.

You may qualify even if you have health insurance, if it does not cover the medication prescribed to you. For expensive medications, the income cut-off is high, so it is worth investigating whether or not you qualify. Several organizations that can help you find and apply to patient-assistance programs are listed in Appendix B, *Resources*. Because the application process takes time and includes obtaining information from your physician, plan ahead so you do not run out of medication.

Our insurance does not cover the growth hormone that my daughter needs. Her physician cannot believe that our insurance company denied coverage for a survivor with a history of radiation to the brain and multiple late effects to the endocrine system, but that's our situation. The medication is incredibly expensive. We applied to a patient-assistance program and were thrilled to find out that we qualified if our adjusted gross income was less than $100,000 a year. The application process the first year was hard and took a few months, but now we just fill in a form and send in our tax return every year, and she is requalified. We get a shipment of growth hormone every 3 months and keep it in the fridge.

Jobs

The population of adults who have survived childhood cancer is growing at a rapid rate. It is estimated that 325,000 young adults in the United States are survivors of childhood cancer.[2] Thousands of survivors are staying well, growing up, graduating from high school or college, and successfully entering the workforce. Survivors of childhood cancers are educators, sports figures, radio announcers, nurses, doctors, social workers, dancers, lawyers, receptionists, computer programmers, and workers of all types.

Work fulfills many needs for adults, including financial security, health insurance, and self-worth. Despite the high numbers of survivors, some still face job discrimination. Cancer survivors' right to work is better protected than ever before by federal and state laws that protect employment rights. However, a cancer history can still create barriers to finding, keeping, or changing jobs.

Interviews

Careful preparation for job applications and interviews can help you avoid job discrimination. Make an honest assessment of your skills and job history when deciding what job to apply for. A job counselor can help you prepare your résumé and practice interviewing skills. Apply only for jobs you are able to do, as employers have the right to reject you if you are not qualified for the job. If you have a choice, work for a company with a large workforce, as it is less likely to discriminate, and it will be easier to get life and health insurance.

> I didn't mention my cancer history in my interview. But, of course, I had to during the physical after they offered me the job. I was petrified I'd lose the job, but I didn't. They didn't say anything about my cancer history and I got the good health insurance with the job. All that worry for naught. In a smaller company, I might not have been that fortunate, because one ill employee can skew the whole plan.

Unless you have specific mental or physical limitations that affect your ability to do the type of work you are applying for, your cancer history should have no bearing on your qualifications for the job. An employer who is covered by anti-discrimination laws such as the Americans with Disabilities Act (ADA) cannot refuse to hire you simply because you are a cancer survivor. Some employers are covered by neither federal nor state laws and therefore could discriminate against someone because of her cancer history. Knowing your rights and preparing strategies for your job interview can make the difference between being hired and being rejected. The following are some suggestions from the National Coalition for Cancer Survivorship about how to conduct yourself during a job interview.

• Do not volunteer information about your cancer history. Employers have the right only to determine if you are capable of performing the job. They do not have the right to ask about personal or confidential information during an interview.

• Under the ADA, employers cannot ask about medical history, require you to take a medical exam, or ask for medical records unless they have made a job offer.

• Do not lie on a job application or during an interview. You can be fired later if your dishonesty is uncovered. Instead, answer only the specific questions asked. Try to steer the conversation toward your current ability to do the job, rather than explaining your past.

• Do not ask about health insurance until you have been offered a job. Before accepting the job, get the benefits information and review it thoroughly.

• If your medical history becomes an issue after the job offer, get a letter from your physician that briefly outlines your treatment and stresses your current good health and ability to do the job. Ask the doctor to let you review the letter prior to giving it to your potential employer. Some survivors who write well prepare these letters themselves and give them to their doctors for a signature.

• Even if you have no disabilities, the ADA and many state laws protect you if you are treated differently because of your cancer history. Courts look to your individual circumstances to determine whether you are covered under the applicable federal or state law.

• You can go to the website of the U.S. Equal Employment Opportunity Commission (EEOC) at *www.eeoc.gov*, and look at its technical assistance documents about Pre-Employment Disability-Related Questions and Medical Examinations. It also has a document about the definition of disability used in federal civil rights (anti-discrimination) laws.

• Both federal contractors and federal aid recipients (e.g., hospitals and universities) are required to provide reasonable accommodations to people with disabilities, including most individuals with a cancer history. When you are seeking a job at one of these employers, you can inquire about their affirmative action program.

> *I've never had a problem during job interviews. I list my experience as a camp counselor for kids with cancer, so they ask about my history and I tell the truth.*

· · · · ·

I've had some problems getting jobs due to my cancer history. I applied for several jobs in the aircraft industry for which I was well qualified. They were enthusiastic until they did a complete medical, then they didn't hire me. It's a form of discrimination. But I didn't want to fight over it so I got another job. After that, I just didn't put it down on the application. If I was directly asked if I had ever had cancer, I said, "Yes, but I was only 9 months old."

Discrimination

Job discrimination can spell economic catastrophe for cancer survivors because most health insurance is obtained from employment. Under federal law and many state laws, an employer who is covered by the relevant law cannot treat a survivor differently from other employees because of a history of cancer except in certain circumstances involving health, life, and disability insurance. A guide to U.S. disability rights laws can be found at *www.ada.gov/cguide.htm.*

Discrimination can take many forms, often appearing in subtle remarks or practices rather than the anticipated overt forms that most often come to mind when we think of the issue. In my case, I found myself in a seemingly "safe" situation—a supervisor with an M.D., no need to mention my history, etc. Yet things began to change after I revealed my history of cancer during a brief illness related to my post-splenectomy status. Since then, I have frequently been called at home or transferred to her line upon calling in sick for close questioning about my symptoms, conversations with my hematologist, tests run or not run, medications, and other personal matters which I feel extremely uncomfortable discussing with someone whom I consider a business colleague.

Despite fantastic performance evaluations and award nominations, since a longer absence for a more severe infection a few months ago and decreased willingness to answer her questions, I have been increasingly criticized, often for seemingly irrelevant matters. Because of the increasingly hostile environment, I'm currently seeking other employment.

I would highly recommend to other survivors that they document everything—details of interview processes, comments about performance, exact hours worked, etc., as the documentation I've had has helped me in this nightmarish situation. In my next job, I don't plan to reveal my history unless absolutely forced to do so, and then I plan to back the discussion with some solid positive evidence on how irrelevant it is to my work.

Americans with Disabilities Act

The ADA prohibits many types of job discrimination by employers, employment agencies, state and local governments, and labor unions. In addition, most states have laws that prohibit discrimination based on disabilities, although what these laws cover varies widely.

The ADA prohibits discrimination based on actual disability, perceived disability, or history of a disability. Any employer with 15 or more workers is covered by the ADA.

The ADA requires that:

- Employers not make medical inquiries of an applicant, unless one of the following situations applies:
  - Applicant has a visible disability, such as amputation.
  - Applicant has voluntarily disclosed his cancer history.
- Such questions be limited to asking the applicant to describe or demonstrate how he would perform essential job functions. Medical inquiries are allowed after a job offer has been made, or during a pre-employment medical exam.
- Employers provide "reasonable accommodations," unless it causes undue hardship. An accommodation is a change in duties or work hours to help employees during or after cancer treatment. An employer does not have to make these changes if they would be very costly, disruptive, or unsafe.
- Employers not discriminate because of family illness. For instance, if an employee has a child who has cancer, the employer cannot treat the employee differently because she thinks the employee will miss work or file expensive health insurance claims.
- If employers offer healthcare, they must do so fairly to all employees. However, employers are not required to provide health insurance.

The EEOC enforces Title 1 (employment) of the ADA. Call (800) 669-4000 for enforcement information and (800) 669-3362 for enforcement publications. Other sections are enforced by, or have their enforcement coordinated by, the U.S. Department of Justice (Civil Rights Division, Public Access Section). The Department of Justice's ADA website is *www.ada.gov*.

> *When my son was in a wheelchair, it really opened my eyes about disability issues because there was no park in our large city that was accessible to him. He couldn't go into the sports arena for baseball or football games, and we had to really check out class field trips to make sure that*

an elevator was available. Now I look at every building that I enter with new eyes. But things are really improving. Now hearing-impaired people can use headsets in the movie theaters. They have started adaptive swimming lessons and are planning T-ball and other programs for disabled kids.

In Canada, the Canadian Human Rights Act provides essentially the same rights as the ADA. The act is administered by the Canadian Human Rights Commission. You can get more information by calling the national office at (613) 995-1151.

I am going to have surgery soon, and expect to be off work for 8 weeks. My business has no provision for medical leave of absence, but I have disability insurance through the Canadian government. So I don't have to quit, just go on medical disability. My boss is very understanding, so I won't have any problems.

If you feel you have been discriminated against due to your disability or a relative's disability, contact the EEOC or the Canadian Human Rights Commission promptly. In the United States, a charge of discrimination generally must be filed within 180 days of when you learned of the discriminatory act. Although you do not need an attorney to file a complaint, an attorney experienced in job discrimination can help you draft the complaint to make it more likely to be successful.

Despite two episodes of discrimination, I have gone through life sort of blithely telling people about my history because it is so much a part of who I am. Since I was diagnosed at 21, being a survivor marks who I am as an adult. I can't separate out the person I am now from the life events that have shaped me. And battling and surviving Hodgkin's disease was in many ways a major influencing factor in my adult life. So for better or worse, I don't hide the fact from people, and overall I would say most have been very accepting and kind, and a few have gone out of their way to help me, finding me (much to my amazement) courageous and strong. Only a few have stood in my way, fearful of my history and past.

The Federal Rehabilitation Act

The federal Rehabilitation Act bans public employers and private employers that receive public funds from discriminating on the basis of disability. The following employees are not covered by the ADA, but are by the Rehabilitation Act:

- Employees of the executive branch of the federal government (Section 501 of the Rehabilitation Act)

- Employees of employers who receive federal contracts and have fewer than 15 workers (Section 503 of the Rehabilitation Act)

- Employees of employers who receive federal financial assistance and have fewer than 15 workers (Section 504 of the Rehabilitation Act)

If you are a federal employee (Section 501), you must file a claim within 30 days of the job action against you. If you are an employee whose employer has a federal contract (Section 503), you must file a complaint within 180 days with your local office of the U.S. Department of Labor, Office of Federal Contract Compliance Programs. If your employer receives federal funds (Section 504), you have up to 180 days to file a complaint with the federal agency that provided funds to your employer, or you can file a lawsuit in a federal court. The federal Rehabilitation Act is enforced by the Civil Rights Division of the Department of Justice, (202) 514-4609. See *www.justice.gov/crt/contact* for more information about how to contact the Civil Rights Division of the Department of Justice.

> *When I applied to graduate school, I was rejected. This was 7 years post-treatment, and I was too dumb to protest. Two years later, the same graduate program did admit me.*
>
> *I hate this sort of stuff. It is all too common and most often quite hidden so we never get the full story. I only know about the grad school because a friend was on the admissions committee. She told me that they wouldn't give one of their precious spots to someone they thought might die. Otherwise I would never have known.*

Family and Medical Leave Act

The Family and Medical Leave Act (FMLA) protects the job security of workers in large companies who must take a leave of absence to care for a seriously ill child, take medical leave when the employee is unable to work because of his or her own medical condition, or for the birth or placement of a child for adoption or foster care. An employee must have worked 25 hours per week for 1 year to be covered. Some states offer paid family leave. The FMLA:

- Applies to employers with 50+ employees within a 75-mile radius.

- Provides 12 weeks of unpaid leave during any 12-month period to care for seriously ill self, spouse, child, or parent. In certain instances, the employee may take intermittent leave, such as reducing her normal work hours.

- Requires employers to continue to provide benefits, including health insurance, during the leave period.

- Allows leave when a health condition renders an employee unable to perform the functions of the position.

- Requires employees to make reasonable efforts to schedule leave so it will not disrupt the workplace.

- Requires employers to return employee to the same or equivalent position upon return from the leave. Some benefits, such as seniority, need not accrue during periods of unpaid FMLA leave.

- Requires employees to give 30-day notice of the need to take FMLA leave when the need is foreseeable.

FMLA is enforced by complaints to the Employment Standards Administration, Wage and Hour Division, U.S. Department of Labor, or by private lawsuit. The nearest office of the Wage and Hour Division may be located by looking in the U.S. Government pages of your telephone directory or through an online search. You have up to 2 years to file an FMLA complaint or a lawsuit.

State laws

The District of Columbia and almost all states have laws banning discrimination against people with disabilities. The type of protection varies from state to state. For information about your state laws, contact the state agency that enforces employment rights, the local bar association, the National Coalition for Cancer Survivorship, or your state chapter of the American Cancer Society. To file a complaint under state law, contact your state division on civil rights or human rights, or call the EEOC Public Information System at (800) 669-4000. The EEOC website has information about filing a charge at *www.eeoc.gov/employees/charge.cfm*.

For more detailed information about laws governing insurance and jobs, read *A Cancer Survivor's Almanac* (2004 edition), edited by Barbara Hoffman, J.D., or contact the National Coalition for Cancer Survivorship listed in Appendix B, *Resources*.

Changing jobs

Survivors are often reluctant to change jobs because they fear that they may lose insurance for themselves and their families. A cancer history requires lifelong medical surveillance that may be impossible to finance without insurance. Survivors often stay in unsatisfying jobs that offer health insurance because they can't risk losing health insurance if they quit and take a better job. This is sometimes called "job lock." Parents of young survivors also face the same dilemma. There will be a bigger safety net under the

Patient Protection and Affordable Care Act as its provisions take effect (if upheld in the courts) over the next several years so that survivors will not need to be without insurance. Still, staying in a job with better coverage may continue to be a real issue.

> I wanted to leave my job for a better paying job as a church secretary (as if that isn't slap enough, a church paying better than a university), and I was told by an independent insurance company that no way would they provide health insurance for Elizabeth, a 5-year survivor of Wilms tumor. Never mind that the doctors say that she is just fine, nothing to worry about, pick out her college—the insurance company says they aren't touching her with a 10-foot pole. I guess I will take the lower pay and stay at the university where I know Elizabeth is covered no matter what.

· · · · ·

> Rachel's neuroblastoma was treated with a bone marrow transplant. When my husband recently transferred to a different university to teach, we were assured that there was no pre-existing condition clause. Since Rachel requires growth hormone, it was essential to have the $6,000 a year cost covered by insurance. We got a call from the pharmacist saying that the new insurance refused to pay. It turns out that a month after our new coverage started, the university elected to use a new prescription insurance coverage, which didn't cover growth hormone. So we are appealing it, but we wouldn't have taken the new job if we'd known. And we are down to one vial.

Armed services, police and fire departments

Some survivors of childhood cancer wish to enlist in the Armed Services; qualify for the Reserve Officers' Training Corps (ROTC), the Reserves, or the service academies; or work for a police or fire department. Applications from survivors for the Armed Services are considered on a case-by-case basis, and you may be eligible for a medical waiver to obtain admission.

Applicants are asked to provide information about their disease, its treatment, and their current health status. The recruiter should also be given the results from a recent medical examination and articles from the latest medical literature. If you are granted a waiver, you must still meet the physical requirements for the position sought. These regulations are outlined in the Department of Defense's Instruction No. 6130.03, called "Medical Standards for Appointment, Enlistment, or Induction in the Military Services" (see *www.dtic.mil/whs/directives/corres/pdf/613003p.pdf*).

*My son was diagnosed with neuroblastoma stage IV when he was
3 years old. He has had no recurrence. He wanted to join the Air Force
ROTC when he entered college. He impressed the commanding officer
of the detachment, who recommended him for the one scholarship he
personally bestows. My son did the paperwork and had the physical and
was rejected solely on his cancer history.*

*He had excellent qualifications, was driven and self-disciplined, and
was extremely goal-oriented. He had his oncologist write a letter stating
that he was "cured" of the neuroblastoma. The commanding officer also
went to bat for him. The Air Force reversed their decision and gave him
the scholarship. He is doing extremely well 3 years later and plans on
becoming a pilot.*

Childhood cancer survivors interested in applying for training or jobs in
police and fire departments will need to check their local department's standards for physical requirements. Generally, though, current physical condition is what matters, and employers cannot ask about health history until
they have made a conditional job offer.[3]

Advocacy

Cancer is a life-transforming experience. After treatment ends, many survivors want to give something back to the cancer community. No matter what
your education, experience, or time restrictions, there is much that can be
done for others if you choose to advocate.

Survivors and their families have the potential to effect individual, institutional, and social change. Advocacy means using this power so that you or other
survivors get what you need to live the healthiest life possible. Sometimes
this consists of educating health professionals, politicians, or society at large.
It can mean setting up a peer support network—from two survivors who
meet for coffee once a week to an organization with thousands of members.
It can take a little time or become a focal point of your life.

Individual advocacy

Individual advocacy means being able to stick up for yourself in order to get
what you need for the rest of your life. You need to learn how to work the
system to get the best healthcare, an appropriate education, and a job that
will not discriminate based on your cancer history.

To be your own (or your child's) best advocate, you need to know everything
you can about what the treatment was, what the risks are, what monitoring

is necessary, and where the resources are. And then you need to go get them. Use the personal health history document at the back of this book to make a permanent record of your treatment. The tables at the end of Chapter 6, *Diseases*, provide basic information about what follow-up is necessary for your particular treatment. Because knowledge is growing daily, you need to be seen by a healthcare provider (preferably in a survivorship clinic) who keeps up with the literature so you will get the most up-to-date follow-up care available.

> *Part of advocating for yourself is knowing what illness and treatment you had. I was diagnosed when I was 8. I found when I went back as an adult that things I'd always assumed were true were not. It had really blurred over the years. When I finally got my records, I was surprised at what I read. I was also kind of sad that I had worried for years about late effects (especially a second tumor) that I was not at risk for. It was really important to get the facts to find out what I was at risk for and what I wasn't (almost everything!). I asked the doctors who treated me for my records, I read them, and then they wrote me a summary for my personal records.*

· · · · ·

> *Getting follow-up is not that easy. Most of us finish treatment and are followed in the pediatric clinic by whoever treated us. When I went to college I wanted to put it all behind me and just be a normal person again. I didn't want to see or hear about cancer. Years later, I went back to get follow-up. Some of us do, and some of us don't. Some who try to go back can't find a place to go that knows anything about late effects.*

· · · · ·

> *Getting good follow-up is frustrating. I was treated at the National Institutes of Health, and I went to their follow-up program until it was closed due to lack of funds. Then I started going to an internist, and I basically tell him what I need and he authorizes it. To find out what I needed, I talked to my treating doctors, took notes of what they said, and got copies of technical articles. I'm an adult so I could talk to them on a more equal basis, which helps. I'm at risk for heart damage so I go for a checkup every year.*

It can be a heavy load to be an advocate in the healthcare system, school, and community. However, much satisfaction can result. The following list contains things you can do as an individual or as a family to advocate for improvements.

- Get copies of your records and/or treatment summary to enable you to advocate for your future healthcare.

Get those records now, including x-rays and other such studies. I need my radiation records from 1972, but they don't exist anymore. I need some earlier chest films, but they have been sold for the silver contained in them. I am out of luck. Collect those records and studies now as you go along. You will care for them far better than the health system.

- Work with the school to get your child an IEP or 504 Plan to get the best possible education. Register with the office for students with disabilities at the college or university.

- Challenge rules that restrict the options of survivors.

    Paige had both eyes removed to treat her bilateral retinoblastoma. I enrolled her in gymnastics and they said she couldn't participate because she was "developmentally handicapped." I disputed that statement and they retracted it, saying instead that there were "safety issues." We had to force the issue through the Human Rights Commission (Canadian), and it took 3 years of fighting to get her reinstated. It's really helped her spatial awareness to walk on the balance beam, jump on the trampoline, and swing from the bars. It's given her a sense of freedom that she wouldn't otherwise have.

- Volunteer to staff a local organization's cancer information line.

- Start a support group in your community or hospital.

- Talk to local civic groups about your experience.

- Write letters to newspapers, magazines, or politicians about survivorship issues.

- Share your experience with the media or legislatures to help shape public opinion or policies about cancer.

- Become a counselor at a camp for children with cancer.

    Ever since I've had cancer, I've felt that I need to make the most of my life, be happy, do things that have meaning for me, and help others who are battling cancer. I've been a camp counselor for the past 15 years at the camp for kids with cancer and their siblings. I enjoy the camp so much I wish I could work there year round. It's so fulfilling. Sometime in the future, I'd like to start a non-profit organization just for children affected by cancer (those who've had it, had parents who had it, or siblings who had it).

- Offer to be a support person for newly diagnosed families.

- Join or start committees to effect changes at your hospital.

I think our follow-up system is inadequate, so I've been appointed to several committees to try to improve services. I sit on one very powerful committee, which dictates protocols for pediatric oncology for our province. We are trying to establish new clinics that will address not only medical but psychosocial needs of survivors. I want to make sure that survivors have information available about their health so that they are not left out in the dark. When I went through the system, there was no such thing.

- Donate to groups that lobby for survivors.
- Help fundraise to start or sustain a comprehensive follow-up clinic.
- Participate in follow-up studies that may be available through a comprehensive follow-up clinic. Information from these studies can have impact through publications, media attention, and public policy change.
- Tell your friends and family your feelings about your cancer journey.

I've never held back information about my illness. I don't look for sympathy in talking about it because I don't need that. I talk about Hodgkin's so that I educate my circle of friends, family, and neighbors. Talking about my cancer and the restrictions it has put on my life is my way to help them learn that "it's not over when it's over." Each person may leave me and share my story with others, and the circle expands to educate those who are not aware of long-term cancer side effects.

I think this is part of the shield that each person has to learn to let go of in order to inform their corner of the world that long-term side effects do exist. If we can't educate the people we know, love, and deal with on a daily basis, how do we expect to educate the medical profession and strangers who may be able to help the cause? We have to be heard, so we have to start with our family, friends, and neighbors.

In telling my story to others, I educate my corner of the world about what it feels like to have cancer and still be alive 22 years later and still dealing with the aftermath. It gives those people who care about me the opportunity to learn compassion for me and others like me.

Advocacy is not for everyone. Sometimes survivors just want to carry on with their lives. Over time, you may have greater or lesser interest in your cancer history.

I've been a survivor of osteosarcoma for a long time and am still quite involved with the cancer world. I am a camp counselor, go to numerous conferences, and have many survivor friends. We have a sense of community and many of us want to give back. In one sense, I want to be an advocate who is proud of who I am and what I went through. But on the other hand, I don't want to get so caught up that I am only identified with cancer. I used to define myself completely by my cancer experience. But I came to realize I shouldn't define my whole life by that. I've grown into a person for whom cancer was a part of my life, not the whole of it.

Group advocacy

Group advocacy can be very effective in encouraging and creating change at the community, state, or national levels. Issues that can be addressed are national funding (e.g., increased monies needed for late effects research), institutional funding (e.g., starting and supporting comprehensive follow-up clinics), political changes (e.g., improving anti-discrimination laws), federal and state programs (e.g., improving insurance options for survivors), and hundreds of others. There are innumerable ways for groups to effect changes.

• Start an online support group.

> *I started an Internet support group for long-term survivors of cancer. Long-term survivors of cancer face unique problems. Most will face social challenges (insurance and employment), some will have emotional challenges, and some will have ongoing health problems related to treatment. This discussion group addresses the unique needs of this group.*

• Organize a conference at a treating facility to educate caregivers about survivorship issues.

• Lobby an institution to provide comprehensive services for survivors.

> *I fly my daughter 1,000 miles to a follow-up clinic because our treating institution doesn't provide comprehensive follow-up care. It really bothered me thinking of the thousands of survivors in our region who didn't know what they were at risk for or had no one to talk to about their medical past. So I wrote a letter to the CEO of the hospital asking that a late effects program be put at the top of the priority list. I asked others in support groups to do the same. I don't know how much impact it had, but the hospital has recently hired a doctor with expertise in late effects to create a follow-up program.*

• Attend local, state, or national gatherings of survivors.

• Encourage family and friends to create or join committees that work for survivor issues.

We need to pressure institutions to reallocate funds and start long-term survivor programs, transitional programs, and adult survivors of childhood cancer programs. There are thousands of survivors out there who have no jobs or are in dead-end jobs who really need help with vocational rehabilitation. Teens with disabilities need help preparing for college. There just doesn't seem to be any corporate interest in funding these programs. I don't think helping survivors is controversial—maybe it just makes people uncomfortable. The flip side of the great cure rates is that a lot of survivors are struggling with late effects, and I think we all need to work to help them out.

Networking with other survivors and advocating for change will help survivors following in your footsteps. A long-term survivor summed it up beautifully:

I guess it comes down to this: We're all in this together. We're all breaking new ground. We're all facing things medical science doesn't yet understand. If we don't talk to each other, who will we talk to? Medical science will continue to move at a snail's pace on long-term survivor issues if we don't speak up. And we can't speak up if we're in a vacuum. It is our collective intelligence that will push the snail a little faster.

I think we have an obligation to go forward, to be as candid as we can be, to protect ourselves, to lessen each other's burdens, to share knowledge and move the cause of long-term survivorship forward. And there's a legion of new survivors behind us, people with cancer living longer lives, who will need the information we are now pioneering.

Chapter 5

Staying Healthy

Science is organized knowledge.
Wisdom is organized life.

—Immanuel Kant

GOOD HEALTH HABITS and regular medical care can protect your health and potentially reduce the impact of late effects from your cancer treatment. Many adult cancers and other illnesses are linked to lifestyle choices that are under your control. Eating a healthy diet, staying physically active, maintaining a healthy weight, limiting alcohol intake, and not smoking all help keep you healthy. Getting regular healthcare exams from someone familiar with your unique history and treatment is crucial to maintaining your health. Other sensible choices that aren't related to cancer risk but contribute to a healthy life are wearing bike or motorcycle helmets, using seat belts, calling a cab instead of getting into a car with a drunk driver, practicing safe sex, and not texting while driving.

Although there are aspects of life over which you have little or no control (such as the genes you got from your parents), the choices you make and how you live your life allow you to direct part of your own destiny. This chapter discusses health-protective choices such as medical follow-up, diet, and exercise. It then discusses health-risk behaviors such as overexposure to sun, smoking, drinking alcohol, and exposure to sexually transmitted diseases. Finally, it shares stories from survivors about ways to take care of your spirit.

Medical follow-up

Until recently, guidelines for comprehensive follow-up care after treatment have not been in general use. With increasing numbers of long-term survivors, it became apparent that these young men and women often faced medical and psychosocial effects from their years of treatment and needed long-term follow-up. As a result, many institutions are establishing follow-up clinics to provide a multidisciplinary team that monitors and supports survivors.

> I was diagnosed with Hodgkin's 10 years ago. I go [to the follow-up clinic] every 6 months. I like going—it makes me feel comfortable and safe. I have a physical exam, a CBC (complete blood count) and differential, thyroid function, electrolytes, liver functions, creatinine, and chemistries. I had a baseline mammogram when I was 23 and now I have one every 2 years. There is no breast cancer on either side of my family, so that's good. I also do monthly breast exams. Nobody ever taught me how to do it properly, so I looked at an instructional video. But once, at a work training session, they passed around one of those practice breasts. I was so glad to be able to actually feel the small lump in it. I wish they'd use them in follow-up clinics to teach every girl diagnosed with Hodgkin's how to examine her breasts.

The first step you can take to ensure you get good follow-up care is to ask the oncologist or clinical nurse practitioner who treated you to fill in the *Cancer Survivor's Treatment Record* at the back of this book. Or you may already have a written summary of your treatment and the complications that occurred during treatment from the institution that treated you. This permanent record will provide all future healthcare providers with the health history they need to work with you to maximize your health. The second step is to use the information in Chapter 1, *Survivorship*, to pick a healthcare provider. Then you should regularly schedule follow-up exams. Your yearly medical care should include the following:

- Physical examination
- Complete blood count (CBC)
- Urinalysis
- Recommended immunizations
- Manual breast examination for women
- Testicular examination for men
- Screening tests (e.g., mammogram, stool check) as recommended by your healthcare provider

Other medical tests you will need for follow-up depend on the treatment you received for your cancer. You and your healthcare provider can consult the tables at the end of Chapter 6, *Diseases*, and the Children's Oncology Group Long-Term Follow-Up Guidelines (*www.survivorshipguidelines.org*) for the type of treatment you had to see what tests may be necessary in the future.

My daughter was diagnosed with Wilms stage II when she was 3 years old. She had surgery and 18 weeks of chemotherapy (actinomycin D and vincristine). The doctor told us the follow-up was primarily to check on the growth and functioning of her remaining kidney. The first year after treatment ended, she had appointments every 3 months that included x-rays, blood work, urinalysis, ultrasound, and a physical exam. The next 2 years she went every 6 months and had the same tests. Her remaining kidney has grown larger and is doing well. Now we've graduated to just a yearly visit that only includes an ultrasound, urinalysis, and exam. She's doing great.

You can safeguard your good health by getting evaluations from experts in treating the late effects of childhood cancer. These experts will know what you are at risk for and will have the most current information. They will give you appropriate tests to ensure early detection and intervention, should a late effect occur. Delayed effects from treatment occur in only some survivors, and they range from mild to severe. Many of these effects are easy to detect and treat, but they can occur years after treatment, so you need lifelong surveillance.

Many survivors do not receive follow-up care from experts in the late effects of childhood cancer. If you leave home to work or attend college, you begin making your own medical decisions. In some cases, you may not know the treatments you had or the medical surveillance you need to check for possible late effects. You may think the chances of developing problems from your treatment are so slight that they don't warrant attention. Or you simply may not want to think about it.

I had Wilms tumor over 20 years ago, and to this day, I take my health for granted. I don't even do monthly breast exams. I also don't go for checkups as often as I should. I think I'm supposed to go twice a year, but I only go once to my regular internist. I think the chances of the cancer coming back are next to nothing. I just don't worry about it, or even think about it. And to tell you the truth, I know very little about Wilms tumor. I've never been interested or even curious to learn about it. However, I'm not that way about other health issues in my life.

• • • • •

I don't go to a follow-up clinic now that I'm in college. I switched to a family practice doctor. I know I had six different drugs in rotating cycles for 18 months, but I don't know what the drugs were. I will never smoke. But I don't eat the right foods—I really don't like vegetables. I guess that's pretty terrible. I also don't exercise regularly.

However, seeing an expert in the late effects after childhood cancer will allow you to receive:

- Help with transitions from treatment to post-treatment and from child to adult care.

- Screening and health promotion to help prevent and manage late effects.

- Education and information needed to maintain health.

After my diagnosis of non-Hodgkin's lymphoma, I went for a yearly chest x-ray, blood work, and physical exam. They would ask me a few basic questions, then I'd leave. Nine years after the initial diagnosis, I developed breast cancer. Now I get a yearly mammogram, pelvic ultrasound, blood work, x-rays, and more questions. They pay a lot more attention to me now.

• • • • •

I had retinoblastoma when I was 2, rhabdomyosarcoma when I was 12, and breast cancer when I was 22. The center where I was treated has no follow-up program, unfortunately. It really disturbs me. I've been trying to find a place to go because I think it's important, and there are issues that bother me that I'd like to talk over with a knowledgeable person.

Many survivors (or their parents) take an active role in their own follow-up care. They search out follow-up programs in nearby or distant cities and travel to get the care they need. They can also arrange to have phone consultations with experts in late effects.

The hospital that treated my daughter does not have a comprehensive program to track survivors. I just relied on our hometown pediatrician. However, as more and more late effects became apparent, we realized we needed someone else to quarterback her care. So now, once a year, we fly to an excellent follow-up clinic. During the year, if any questions arise, our pediatrician can call them for expert advice.

Some survivors keep copies of their key medical records. Many hospitals are merging with other healthcare institutions, and some are being bought by large corporations. Finding records at these institutions years after your treatment for cancer may become increasingly difficult, so request a copy of yours as soon as possible.

I have copies of my complete medical records. I have all the doctors' notes, the pathology reports, treatment records, and CT (computed tomography) and MRI (magnetic resonance imaging) reports. My parents asked me why I was gathering all that up. I told them that when I went in for a liver biopsy, the doctor had not been sent the report from the CT scan. So I pulled my copy out and he said, "Oh, good." He was able to determine the specific area to take the sample from. Sometimes the records don't get sent to the proper place, and sometimes they get lost. The first two volumes of my records are in a vault 20 miles away from Children's. Once I waited 3 hours for treatment while they couriered them over. So now, I always carry my own.

Doctors, researchers, nurse practitioners, and psychologists are learning more about the late effects from treatment for childhood cancer, although there are still many gray areas. Recommendations for your follow-up care will change over time as more is learned about late effects. For this reason, it is very important to keep in touch with a center that specializes in follow-up care.

Diet

The typical American diet contains plenty of meat, but few fruits and vegetables. Changing to a healthier diet can cut your risk of cancer and provide other benefits, such as more energy and lower weight. While genetics and environment play a role, you control the rest. Eating a varied diet rich in fruits and vegetables and low in fat, salt, and sugar is a good general health practice.

I'm 44 and I had retinoblastoma when I was 2. For the last few years I've been trying to keep my cholesterol down. My dad had a stroke in 1973. I don't know if he had high cholesterol or not. All of his brothers and his father died of heart attacks. My 50-year-old brother also experienced heart problems, which ultimately led to a bypass. None of the men in the family seem to worry about it until it happens. To lower my cholesterol, I've been eating well and taking vitamin supplements. I've lost 15 pounds in the last 4 months. I also walk at least 20 minutes every day. I have a guide dog, which helps me maintain a consistent pace.

• • • • •

I'm looking into nutrition because it's instrumental in prevention of cancer as well as just having a healthy lifestyle. I'm hypoglycemic, which might have been caused by radiation to my pituitary. I need to eat frequent small meals that have a balance of protein and carbohydrates. That was hard to do at college. Plus, I'm an athlete so I need lots of fuel. I eat a very healthy diet.

• • • • •

In an ideal world I'd think about my diet, but really, I don't too much. I try to keep my fat intake low and my fruit and veggie consumption high.

But it doesn't always happen. As a kid, when I was upset I would eat. Then I was conditioned during treatment to eat even if I didn't feel like it. So it's been hard to develop and keep good habits.

A healthy diet includes small portions of meat, fish, poultry, eggs, and dairy products. Most of your meals should be made up of:

- Vegetables and fruits.
- Whole grains.
- Tubers such as potatoes, turnips, and sweet potatoes.
- Legumes such as peas, beans, and lentils.

A nurse at a follow-up clinic explains the following to her patients about their diets:

I tell my patients to try to lower their fat intake (eat fewer French fries and other fast foods), increase fiber (more grains and veggies), and get plenty of calcium. It doesn't do any good to eat a salad if you slather on the Thousand Island dressing. One tablespoon of that has 100 calories, and some people use a quarter of a cup! Drinking water is better than drinking soda. I also tell parents who are worried about their child's eating habits to give them a daily vitamin, provide healthy food, and try to stop nagging. Older survivors with weight problems should avoid binge dieting and seek help from organized programs like Weight Watchers®.

Cancer prevention is not the only benefit of a healthy diet. Eating an abundance of fruits, vegetables, and grains may protect against stroke, high blood pressure, diabetes, and heart disease. Fiber from legumes and grains may help keep your cholesterol low. And antioxidants contained in plants help prevent cataracts and other eye diseases.

There is so much we can do for ourselves to keep ourselves healthy, energized, and living a fulfilling life. Nutrition and exercise are two of them. I do stay very mindful of what I eat, eating as fresh, toxic-free, and varied as I can. Living in California makes that a pretty easy thing to do. I have also done some self-educating on some of the complementary therapies that can strengthen me, and have pursued massage, acupuncture, chiropractic, yoga, meditation, and daily relaxation in the hot tub (works wonders on fibrosis). These have been immensely supportive to my continued well-being. I incorporate many vitamin and herbal supplements in my diet. I also follow all of my medical doctors' advice and inform them of all I am doing for myself.

I think we need to find out what works best for each of us. I know for myself that it did not work for me to be a vegetarian. With all of the

*radiation-related swallowing and stomach problems, I could not eat
enough strictly vegetarian food to maintain myself. It was easier to
incorporate some animal protein to give my diet the balance it needed
in a more "compact" food. I'm sure that having a healthy lifestyle is one
reason I am still here 32 years after Hodgkin's and radiation.*

If you are overweight or underweight, consider consulting a nutritionist.
Most hospitals have a registered dietitian on staff, or you can ask to meet
with one through your healthcare provider or follow-up clinic. If you combine the visit with an appointment in the hospital, your insurance may be
more likely to cover the costs. If you are looking for a dietitian on your own,
ask about credentials (usually a master's degree) and experience. Beware of
anyone who tries to sell nutritional products during a consultation.

Obesity is a possible late effect from treatment for childhood cancer. To
learn more about this, see Chapter 17, *Muscles and Bones*.

Exercise

Regular exercise helps you look better and feel better. It helps your heart
work efficiently, helps your muscles and bones stay stronger, and keeps
your brain agile. It can also reduce depression. Briskly walking for 30 minutes a day can make remarkable changes in your level of health.

*I had both eyes removed when I was 2 because of bilateral retinoblasto-
ma. My mom always told me I could do whatever I wanted. She enrolled
me in tap dancing when I was 4. She later read in a magazine that roller
skating was good for blind children's balance. My sister was already a
roller skater so she asked the coach if he would teach me also. I started
skating when I was 7. We went on to the competitive level and later
qualified for the junior Olympic nationals.*

When picking what exercises to do, choose things you enjoy. You are much
more likely to stick with something fun. Exercising with a friend also helps
make the time pass quickly and more enjoyably.

*I had scoliosis prior to my Hodgkin's diagnosis, and never followed up
on it because of the cancer. Now, 10 years later, I have a lot of back pain,
and I've had to follow a pretty rigorous exercise program designed by
a physical therapist. I work out with weights 3 times a week, and I do
aerobics (swimming, walking) 6 days every week. I do mostly swimming, though, because it is something I enjoy so it's easier to stick with
for the long run.*

We have a saying in my family: Shoulda, woulda, coulda. I'm 30 pounds overweight and not doing a thing. I have a NordicTrack® right here which is a great clothes hanger. I went in and had a stress echocardiogram and I was fine, but I am starting an exercise program through the wellness program at work. I'm going to use the treadmills and start a low-fat diet. I also like to cross-county ski and bicycle. I know, though, that the theory is great, but the implementation is hard.

• • • • •

My favorite time of year is autumn. Our hills aren't covered in colors, but I like the crisp air so I never have trouble motivating myself to go outdoors whether the sun's out or not. Usually once I get out the door, I go for 5 or 6 miles. I enjoy the quiet time for personal reflection, and the exercise makes me feel good mentally.

I wear a Walkman® with rock and roll to keep my pace. I started by walking around the block and built up the distance over a period of years. Walking increases aerobic fitness of your heart, lungs, and circulatory system. It strengthens muscles in your lower body, helps control weight, and improves sleep, mood, and resistance to cold and heat. It doesn't cost anything. It's easy to do any time of day. Once you do it for 3 weeks, it becomes routine.

If you are at risk for heart problems, or you have another physical limitation, exercise can make a big difference in your long-term health. Incorporating exercise into your life can help you stay healthier as well as feel better. One way to start exercising more is to use a pedometer (a device that you strap on your leg, wrist, waistband, or access on a smartphone) to learn how many steps you are taking every day; then set reasonable goals to increase the number of steps you take each day. Before starting an exercise program, check with a healthcare provider experienced in follow-up for survivors of childhood cancer.

My main concern is my heart. I work out religiously. Part of it is to keep my sanity, but the major part is to keep my health and youth. I want to enjoy my family and friends for as long as I can. Your heart can go to pot if you don't take care of it. I used to swim competitively before cancer and I've continued to swim and run every day.

For reasons that are not well understood, many survivors (especially those who had cranial radiation at a young age) exercise less than other people their age. Researchers who recently reviewed 26 studies on diet and exercise in survivors stressed the importance of interventions to increase the physical activity of survivors.[1]

Taking risks

Some people are cautious by nature, and others are adventurous. Survivors of childhood cancer sometimes change their attitudes toward risk after treatment ends. One study found that 30 percent of survivors reported changes in their risk-taking behaviors—half became more cautious and half increased their risky behaviors.[2] Another study found that 25 percent of teenaged cancer survivors used cigarettes, 49 percent used alcohol, and 16 percent used marijuana.[3] These rates are slightly lower than those in the general population, but they are high given the health vulnerability of cancer-surviving adolescents.

These tendencies are important because, unlike other teens or young adults, survivors may be at increased risk for serious health problems, such as cancer and heart disease, due to treatments they received.

> I had osteosarcoma when I was a teen. I have a friend who also had osteosarcoma, and he does all sorts of things he's not supposed to do like running and playing basketball. He says, "Live for today, tomorrow you might get hit by a bus." But me, I think ahead. If I take care of my knee now, I won't have to replace it too soon. I baby that plastic thing so it won't wear out.

$$\cdot\ \cdot\ \cdot\ \cdot\ \cdot$$

> I go out with my friends and party. I smoke cigarettes and drink some. I beat cancer, and I really don't think anything else bad is going to happen to me. I'm going to be fine.

$$\cdot\ \cdot\ \cdot\ \cdot\ \cdot$$

> Some risks are worth taking (not drugs or alcohol, of course) because they make for a more complete life. My daughter is an osteosarcoma survivor who had her knee replaced. I never want her to sit back and be an observer. Having her knee replaced (which will eventually happen anyway) is worth the adventures she has in the meantime. Besides, her surgeon agreed that her activities (horseback riding, diving, cheerleading) have given her a far better range of motion in her knee and leg than any of his other patients. Because of this, he has revised the precautions he gives patients.

$$\cdot\ \cdot\ \cdot\ \cdot\ \cdot$$

> I live for adventures. Life is too short and there is so much to soak up out there. This summer I was invited to travel to Costa Rica in October to compete in a tough mountain bike race. It was a 3-day race covering 300 miles and climbing over 26,000 feet. Even though I had never taken

one single pedal stroke on a mountain bike, I couldn't turn down the opportunity. I trained on the road by riding 300 miles a week.

We had relentless hills to climb and in some places we had to paperboy (zigzag) back and forth. There were rugged stretches through the steaming jungle where the terrain was so rugged with ruts and washouts and so steep that we had to hike and push the bike for 45 minutes. The rewards came with the downhills—40 miles an hour at times on root-infested dirt trails.

I rode 8 hours straight and climbed 11,000 feet. I overdid it and ended up in the hospital. Next year, I'll prepare more and hopefully go back to conquer the route of the conquistadors. Mountain biking is the ultimate!

Some survivors become much more cautious and worry about what the future might hold.

Cancer has changed my daughter Elizabeth's personality drastically. Before cancer she was so terribly shy and introverted that she was afraid of her own grandfather. Boy, is she over that! Outspoken, opinionated, aggressive, and bossy—yep, those are all words that fit my little one now.

However, I have to say that she is so very far away from being a risk taker. She can spot danger a mile away and will move heaven and earth to avoid it. A week ago she had heard on some trivia show that 300 people die every year from accidentally swallowing pen caps. She saw her grandfather with a pen cap in his mouth and was very upset until he removed it. She is that way about every little thing. It is odd because I have tried to stress to her the importance of "enjoying the day" and not worrying about things that might never happen. We have repeatedly had a conversation that includes me saying, "I have lived 40 years without ever seeing a tornado. I'm not going to worry every single day about what I will do if it comes." For Elizabeth, tornadoes are a daily worry. She tends to remain very focused on the idea that you never know what bad thing might happen next.

Cancer causes some young people to reprioritize their values. During their cancer treatment, they may have spent months or years avoiding crowds, forcing themselves to eat when they weren't hungry, and fighting for their lives. Some survivors have lost friends to the disease and view engaging in risky behavior as taking a chance with something that is precious—one's life.

I think teens who have walked the cancer road have a greater appreciation of life for having faced cancer. My son is less a risk taker than his older brother. He's a very careful driver. He also has no time for a lot of dumb immature stunts that teens usually enjoy. He will come home early on a weekend night and tell us that his friends are doing stuff that he doesn't want to do (this is code for drinking), so he comes home. I can tell that he's different in some ways due to his experience, but he would tell you it hasn't affected him much.

· · · · ·

Luc doesn't relate well to kids his own age because he thinks they take too many risks. He is a very cautious driver—much different than my older son. We would have never allowed our oldest son to take the family van to travel any significant distance when he was 17, but we let Luc go to Rochester, about 120 miles west, for a weekend with kids he had been at camp with. I just knew that he would drive like a responsible adult and he wouldn't drive the car after 9 p.m. He also acts as though not much is different, but I know his attitude is significantly different than teens who have never experienced the severity of what kids go through with cancer.

Smoking

Almost half a million people in the United States die each year from tobacco-related illnesses such as cancer of the lung, mouth, neck, esophagus, bladder, and pancreas.[4] Many adult Americans have stopped using cigarettes, pipes, and chewing tobacco because of health warnings on packages, increased awareness of the dangers, and increased cost.

Survivors of childhood cancer shouldn't smoke because of their risk of cardiac problems, premature emphysema, and lung fibrosis (scar tissue buildup), and, in some cases, increased risk for second cancers. But many survivors do. It's not surprising that survivors smoke, given that more than a million teens and preteens start smoking every year. Learn about the dangers of smoking at the American Cancer Society's Tobacco and Cancer website (*www.cancer.org/Healthy/StayAwayfromTobacco/index*).

Survivors who don't smoke tend to have strong feelings about it.

I had retinoblastoma as an infant a long time ago. I never smoked, although all of my brothers and sisters do. My dad smoked, too, until he died of cardiac arrest.

· · · · ·

I have a 15 times higher chance of getting lung cancer because of the mantle radiation I had to treat my Hodgkin's disease. My doctor specifically asked me about smoking and drinking. I guess I'm an odd character—I'm a Pentecostal. I was raised never to use alcohol or tobacco, so it's just against my principles. It's made a lot of things like this very simple—I just don't do it.

• • • • •

I will never smoke. I don't like to even be around smoke. Having cancer once is enough. I don't want to do anything to increase my risks.

• • • • •

I'm an ALL (acute lymphoblastic leukemia) survivor who relapsed three times. I do not smoke and do not like to be around anyone who is smoking. When I was in junior high, it was cool to smoke. I remember the kids dashing across the street during breaks to smoke. I would say, "I've already had one type of cancer, why would I want another? You people don't realize what you're doing." My dad is a heavy smoker who smokes two packs a day, and my three brothers and sisters all smoke. I also worry about secondhand smoke. I think if people won't stop for themselves, they should stop to protect the people around them. I'm very anti-smoking.

Some survivors smoke because they never learned that they have an increased risk for a second cancer, while for others, the cancer treatment was so long ago they don't consider it in their everyday decisions. Still others have impaired decision-making abilities due to surgery, radiation, or chemotherapy to the brain. Some start to smoke due to peer pressure or advertising, become addicted, and can't stop.

My teenage son Jeremy is finished with his treatment, but he still doesn't get the fact that he's still susceptible to infection, and also at a higher risk for other cancers. Not only does he hang out with kids who smoke, but he smokes, and makes no bones about it. I know it is his way of having control over something. The other night I actually said to him that if he had mets (metastases) to his lungs on his January chest x-ray that he could make the funeral arrangements himself. He got mad at me for yelling at him, but he has started taking his Zyban® again (anti-smoking medication) and is no longer going outside in the evening to smoke.

• • • • •

I had Wilms tumor when I was a toddler and started smoking cigarettes in college. Because I don't remember much of my treatment for cancer, I just went on with the rest of my life as if I hadn't had it. I did stop smoking when I started dating my future husband. He was a nonsmoker and a friend told me that he would think kissing me was like kissing a dirty ashtray. That did it. I stopped.

One component of good follow-up care is education about the effects of tobacco use. Part of the discussion should focus on your increased vulnerability to the cancer-causing aspects of tobacco use. For instance, if you were treated with the drugs bleomycin, carmustine (BCNU), or lomustine (CCNU) and/or had chest radiation, you have an increased risk of lung problems. It is very dangerous to smoke if your lungs might already be damaged from these drugs or radiation. Smoking is also sometimes used as a self-medication for depression. If you think this may be the reason you smoke, get information and help for the underlying depression.

If you don't smoke, don't start. If you do smoke, try to stop. By smoking, you may be doing worse things to your body than all of the surgeries, radiation, and chemotherapy you had to treat your cancer. The one thing you can do that will make the biggest difference in your health is to stop smoking. Ask for help from your follow-up clinic or a healthcare provider. You can find motivation and tips about how to stop smoking at *www.smokefree.gov*. It is very important to remember that no matter how long you have smoked, you can always improve your health by stopping.

Alcohol

When used in moderation (one drink or less a day), alcohol can be part of a healthy life. Many adults enjoy a glass of wine with meals or with friends. However, alcohol is frequently abused.

Alcohol is a depressant that affects the central nervous system. Just two beers or drinks can impair coordination and thinking. Excessive drinking can cause liver damage and increase your risk of mouth and liver cancer. This number of drinks can also cause high blood pressure, stroke, decreased fertility, and miscarriages in women.[5] If you drink at all while pregnant, your baby can be harmed. Excessive drinking can also dramatically lower the quality of your life.

Some survivors have seen firsthand the effect of drinking on their families:

> I'm a long-term leukemia survivor. My father's an alcoholic and I drank way too much in my 20s to escape my feelings. But I decided I wasn't going to raise my children the way I was raised. I got some counseling and now I only drink socially, and I'm very careful with how much I drink.

Many adults and adolescents think drinking beer is somehow not the same as drinking wine or liquor. But one beer contains the same amount of alcohol as a glass of wine or a shot (ounce) of hard liquor. Binge drinking (drinking several drinks at one time followed by periods of no drinking) is just as dangerous to your body as daily, heavy drinking. Binge drinking is especially prevalent in high schools and on college campuses. Rather than being swayed by peer pressure to engage in these activities, avoid them altogether or think of strategies ahead of time to avoid excessive drinking. You could drink a soft drink at parties instead of alcohol, or sip one weak alcoholic drink throughout the entire evening.

I drink beer and wine, and I have a fondness for single malt scotch. I probably like beer too much. I think I probably drink too much and need to find a happy medium. When I was a kid, my dad came home from work and had two or three beers every night. I'm in that mode now and it bothers me. I feel like I'm becoming my father.

Scientific evidence of the healthful effects of alcohol use has frequently been in the news, causing confusion about the risks and benefits of drinking. Although a daily glass of wine may slightly lower the risk of heart disease, better ways to accomplish this are to exercise, eat less fat, and maintain a normal weight. Survivors of childhood cancer may already have damaged organs from radiation or chemotherapy treatments. Excessive alcohol can increase that damage. In addition, if you are infected with the hepatitis C virus, you should not drink any alcohol.

I am the parent of a teen who had cancer. He doesn't talk about it much, and only occasionally do I get an inkling of what he is thinking. I know he believes so strongly both in science and in his own strength that he feels he will survive and live to a ripe old age. I may complain because he is not a social butterfly, but it has made all of this easier. He has yet to date or even go out with "the guys." When I told him as he went off to college that drinking on a chemo-liver would be deadly, he said, "Good, now I have an excuse not to drink."

To get help for problem drinking, join Alcoholics Anonymous® (to find a meeting near you visit *www.aa.org*) and talk with your healthcare provider.

Sexually transmitted diseases

As with all teens and young adults, cancer survivors should be counseled about safe sexual practices. Despite the prevalence of sexual messages in our culture, most teens are woefully under-informed about the facts. Many survivors think, erroneously, that if they are infertile, they do not have to use condoms. However, all sorts of diseases, some potentially fatal (e.g., hepatitis C, AIDS) and some life-altering (e.g., genital herpes, genital warts, gonorrhea), can be transmitted through sexual activity. Sexually transmitted diseases can also reduce fertility.

> *No one in the follow-up clinic has ever mentioned sexually transmitted diseases. I just can't imagine my strait-laced doctor talking about it.*

One nurse practitioner at a large follow-up clinic said:

> *I tell every teenager who comes through the door, regardless of his or her medical background, that I think he or she is too young to have sex and I explain why. But then I say, in the event that you do choose to become sexually active, you always need to use a condom, and not just any condom. I tell them to use a latex condom with a spermicide, because it is the most barrier-protective. I explain that no sex is the only guarantee to avoid the many diseases out there, but a latex condom with spermicide offers the next best protection. And I really stress that this should be done whoever the partner is, and for whatever type of sex. So many teenagers think that diseases only happen to other types of kids.*

Sun exposure

Skin cancer is very common, but your likelihood of getting it is, to an extent, in your control. Most skin cancers are caused by exposure to the sun. A lifetime of tans and burns increases your cancer risk and can also cause wrinkles and brown spots on your skin. Hazards of overexposure to the sun include:

- **Skin cancer.** The risk of skin cancer increases the more your skin is exposed to sunlight or UV (ultraviolet) light from sun lamps, especially in areas that received radiation. Most skin cancers can be removed, but they can be life-threatening if not diagnosed and treated early.

- **Sunburns.** These can occur to both skin and eyes.

- **Premature skin aging.** Years of overexposure to the sun can result in dry, wrinkled, and leathery skin.

- **Cataracts.** The risk of developing cataracts is increased by long-term exposure to the sun's UVB (ultraviolet B) rays.

> *I'm not a sun buff, that's for sure. I think having cancer is the reason why. Why tempt fate? If I go out, I always put sunscreen on. But mostly I just limit my exposure.*

Those at highest risk for damage from the sun are people with fair skin, blond or red hair, and blue eyes. However, anyone can be damaged by excessive exposure to the sun or to the lights used in tanning beds or booths. In addition, any skin that has been irradiated is at risk for developing skin cancer. You can prevent these problems by:

- Limiting the amount of time you are in the sun, especially during the middle of the day. Sun exposure at high altitudes and in places near the equator increases your exposure to harmful rays.

- Wearing sunscreen with an SPF (sun protective factor) of 15 or higher. It should be applied at least 30 minutes before going outdoors and periodically throughout the day. Wear sunscreen even on cool or cloudy days, especially if you are around surfaces such as snow or water that reflect the sun's rays. If you have acne, use an alcohol-based and non-waterproof product.

- Covering your skin (especially irradiated areas) with clothing, sunglasses, or hats.

- Avoiding tanning beds or booths. The UVA (ultraviolet A) light used in these places damages the skin.

When you use sunscreen, you may not absorb enough vitamin D. Therefore, it is a good idea to make sure you take a vitamin D supplement (*www.nlm.nih. gov/medlineplus/druginfo/natural/929.html*). Also, routinely check any areas of skin that were irradiated and ask someone else to check areas you can't see well. If you have numerous moles, see a dermatologist on a regular basis. If you develop any of the following symptoms, bring them to the attention of your healthcare provider:

- A bump or mole that has different colors rather than being a uniform color

- A bump or mole that changes size or bleeds

- A bump or mole that is red or sore

- Any freckling or color changes in the skin

In addition, some medicines, foods, and cosmetics may increase your sensitivity to sunlight.

Nurturing your spirit

The mind and body are intertwined. Many survivors were raised to be tough, to soldier on through difficult and painful experiences. Not releasing strong emotions can cause all sorts of physical and psychological problems. It's simply not healthy to try to stuff uncomfortable feelings deep inside. As one survivor remarked, "It's like not taking the trash out. Pretty soon it starts to pile up and stink."

Survivors, just like other people, need to recognize stress, anxiety, and depression and get appropriate help, if necessary. Some survivors find exercise, religion, reading, counseling, or spending time with other survivors to be a good way to reduce stress. Others need more intensive support and possibly medication. Seeking help is an action of an individual who has great strength and is willing to obtain whatever help is necessary for a healthy mind and body.

I take time to explore feelings rather than shove them into a back corner. It took me a long time to realize that it's okay to be sad about it. I've had to learn to give myself permission to stand and look out the window for 15 minutes and cry because I'm scared of my future. Not everybody has a crystal ball put in front of them. For me, all my Hodgkin's survivor friends are crystal balls. And I've seen too many of them die. To deal with that, sometimes I just need to sit with that feeling and be scared. I just need to drain out the emotion that's absorbing every bit of my energy.

I try to see the positive side, too. Yes, it's horrible to live with this hanging over my head, but there are people who get to the end of their life and have never lived. If I died tonight, nobody could say I didn't really live.

• • • • •

I've really gotten into a mind/body/spirit approach to health maintenance and prevention of disease. I don't need any more stress in my life. I can't control outside influences and that's hard. But I can control my eating, exercising, and relaxation. I'm the picture of health.

Some survivors find that writing about their feelings is very cathartic. Others talk to loved ones, get comfort from faith, or give back to the cancer community. Many start or join support groups for survivors of cancer.

Certain periods of life are harder than others. Survivors are sometimes surprised when intense feelings surface many years after treatment ends.

There are several things that I do to cope. First, I believe that laughter can boost the spirit. I watch cartoons rather than the news when I get home from work. Laughing hard is a big stress reducer. I try to regularly do fun, relaxing, and entertaining things.

I try to take breaks and work on non-cancer-related projects. I try to keep up with things that interested me prior to the cancer. It helps me to maintain my identity. I also write a lot—fiction, nonfiction, poetry. I really calm down when I express my emotions in my writing.

· · · · ·

I went to therapy to learn how to get rid of the anger I've carried around for years. I really thought that when the cancer ended, the world would open up to me and everything would be great. I imagined that my life after cancer would be perfect. I have two beautiful healthy kids and a great husband. I thought, what's the matter with me—why aren't I happy? The therapy that I go to has been just fabulous.

· · · · ·

One thing that I do for myself is try to give back to the cancer community. I was a co-leader of a cancer awareness group in college called "Students Striving Against Cancer." For breast cancer awareness month we distributed ribbons and literature on campus. Next we're planning some activities associated with the Great American Smokeout®. We also help plan and participate in the Relay for Life. I'm also a counselor each year at the camp for kids with cancer and their siblings. I've been growing my hair ever since losing it twice 13 years ago, and just last week I had 12 inches cut off to send to a place that makes wigs for kids who have no hair. These are things that I need to do and I want to do. I feel like I've been given so much and I want to give back.

Although cancer may alter the lives of young survivors and their families, accepting that life is different allows them to move forward. Parts may be better, and parts may be worse. Surely, it is not what anyone in the family expected or wanted. But what is done with the new life is the important thing. Finding meaning in the altered circumstances and living life to the fullest can bring satisfaction and fulfillment.

Chapter 6
Diseases

The world breaks everyone and afterward many
are strong at the broken places.

—Ernest Hemingway
A Farewell to Arms

SURVIVORSHIP continues throughout your life. Whether you develop any late effects from your treatment for childhood cancer depends on your disease, your age at diagnosis, your sex, the treatment received, genetic predisposition, and complications you had during treatment. For many cancers, treatment toxicity has lessened over the years; for others, eliminating the cancer comes at a higher price.

This chapter is divided into sections that describe the major cancers of childhood and adolescence in alphabetical order: acute lymphoblastic leukemia (ALL), acute myelogenous leukemia (AML), brain tumors, Ewing sarcoma, Hodgkin lymphoma (formerly called Hodgkin's disease), neuroblastoma, non-Hodgkin lymphoma (NHL), osteosarcoma, rare cancers, retinoblastoma, rhabdomyosarcoma, and Wilms tumor. Brief descriptions of the cancers, their treatments, and possible late effects are included. Because many diseases are now treated with stem cell transplants (which includes bone marrow, stem cell, and cord blood transplants), a separate section about this topic is included after the disease sections. At the end of the chapter are tables listing the treatments used and some of the tests you may need to monitor your health.

These tables and the Children's Oncology Group's follow-up guidelines (*www. survivorshipguidelines.org*) will help you better understand your risks based on the treatment you received and can help you make choices that lessen your chances of developing a particular problem. For instance, if you are at increased risk for heart disease, you can decrease the full impact of this risk by eating a healthy diet, doing the right kinds of exercise, and not smoking.

The tables will help you keep all medical caregivers updated on the follow-up necessary to maximize your health. For this information to be most helpful, ask your oncologist or nurse practitioner to fill in the *Cancer Survivor's Treatment Record* (at the back of this book) or give you a treatment summary so you know which sections of the tables apply to you.

Adult survivors of childhood cancer are pioneers; researchers are still learning about effects of earlier treatments as survivors grow and age. The late effects from current protocols may not be completely understood for decades. Therefore, at the time of diagnosis, it is not possible to predict all potential long-term effects. Even with known late effects, there is considerable variation from person to person. Just because it may happen does not mean it will happen.

> Heather was diagnosed with stage IV neuroblastoma, a very, very aggressive type of solid tumor, when she was 14 months old. They only gave her a less than 10 percent chance to live. Given this, we opted to take the most aggressive route, toxicities, risks, and all. Basically, we were more afraid of that neuroblastoma than anything else. Well, miraculously, 6 years later, Heather is with us today. They told us that she would have severe hearing loss (her hearing is perfect), she would be very short (she's not), she would have cardiac problems (she doesn't), and she would have learning disabilities and be socially delayed (she is superior in all intelligence tests, in all advanced classes, and very outgoing and well-adjusted). They also said that she would probably be sterile, but I'm not going to count on that one, either, and I'll make sure that neither does she.

· · · · ·

> Joan was diagnosed with high-risk ALL when she was 3 years old. She was treated with high-dose chemo and cranial radiation. We are grateful that she survived, but she has many late effects. She had problems with growth and an early puberty, and currently has endocrine problems, learning disabilities, and social difficulties (because she doesn't process verbal communication very quickly and she doesn't understand nonverbal communication very well).

Certain groups of children, adolescents, and young adult survivors are more at risk for side effects than others. Reading the following sections for details about late effects and getting thorough follow-up care will maximize your chance for a long and healthy life and prepare you to talk over any questions or concerns with your healthcare provider. All of the statistics in the following sections are from the National Cancer Institute (NCI) website (*www. cancer.gov/cancertopics/pdq/pediatrictreatment*) and an NCI publication titled *Cancer Incidence and Survival Among Children and Adolescents*.[1]

Acute lymphoblastic leukemia

Leukemia is the most common cancer in children less younger than age 15. Eighty percent of children and teens diagnosed with leukemia have acute lymphoblastic leukemia (also called acute lymphocytic leukemia or ALL). Approximately 2,900 children and teens in the United States are diagnosed with ALL each year, and today approximately 90 percent of children younger than age 15 survive the disease.[2]

Childhood ALL is most commonly diagnosed in children ages 2 and 3. In the United States, ALL is more common in Hispanic children than in other racial and ethnic groups, and boys have a slightly higher incidence than girls.

Description

ALL is a cancer that begins in the blood-forming tissues of the bone marrow—the spongy center of the bones that produces blood cells. In ALL, the bone marrow creates too many immature lymphocytes (a type of white blood cell) that cannot perform their normal function of fighting infection. As the bone marrow floods the bloodstream with these white blood cells, production of healthy white cells, red cells (which carry oxygen), and platelets (which form clots to stop bleeding) slows and stops. The blood carries the leukemic cells to organs such as the lungs, liver, spleen, kidneys, and testes. Leukemic cells can also cross the blood-brain barrier and invade the central nervous system (CNS)—made up of the brain and spinal cord.

Treatment

Treatment of childhood ALL is one of the major medical success stories of the last 3 decades. In the early 1960s, children with ALL usually lived for only a few months, but by 2010, about 90 percent of children younger than age 15 who receive optimal treatment survive. The appropriate treatment for each child with ALL is determined by an analysis of a multitude of clinical, biologic, and clinical features. Most childhood cancer treatment centers describe a child's risk of relapse using the terms "standard risk," "high risk," or "very high risk," and children with high-risk or very high-risk disease receive the most intensive therapy.

To determine the risk level, the following prognostic factors are considered:

- Initial white blood cell count
- Age at diagnosis
- Presence of CNS leukemia or testicular leukemia at diagnosis

- Presence or absence of chromosomal changes in the leukemic cells

- Response to treatment

Chemotherapy

The most common treatments for ALL are chemotherapy and CNS prophylaxis (i.e., chemotherapy and/or radiation to the CNS to prevent the spread of cancer to the brain). For standard-risk patients, treatment is typically divided into three phases: induction, consolidation/intensification, and maintenance.

Induction is the most intensive phase of treatment because its purpose is to kill as many leukemia cells in the shortest amount of time possible. The majority of ALL induction programs include the following chemotherapy drugs: methotrexate, cytarabine (ARA-C), vincristine (Oncovin®), prednisone and/or dexamethasone (Decadron®), cyclophosphamide (Cytoxan®), asparaginase, and sometimes daunorubicin (Cerubidine®) or doxorubicin (Adriamycin®).

CNS treatment is an essential component of treatment for ALL. Because leukemia cells can hide in the brain and spinal cord, the CNS was a frequent site for relapse prior to the use of cranial radiation, high-dose systemic chemotherapy, or chemotherapy injected directly into the cerebrospinal fluid (called intrathecal or IT). Standard-risk patients usually receive several doses of intrathecal methotrexate or triple IT therapy—methotrexate, hydrocortisone, and ARA-C—to prevent the spread of leukemia to the CNS.

Consolidation/intensification is begun after remission is achieved to destroy any remaining cancer cells. A combination of some of the following drugs is used: methotrexate, cyclophosphamide, cytarabine, mercaptopurine (6-MP, Purinethol®), asparaginase, prednisone, dexamethasone, vincristine, thioguanine, etoposide, and doxorubicin. A delayed intensification phase is administered prior to maintenance in current protocols.

Maintenance therapy consists of daily low-dose chemotherapy and continues for 2 to 3 years. The backbone of maintenance therapy in most protocols is daily mercaptopurine and weekly methotrexate. In addition, monthly doses of vincristine and prednisone (or dexamethasone) may be given. ALL protocols also include intrathecal methotrexate during maintenance.

Radiation

For very high-risk patients, cranial radiation is sometimes needed to prevent the spread of leukemia to the CNS. Children who have leukemia in the cerebrospinal fluid at diagnosis require cranial and spinal radiation. Infants who are in the high-risk group are not given radiation to the brain, or it is delayed until they are older. Boys with disease in their testes are treated with testicular radiation.

Late effects

Children with standard-risk ALL often have few or no long-term effects. Children with high-risk ALL, or those who have relapsed and require more intensive treatment, sometimes pay a higher price. The following information briefly outlines some common and uncommon late effects from treatment. Remember that you may develop none, a few, or several of these problems in the months or years after treatment ends. Your individual risk depends on a number of different factors.

Learning disabilities. Treatment for childhood ALL may result in learning disabilities. Radiation and/or methotrexate can damage children's central nervous systems. The degree of damage depends on the dose of radiation, the child's age, and the child's sex, with younger female children more at risk than older children or teens. These cognitive difficulties can develop years after treatment ends. Typically, areas of difficulty are mathematics, memory, organization, planning, spatial relationships, problem solving, attention span, concentration skills, and social skills. For more information, see Chapter 8, *Brain and Nerves*.

Growth. Radiation can affect growth. Children who receive 2400 centigray (cGy) or more of cranial radiation or spinal radiation often fail to grow to their potential height. Some children (most often girls) who receive 1800 cGy or more at an early age may also have shortened stature as adults. Radiation can cause early, delayed, or accelerated puberty. For more information, see Chapter 9, *Hormone-Producing Glands*.

Female fertility. Female fertility usually is not affected by treatment for leukemia unless a girl had spinal radiation that included the ovaries or had very high doses (more than 7.5 grams/m^2) of cyclophosphamide. In the vast majority of cases, girls treated for leukemia exhibit normal sexual development and fertility. The chances of having a normal pregnancy and birth are the same as in the general population. For more information about growth, sexual development, and fertility, see Chapter 9, *Hormone-Producing Glands*, and Chapter 3, *Relationships*.

Male fertility. Cyclophosphamide causes a rapid decrease in sperm count in males who have entered puberty. Normal sperm production and motility generally return during maintenance or after treatment. Boys who go through puberty after leukemia treatment usually experience a normal puberty. However, boys who received very high doses of cyclophosphamide (more than 7.5 grams/m²) and/or radiation to the testes should have testosterone levels and sperm count checked. Most males treated for leukemia with chemotherapy alone have normal growth, sexual development, and fertility. For more information about growth, sexual development, and fertility, see Chapter 9, *Hormone-Producing Glands,* and Chapter 3, *Relationships.*

Heart problems. Heart problems can occur months or years after treatment with anthracyclines (i.e., doxorubicin, idarubicin, or daunorubicin) or mitoxantrone. Symptoms include shortness of breath, fatigue, wheezing, anxiety, poor exercise tolerance, rapid heartbeat, and irregular heartbeat. The number of leukemia survivors who develop this late effect is small, but regular checkups are crucial. Survivors often have no symptoms, but problems may be found on cardiac tests such as echocardiograms, electrocardiograms (EKGs), and Holter monitors. For more information, see Chapter 12, *Heart and Blood Vessels.*

Hepatitis C. Infection with the hepatitis C virus can develop in survivors who had blood transfusions prior to July 1992. For more information, see Chapter 15, *Liver, Stomach, and Intestines.*

Fatigue. After treatment for leukemia, most children resume normal activities at age-appropriate levels, but some children have persistent weakness and/or fatigue. This late effect usually only occurs in survivors who received cranial radiation. For more information, see Chapter 7, *Fatigue.*

Obesity. A small number of survivors of ALL become overweight during or after treatment. An association has been noted between learning disabilities and obesity in ALL survivors—both effects are probably related to the effects of radiation on the brain. Some ALL survivors develop osteopenia or osteoporosis (low bone density). For more information, see Chapter 17, *Muscles and Bones.*

Dental problems. Dental abnormalities, such as failure of the teeth to develop, arrested root development, unusually small teeth, increased periodontal disease, and enamel abnormalities may occur after chemotherapy or radiation. For more information, see Chapter 11, *Head and Neck.*

Less common problems. Less common late effects include osteonecrosis (death of blood vessels that nourish bones) from high-dose steroids, especially dexamethasone; bladder problems (i.e., hemorrhagic cystitis and bladder fibrosis) from cyclophosphamide; hypothyroidism (from cranial radiation); cataracts (from cranial radiation); and secondary cancers (from cranial radiation).

Information about the late effects from stem cell transplants (including bone marrow transplants) is found at the end of this chapter.

Acute myelogenous leukemia

Acute myelogenous leukemia (also called acute myeloid leukemia, acute non-lymphocytic leukemia, or AML) is cancer of the granulocytes (a type of white blood cell). Approximately 500 cases of AML are diagnosed in the United States each year. The incidence is highest in the first 2 years of life. Incidence rates gradually decrease until 9 years of age and then slowly increase during adolescence.

Description

AML is a cancer that begins in the blood-forming tissues of the bone marrow—the spongy center of the bones that produces blood cells. In AML, the bone marrow creates too many immature granulocytes (a type of white cell) that cannot perform their normal function of fighting infection. As the bone marrow floods the bloodstream with immature white cells, production of healthy white cells, red cells (which carry oxygen), and platelets (which form clots to stop bleeding) slows and stops. The blood carries the leukemic cells to organs such as the lungs, liver, spleen, and kidneys. The cancer can also cross the blood-brain barrier and invade the central nervous system (CNS)—made up of the brain and spinal cord.

AML is grouped into subtypes by the presence of genetic abnormalities in the leukemia cells. AML that doesn't fall into these categories is grouped into eight different subtypes of AML—M0 to M7—based on cell shape and chemical properties.

Treatment

Treatment for AML is intensive. Treatment is ordinarily divided into two or three phases: induction (to attain remission), stem cell transplantation or post-remission consolidation, and/or post-remission intensification. Maintenance therapy is no longer used in most current protocols. Intrathecal (through a needle into the spine) chemotherapy is used to prevent leukemia in the CNS.

Chemotherapy

Chemotherapy for AML includes combinations of drugs that may include cytarabine (ARA-C), fludarabine (Fludara®), cladribine (Leustatin®), azacytidine, clofarabine (Clolar®), daunorubicin (Cerubidine®), etoposide

(VP-16 or Vepesid®), idarubicin (Idamycin®), mitoxantrone (Novantrone®), and amsacrine (Amsidine®). More recently, biological response modifiers such as sorafenib (Nexavar®) have been used to treat AML. Intrathecal chemotherapy includes cytarabine, methotrexate, and hydrocortisone to treat or prevent leukemia in the CNS.

All types of AML except M3 (called promylocytic leukemia or APML) are treated similarly. The inclusion of all-trans-retinoic acid into M3 protocols has doubled the remission rates for this subtype of AML.

Stem Cell Transplantation

After obtaining a remission, treatment with additional chemotherapy or stem cell transplantation is necessary. Information about the late effects of stem cell transplants is available at the end of this chapter under "Stem cell transplantation."

Late effects

Some children who were treated with chemotherapy alone have few or no long-term effects. Children who had stem cell transplants or children who relapsed and require more intensive treatment sometimes pay a higher price. The following information briefly outlines some common and uncommon late effects from treatment. Remember that you may develop none, a few, or several of these problems in the months or years after treatment ends.

Heart problems. Heart problems can occur months or years after treatment with anthracyclines (i.e., doxorubicin, idarubicin, or daunorubicin), high-dose cyclophosphamide, and chest radiation. Symptoms include shortness of breath, fatigue, wheezing, anxiety, poor exercise tolerance, rapid heartbeat, and irregular heartbeat. The number of AML survivors who develop this late effect is small, but regular checkups are crucial. Survivors often have no symptoms, but problems may be found on cardiac tests such as echocardiograms, electrocardiograms (EKGs), and Holter monitors. For more information, see Chapter 12, *Heart and Blood Vessels*.

Fatigue. After treatment for AML, most children resume normal activities at age-appropriate levels, but some children have fatigue. These children, usually those who have received cranial radiation and/or had stem cell transplants, may have long-term troubles with strength, coordination, and weakness. For more information, see Chapter 7, *Fatigue*.

Hepatitis C. Infection with the hepatitis C virus can develop in survivors who had blood transfusions prior to July 1992. For more information, see Chapter 15, *Liver, Stomach, and Intestines.*

Dental problems. Dental abnormalities such as failure of the teeth to develop, arrested root development, unusually small teeth, and enamel abnormalities occasionally occur after chemotherapy or radiation. For more information, see Chapter 11, *Head and Neck.*

Less common problems. Less common late effects include bladder problems (i.e., hemorrhagic cystitis and bladder fibrosis) from cyclophosphamide and osteonecrosis (death of blood vessels that nourish bones) from high-dose steroids. Children who receive cranial radiation have a small risk of developing a secondary cancer. Those treated with VP-16 have a slight chance of a second leukemia, which usually develops within 3 to 5 years after treatment. For more information, see Chapter 19, *Second Cancers.*

Descriptions of stem cell transplants and their late effects are at the end of this chapter.

Brain tumors

Primary brain tumors are the most common solid tumors occurring in children. Between 2,500 and 3,500 children and teens are diagnosed with brain tumors in the United States each year. Because there are many different kinds of brain tumors, the number of children diagnosed with each particular type is small. The incidence of brain tumors is higher in males than females and higher among white children than black children.

Description

Describing the various brain tumors is difficult because there is no universally accepted system for categorizing them. Generally, however, most tumors are named for the type of cell from which the cancer originated and the location of the tumor in the brain. The most common pediatric brain tumors are astrocytoma, medulloblastoma, brain stem gliomas, ependymomas, and optic nerve gliomas.

• **Astrocytomas.** Astrocytomas are tumors that arise from star-shaped cells called astrocytes. Low-grade astrocytomas grow slowly, and many types have a favorable prognosis. High-grade astrocytomas grow quickly and are more difficult to treat.

- **Medulloblastomas.** Medulloblastomas are fast-growing, malignant tumors that are usually located in the cerebellum. They are diagnosed most often in children between the ages of 4 and 8 and are more common in boys than girls.

- **Brain stem gliomas.** Brain stem gliomas are slow- or fast-growing tumors that occur equally in both sexes and are most common in children between the ages of 5 and 10.

- **Ependymomas.** Ependymomas are tumors that usually grow on the internal surfaces of the brain and spinal cord and are often benign. Ependymomas in the brain occur most often in children younger than age 10; those of the spinal cord usually strike children older than age 12.

- **Optic nerve gliomas.** Optic nerve gliomas are tumors located along the optic nerves, the optic chiasm, and the hypothalamus.

Brain tumors can be benign (noncancerous) or malignant (cancerous). Treatment of both benign and malignant brain tumors can result in numerous late effects.

Treatment

Treatment for brain tumors usually is some combination of surgery, radiation, and chemotherapy. In some cases, stem cell transplantation is also used. If the tumor is benign, surgery may remove it completely. Whether the tumor is benign or malignant, its location in the brain usually determines how it is treated.

Surgery

Surgery has many uses in the treatment of brain cancers. It is used to get a sample of tissue to confirm the diagnosis, remove as much of the tumor as possible, or alleviate symptoms. For some brain tumors, surgery is used to place a shunt to drain fluid from the brain. There are some instances when surgery is not possible due to the location of the tumor and the damage that would be done to the child's ability to function by trying to remove it.

After surgery for brain tumors, physicians classify, grade, and stage the tumor before deciding on what further treatment, if any, is necessary. Each step of this process is explained in the following list:

- **Classification.** A pathologist looks at a sample of the tumor under a microscope to determine the origin of the tumor cells. For instance, tumors that arise from glial cells in the brain are ependymomas, astrocytomas, and oligodendrogliomas.

- **Grading.** The pathologist estimates the degree of the malignancy by studying many different features of the tumor cells. Numbers are used to describe the aggressiveness of the tumor, with the higher numbers being the more aggressive. Tumors are assigned a grade of I, II, III, or IV. Some brain tumors do not get a grade because they are always considered to be aggressive (for instance, medulloblastoma). Aggressive means they will grow and spread if left untreated.

- **Staging.** Before surgery, the extent of the tumor spread is evaluated using scans. During surgery, the neurosurgeon decides whether the tumor can be completely removed (called resected) and whether other tumors are present. For most tumors, doctors recommend a lumbar puncture to check for cancer cells in the cerebrospinal fluid. The doctor will determine how many additional studies, if any, are needed after surgery to stage the tumor.

After the tumor has been classified, graded, and staged, the oncologist gives recommendations for treatment.

Radiation

Radiation therapy—directing high-energy x-rays at tissue—is frequently used for brain tumors. In most cases, the radiation is directed at the tumor itself, sparing surrounding healthy tissue as much as possible. To minimize damage to healthy brain cells, 3-dimensional conformal radiation therapy or charged-particle radiation therapy (such as proton beam therapy) are being used at many cancer treatment centers around the country. Research is currently underway with children to examine the acute and long-term effects associated with this new way to deliver radiation. For extremely malignant tumors, the entire cranium and sometimes the spine are irradiated to destroy any cancer cells that have broken off from the main tumor and lodged elsewhere.

Radiation is generally given in many doses (called fractions) over a period of time. The length of radiation treatment and the amount of radiation given varies depending on the type of tumor, its location in the brain, and the child's age. Because of the critical brain growth that would be disrupted in young children, doctors try to postpone or avoid using radiation until children are at least 2 years old.

Chemotherapy

Chemotherapy has variable effectiveness against brain tumors because the blood-brain barrier prevents many types of chemotherapy from penetrating brain tumors. In some cases, chemotherapy is used in very young children to slow the progression of their disease until radiation can be given with fewer long-term side effects. In other cases, chemotherapy is one of the front-line treatments used to cure disease.

Stem Cell Transplantation

Autologous bone marrow transplants and peripheral blood stem cell transplants have been used with increasing frequency to treat children with high-risk or relapsed brain tumors. Descriptions of the types of stem cell transplants and their late effects are at the end of this chapter under "Stem cell transplantation."

Late effects

This section briefly outlines some common and uncommon late effects from treatment. Remember that you may develop none, one, or several of these problems in the months or years after treatment ends.

The brain is the master of thoughts, emotions, and actions. All treatments for brain tumors can result in major effects on thinking and functioning. Following are brief descriptions of some of the more common known late effects after treatment for brain tumors. Of course, the specific treatment used (i.e., surgery, radiation, chemotherapy), the age of the child, and the location of the tumor determine the types of late effects that are likely to develop.

Learning disabilities. Both surgery and radiation can damage a child's CNS. When whole brain radiation is used, it can have profound effects on how well the brain functions. The amount of damage depends on the child's treatment, age, and sex, with younger female children more at risk than males and older children or teens. Learning disabilities can develop years after treatment ends, and social functioning is often impacted as well. For more information, see Chapter 8, *Brain and Nerves*.

Growth and hormonal problems. Radiation can also affect growth. Children who receive more than 2400 cGy of cranial radiation or spinal radiation often fail to grow normally. Radiation can cause early or delayed puberty, thyroid problems, and other hormonal imbalances. For more information, see Chapter 9, *Hormone-Producing Glands*.

Hearing loss and kidney damage. Cisplatin can cause significant hearing loss and kidney damage. For more information, see Chapter 10, *Eyes and Ears,* and Chapter 14, *Kidneys, Bladder, and Genitals.*

Hepatitis C. Infection with the hepatitis C virus can develop in survivors who had blood transfusions prior to July 1992. For more information, see Chapter 15, *Liver, Stomach, and Intestines.*

Other late effects. Radiation to the head can also cause cataracts and, rarely, secondary cancers. For additional information, see Chapter 10, *Eyes and Ears* and Chapter 19, *Second Cancers.*

Ewing sarcoma

Ewing sarcoma gets its name from the physician who first described it in 1921, Dr. James Ewing. For many years it was believed that Ewing sarcoma occurred only in the bone; however, other tumors within soft tissues have since been found to be similar. These include extraosseous Ewing sarcoma (EES) and peripheral primitive neuroectodermal tumor (PNET). Together, these malignancies are called the Ewing sarcoma family of tumors (ESFT).

Each year in the United States, about 500 children and adolescents younger than age 20 are diagnosed with an ESFT malignancy. The majority are diagnosed with Ewing sarcoma of the bone.

ESFT tumors can occur from ages 5 to 10, but the incidence rate sharply increases at age 11. The peak incidence occurs at age 15. Boys tend to be diagnosed with this disease more often than girls, and there is a much higher incidence in white children than children of other races.

The treatment and late effects are similar for both types of tumors and are addressed together in this section.

Treatment

ESFT tumors usually require surgery, radiation, and chemotherapy.

Surgery

Before the development of limb-salvage surgery and newer radiation techniques, most children with extremity tumors had the affected limb amputated. Many children now are treated with state-of-the-art radiation therapy and/or have limb-salvage procedures that use autologous grafts, allografts, or endoprostheses. In some cases, orthopedic reconstruction is required after removal of the tumor.

Radiation

Radiation is needed to treat children diagnosed with ESFT tumors that cannot be completely removed. Some chest wall tumors are treated with whole-lung radiation. ESFT tumors are generally treated with doses ranging from 4000 to 5600 cGy, fractioned over a period of 4 to 6 weeks.

In the past, cranial radiation was used to prevent central nervous system (CNS) relapses in patients with Ewing sarcoma. Since then, studies have shown this is unnecessary for patients who have no tumor in the bones of the skull. Whole-lung radiation also was used in some studies to reduce the number of pulmonary relapses; however, this resulted in significant toxicity when combined with systemic chemotherapy. Currently, lung radiation is used only for some chest wall tumors.

Chemotherapy

Before chemotherapy became a standard weapon against ESFT tumors in the 1960s, very few children survived. Chemotherapy improved the long-term survival rate and made it easier to remove the tumor by making it smaller before surgery. Treatment of Ewing sarcoma now includes chemotherapy for all children. This is necessary even for children with localized disease. The most commonly used combinations of chemotherapy drugs include vincristine (Oncovin®), doxorubicin (Adriamycin®), cyclophosphamide (Cytoxan®), ifosfamide (Ifex®), and etoposide (VP-16 or Vepesid®).

Late effects

This section briefly outlines some common and uncommon late effects from treatment. Remember that you may develop none, one, or several of these problems in the months or years after treatment ends.

Damage to soft tissues and bones. One of the most common and troublesome late effects from radiation treatment for ESFT tumors is damage to soft tissues and the underlying bones. If the leg of a young child gets high doses of radiation, it stops growing and will be shorter than the unirradiated leg. Radiation around the arm or leg can result in fibrosis (meaning scarring), swelling, and poor function. Most of these changes happened with older radiation techniques.

Currently, many patients are given up to 5000 cGy using shaped fields to help protect normal appearance and function. Loss of function can also be minimized or prevented by a comprehensive physical therapy program during and after treatment. For more information, see Chapter 17, *Muscles and Bones.*

Heart problems. Heart problems can occur months or years after treatment with anthracyclines (i.e., doxorubicin, idarubicin, or daunorubicin), high-dose cyclophosphamide, or chest radiation. Symptoms include shortness of breath, fatigue, wheezing, anxiety, poor exercise tolerance, rapid heartbeat, and irregular heartbeat. The number of ESFT tumor survivors who develop this late effect is small, but regular checkups are crucial. Survivors often have no symptoms, but problems may be found on cardiac tests such as echocardiograms, electrocardiograms (EKGs), and Holter monitors. For more information, see Chapter 12, *Heart and Blood Vessels.*

Hepatitis C. Infection with the hepatitis C virus can develop in survivors who had blood transfusions prior to July 1992. For more information, see Chapter 15, *Liver, Stomach, and Intestines.*

Fertility. Abdominal radiation and high doses of cyclophosphamide and/or ifosfamide can affect fertility. For more information, see Chapter 9, *Hormone-Producing Glands,* and Chapter 3, *Relationships.*

Digestion. Abdominal radiation can also cause problems with digestion and absorption of food. For more information, see Chapter 15, *Liver, Stomach, and Intestines.*

Second cancers. There is a very small chance of developing a second cancer in the radiated area. For more information, see Chapter 19, *Second Cancers.*

Hodgkin lymphoma

Hodgkin lymphoma (which used to be called Hodgkin's disease) accounts for 6 percent of all cancers in children in the United States. Approximately 800 children and teens are diagnosed in the United States each year. The disease, very rare in children younger than age 5, is most commonly diagnosed in 15 to 19 year olds. It occurs more often in boys than girls in patients younger than age 10, but, in adolescence, the incidence is slightly higher in females than males. Approximately 90 to 95 percent of children and adolescents treated with modern methods survive their disease.

Description

Hodgkin lymphoma, first described by Thomas Hodgkin in 1832, is a cancer of the lymph system. This system is made up of lymph vessels throughout the body that carry a clear liquid called lymph. Throughout this network are groups of small organs called lymph nodes that make and store lymphocytes—cells that fight infection. Lymph tissue is found throughout the body, so Hodgkin lymphoma can be found in almost any organ or tissue, such as the liver, bone marrow, or spleen.

Treatment for Hodgkin lymphoma is risk based, and it usually involves multiagent chemotherapy with or without low-dose radiation. Risk is determined by the stage of the disease, symptoms, and/or the presence of bulky disease (i.e., a large mass).

Treatment

The goal of treatment for Hodgkin lymphoma is to eliminate the disease with the smallest number of long-term problems. The method of treatment is based on stage of the disease, the age of the child or teen, and possible long-term effects. Historically, children and teens diagnosed with Hodgkin lymphoma were treated with surgery (i.e., removal of the spleen), chemotherapy, and high-dose radiation. Now, radiation often is used in low doses, surgery is almost always omitted, and treatment with chemotherapy alone is done in certain circumstances. Some clinical trials include stem cell transplantation for recurrent disease. The intensity and duration of chemotherapy and the location and amount of radiation used are based on risk factors.

Radiation

Figure 6-1 shows the areas of the body that may be irradiated in children or teens with Hodgkin lymphoma. Typically, only one field is used for localized disease. However, for patients with stage IIB or IIIB disease, both the mantle and the inverted-Y field are irradiated.

Higher doses of radiation were given to children and teens treated in the 1960s and 1970s. Researchers have worked diligently to fine-tune protocols to give children and teens only the amount of treatment they need for cure and to minimize late effects. Currently, it is much more common to get lower doses of radiation than it was long ago. Thus, survivors treated prior to the 1990s have very different late effects than do those treated more recently.

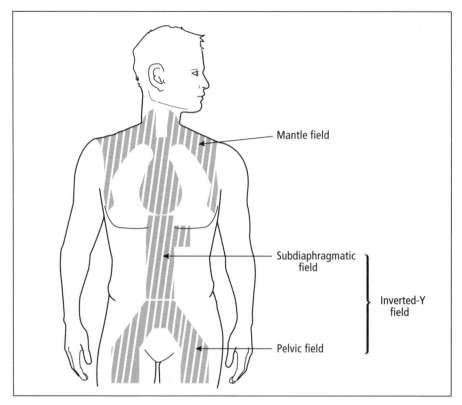

Mantle field

Subdiaphragmatic field

Inverted-Y field

Pelvic field

Figure 6-1. Radiation fields for Hodgkin lymphoma

Chemotherapy

For decades, the traditional chemotherapy for Hodgkin lymphoma was MOPP—mechlorethamine (Mustargen®), vincristine (Oncovin®), procarbazine (Matulane®), and prednisone. This combination of drugs provides excellent disease control, but can cause a variety of late effects. Other chemotherapy regimens used for treating Hodgkin lymphoma are:

- ABVD—doxorubicin (Adriamycin®), bleomycin (Blenoxane®), vinblastine (Velban®), and dacarbazine (DTIC®)

- ABVE—doxorubicin (Adriamycin®), bleomycin, vincristine, etoposide

- VAMP—vincristine, doxorubicin, methotrexate, prednisone

- COP(P) (with or without prednisone)—cyclophosphamide, vincristine, procarbazine, prednisone

Other drugs that are sometimes given, depending on risk, are irinotecan, ifosfamide, and mechlorethamine.

Late effects

Much is known about possible late effects of treatment for Hodgkin lymphoma because so many children and teens survive the disease. The following information briefly outlines some common and uncommon late effects from treatment. Remember that you may develop none, a few, or several of these problems in the months or years after treatment ends.

Obstructions and infections. Late complications after a splenectomy (surgery to remove the spleen) are adhesions and intestinal obstruction. In addition, bacterial sepsis (massive infection) occurs in some patients who had their spleen removed or irradiated. For more information, see Chapter 16, *Immune System*.

Growth. Radiation can also cause significant late effects in survivors. The growth of prepubertal children who receive more than 3000 cGy of spinal radiation is markedly slowed. Children who are past puberty are usually not as affected as younger children. For more information, see Chapter 17, *Muscles and Bones*.

Dry mouth and narrowed esophagus. If the jawbone is in the radiation field, malfunctioning salivary glands can cause dry mouth and tooth decay. Mantle radiation can also result in delayed or arrested tooth development. Another effect that can occur several years after mantle radiation is esophageal strictures (which is narrowing of the tube between the mouth and the stomach). Symptoms are difficulty swallowing or needing to drink liquid to help swallow solid food. For more information, see Chapter 11, *Head and Neck*.

Thyroid problems. Hypothyroidism in Hodgkin lymphoma survivors treated with mantle radiation is common. Other possible problems are thyroid nodules, hyperthyroidism, and thyroid cancer. For more information, see Chapter 9, *Hormone-Producing Glands*.

Osteonecrosis. Some patients who were irradiated and also received chemotherapy that included prednisone develop osteonecrosis (destruction of blood vessels that go to the bones). Osteonecrosis can develop during treatment, but it also can occur years after treatment ends. This condition weakens bones and increases the risk of fractures. Children and teens who receive mantle radiation may also have short collarbones and underdeveloped tissues of the neck and chest. For more information, see Chapter 17, *Muscles and Bones*.

Lung damage. Radiation to the chest can damage the lungs, especially in survivors who also received bleomycin. The extent of the injury depends on the total amount of radiation, the amount given each day (fraction size), and the amount of lung tissue in the radiation field. For more information, see Chapter 13, *Lungs*.

Heart problems. Chest radiation (especially in combination with doxorubicin) can affect how well the heart works. Children or teens who received high-dose mantle radiation (more than 3000 cGy) are at risk for cardiac problems ranging from EKG changes (with no symptoms) to life-threatening pericarditis (which is inflammation of the pericardium, the sac surrounding the heart). Other injuries to the heart include underdevelopment of the blood vessels, coronary artery disease, thickening of the pericardium, valve damage, and accelerated atherosclerosis. Treatment with anthracyclines also increases the risk for heart problems. For more information, see Chapter 12, *Heart and Blood Vessels*.

Fertility. After pelvic radiation, sterility or changes in fertility can occur in girls. A young ovary can tolerate more radiation than can an older ovary. Prepubescent girls still retain good ovarian function after 600 to 800 cGy, and some still retain function after 1000 cGy. Girls whose ovaries are radiated during puberty or after are more at risk for ovarian problems, including infertility and early menopause.

In males, functioning of the testes may be affected by pelvic radiation. Pelvic radiation can cause temporary oligospermia (a decrease in the number of sperm) or azoospermia (no sperm). If the testes are not in the field of radiation, they are usually unaffected.

Chemotherapy can also affect fertility in males. MOPP therapy (six courses) usually causes males to become permanently sterile, although after three courses up to 50 percent of patients retain fertility. ABVD treatment appears to cause less gonadal damage to males than MOPP. Usually, hormone-producing cells of the testes function well after therapy, so boys continue to grow and have a normal puberty. For more information about fertility, see Chapter 9, *Hormone-Producing Glands*, and Chapter 3, *Relationships*.

Reynaud's syndrome. Reynaud's syndrome (when fingers and toes become icy, white, and plump when exposed to cold) is a rare late effect of patients treated with vinblastine (Velben®) and bleomycin.

Hepatitis C. Infection with the hepatitis C virus can develop in survivors who had blood transfusions prior to July 1992. For more information, see Chapter 15, *Liver, Stomach, and Intestines*.

Second cancers. One of the most serious late effects of treatment for Hodgkin lymphoma is second cancers. Some survivors develop either AML (acute myelogenous leukemia) or its precursor—pancytopenic myelodysplastic syndrome. The highest incidence of secondary leukemia is 5 to 10 years after treatment with chemotherapy. After 10 years, it is rarely seen. Solid tumors in the lungs, genitourinary tract, breasts, and thyroid sometimes occur after treatment of these areas with radiation. The risk of developing these cancers increases with time. The risk of developing breast cancer after chest radiation for Hodgkin lymphoma has been estimated to be as high as 35 percent at 40 years of age, depending on radiation dose and age at diagnosis.[3] The greatest risk of breast cancer appears to be in girls treated between the ages of 10 and 16. Thus, all female survivors of Hodgkin lymphoma should have routine mammograms starting 8 years after radiation or at age 25 (whichever occurs last) and have regular breast exams by their healthcare provider. For more information, see Chapter 19, *Second Cancers*.

Neuroblastoma

Neuroblastoma is cancer of the sympathetic nervous system—a network of nerves that carries messages from the brain to all parts of the body. Primary neuroblastoma is a solid, malignant tumor that usually first appears as a mass in the abdomen (most often in the adrenal glands) or near the spine.

Approximately 700 children are diagnosed with neuroblastoma each year in the United States, and an additional 65 are diagnosed in Canada. The average age at diagnosis is 2, and two-thirds of newly diagnosed children are younger than age 5. Neuroblastoma occurs slightly more often in boys than in girls. A very small number (1 to 2 percent) of children who are diagnosed with neuroblastoma have a family history of the disease.

Treatment

Treatment of neuroblastoma is based on age, stage of disease, and biologic features and usually includes surgery, chemotherapy, and radiation. The International Neuroblastoma Staging System (INSS) categorizes neuroblastoma into six distinct stages. Most oncologists now also categorize patients into low-risk, intermediate-risk, or high-risk groups and tailor the treatments accordingly.

Surgery

Surgery is used to treat virtually all neuroblastomas and has many important roles. It is used to establish the diagnosis, to obtain tumor tissue for examination, to stage the disease, and for second-look procedures. If the tumor is localized and appears to be removable, surgery is performed soon after diagnosis, before further therapy is begun. Most often, however, this is not possible and chemotherapy is used to shrink the tumor prior to surgery. Even after chemotherapy, surgical removal is often incomplete, and radiation is required to ensure that all tumor cells are destroyed.

The goals of initial surgeries are developed on an individual basis. Factors considered include tumor location, whether it can be removed, relationship to major blood vessels, and the child's prognosis. Lymph nodes in the area of the tumor usually are sampled to determine whether the disease has spread.

Chemotherapy

Chemotherapy is used to treat almost all children with neuroblastoma. Response rates have improved considerably by using combinations of chemotherapy drugs. The most commonly used chemotherapy drugs include cyclophosphamide (Cytoxanv), carboplatin, cisplatin (Platinol®), doxorubicin (Adriamycin®), vincristine (Oncovin®), ifosfamide, etoposide (VP-16 or Vepesid®), and topotecan. For high-risk neuroblastoma, a combination of 13-cis-retinoic acid and GM-CSF is also used.

Radiation

Neuroblastoma is very sensitive to radiation. The primary role for radiation is for local control of tumors that cannot be removed surgically, even after several courses of chemotherapy. Radiation can be used for symptomatic relief of painful bony lesions at any time.

In the past, patients with spinal cord compression were treated with radiation doses of 750 to 3000 cGy. Currently, chemotherapy is used instead, as it has proven to be just as effective with fewer side effects.

Stem cell transplantation

In the last decade, stem cell transplants (i.e., bone marrow, stem cell, cord blood) have been used with increasing frequency to treat children with high-risk or relapsed neuroblastoma. Various regimens are used to prepare the child for transplant. Descriptions of the types of stem cell transplants and their late effects are at the end of this chapter under "Stem cell transplantation."

Late effects

This section briefly outlines some common and uncommon late effects from treatment. Remember that you may develop none, one, or several of these problems in the months or years after treatment ends.

Surgery for neuroblastoma results in complications in 5 to 25 percent of young patients. The highest rates occur after aggressive attempts to remove abdominal tumors at diagnosis. Long-term effects from these surgeries may include adhesions, injuries to vessels to the kidneys resulting in kidney failure, and neurologic deficits. Surgeries after tumor shrinkage by chemotherapy have much lower complication rates. For more information, see Chapter 15, *Liver, Stomach, and Intestines.*

Heart problems. Heart problems can occur months or years after treatment with anthracyclines (i.e., doxorubicin, idarubicin, or daunorubicin), high-dose cyclophosphamide, or chest radiation. Symptoms include shortness of breath, fatigue, wheezing, anxiety, poor exercise tolerance, rapid heartbeat, and irregular heartbeat. Survivors often have no symptoms, but problems may be found on cardiac tests such as echocardiograms, electrocardiograms (EKGs), and Holter monitors. For more information, see Chapter 12, *Heart and Blood Vessels.*

Hepatitis C. Infection with the hepatitis C virus can develop in survivors who had blood transfusions prior to July 1992. For more information, see Chapter 15, *Liver, Stomach, and Intestines.*

Hearing loss. Cisplatin can cause mild to profound hearing loss in some children. For more information, see Chapter 10, *Eyes and Ears.*

Second cancers. An uncommon side effect from treatment of neuroblastoma is developing secondary cancers. For more information, see Chapter 19, *Second Cancers.*

Opsoclonus-myoclonus syndrome. Patients with neuroblastoma and a syndrome called opsoclonus-myoclonus (also called dancing eyes-dancing feet) have an excellent response to treatment, but they tend to have severe long-term neurologic deficits, including cognitive and motor delays, language problems, and behavioral abnormalities. Although these are not treatment-related effects, they affect quality of life.

The possible long-term effects of stem cell transplants are listed at the end of this chapter under "Stem cell transplantation."

Non-Hodgkin lymphoma

Non-Hodgkin lymphoma (NHL) is the third most common childhood cancer (after leukemia and brain tumors). Approximately 800 children younger than age 20 are diagnosed with NHL in the United States every year. It is rare in very young children, and the incidence increases with age. There is an increased risk of NHL in children diagnosed with AIDS. Childhood NHL is more common in males than in females, and slightly more white children than black children are diagnosed with NHL. The 5-year survival rate for children younger than age 15 is 88 percent, and for 15 to 19 year olds is 77 percent.

Description

Lymphomas are cancers of the lymph system. This system is made up of lymph vessels throughout the body that carry a colorless liquid called lymph. Throughout this network, groups of small organs called lymph nodes make and store lymphocytes—cells that fight infection. Lymph tissue is found throughout the body, so NHL can be found in almost any organ or tissue, such as the liver, bone marrow, or spleen. Hodgkin and NHL are differentiated by cell type and require different treatments.

Although there are many different types of NHL, the three most common in children are lymphoblastic, small noncleaved cell lymphoma (Burkitt's and non-Burkitt's), and large cell lymphoma.

Treatment

Treatment for NHL is based on histology (meaning how the tissue and cells look under a microscope) and clinical stage. Several staging systems are used.

Radiation

In the past, radiation was given to most children with NHL, and its use significantly increased the toxicity of treatment. Currently, radiation is used only for tumors in the chest that cause trouble breathing, compression of major blood vessels, testicular tumors, or primary NHL of bone. The use of radiation in even these situations is in dispute in scientific circles. Many experts now believe radiation should be used only in exceptional circumstances for children or teens with NHL.

Chemotherapy

The mainstay of treatment for NHL is combination chemotherapy. Drugs used to treat this disease include vincristine (Oncovin®), doxorubicin

(Adriamycin®), cyclophosphamide (Cytoxan®), prednisone, mercaptopurine (6-MP or Purinethol®), methotrexate, daunorubicin (Cerubidine®), cytarabine (ARA-C), thioguanine (6-TG), and asparaginase.

Almost all children and teens with NHL stage III and stage IV receive intrathecal methotrexate regardless of the tumor location to prevent the spread of the tumor into the cerebrospinal fluid and brain.

Late effects

This section briefly outlines some common and uncommon late effects from treatment. Remember that you may develop none, one, or several of these problems in the months or years after treatment ends.

Children with stage I or II NHL may have few or no long-term effects. Children with stage III or IV NHL, or those who have relapsed and require more intensive treatment, sometimes pay a higher price.

Fertility. Female fertility usually is not affected by treatment for lymphoma unless the girl had spinal radiation that included the ovaries or had very high doses of cyclophosphamide—more than 7.5 grams per square meter (grams/m²). In the majority of cases, girls treated for lymphoma have normal growth, sexual development, and fertility. The chances of having a normal pregnancy and birth if fertility is not affected are the same as for the general population.

The use of methotrexate, vincristine, cyclophosphamide, and prednisone cause a rapid decrease in sperm count in male teens who have passed puberty. Normal sperm production and motility generally return after treatment. Boys treated for lymphoma before puberty usually experience a normal puberty. However, patients who received very high doses of cyclophosphamide (more than 7.5 grams/m²) or radiation to the testes should have testosterone levels and sperm count checked. Most males treated with chemotherapy alone have normal growth, sexual development, and fertility. For more information about growth and fertility, see Chapter 9, *Hormone-Producing Glands*.

Heart problems. In a small number of survivors, heart problems can occur months or years after treatment with anthracyclines (i.e., doxorubicin, idarubicin, or daunorubicin), high-dose cyclophosphamide, or chest radiation. Symptoms include shortness of breath, fatigue, wheezing, anxiety, poor exercise tolerance, rapid heartbeat, and irregular heartbeat. Survivors often have no symptoms, but problems may be found on cardiac tests such as echocardiograms, electrocardiograms (EKGs), and Holter monitors. For more information, see Chapter 12, *Heart and Blood Vessels*.

Hepatitis C. Infection with the hepatitis C virus can develop in survivors who had blood transfusions prior to July 1992. For more information, see Chapter 15, *Liver, Stomach, and Intestines*.

Learning disabilities. Cranial radiation, intrathecal methotrexate, and/or high-dose methotrexate may cause cognitive problems. Learning disabilities can develop years after treatment ends. Typically, problems develop in the areas of mathematics, spatial relationships, problem solving, organization, planning, attention span, concentration skills, and social skills. For more information, see Chapter 8, *Brain and Nerves*.

Dental problems. Dental abnormalities can occur after chemotherapy or radiation to the jaw area. The most frequent problems are failure of the teeth to develop, arrested root development, unusually small teeth, and enamel abnormalities. For more information, see Chapter 11, *Head and Neck*.

Uncommon late effects. Extremely rare late effects include bladder problems (i.e., hemorrhagic cystitis and bladder fibrosis) from cyclophosphamide, osteonecrosis (death of blood vessels that nourish bones) from high-dose steroids, and second cancers.

Osteosarcoma

Malignant bone tumors account for approximately 5 percent of all childhood cancers. Fifty-six percent of all bone tumors diagnosed are osteosarcoma, most of which occur during the adolescent growth spurt. Males are affected more than females, and more black children are diagnosed than are white children.

Description

Osteosarcoma is a primary malignant cancer of the bone. It typically occurs at the ends of the long bones, usually at the knee. Other, less common sites are the upper arm (close to the shoulder), the pelvis, and the skull.

Treatment

During the last 25 years, treatment for osteosarcoma has greatly improved. Today, the majority of young patients with a primary tumor in a limb and no metastases will survive. Advances in surgical techniques have also markedly improved the quality of life for survivors.

When osteosarcoma is diagnosed in a bone, more tests are done to determine if the cancer has spread to other parts of the body. A biopsy is required to determine the type and stage of the tumor. Imaging studies that may be performed to check for metastases are magnetic resonance imaging (MRI), computed tomography (CT) of the chest, a bone scan, and sometimes a positron emission tomography (PET) scan.

There are two stages for osteosarcoma at diagnosis:

• **Localized.** Tumors limited to the bone of origin.

• **Metastatic.** Tumors found in other parts of the body, including the lungs, other bones, or distant sites.

Surgery

Surgery usually is performed after a period of chemotherapy. Successful surgical removal of the primary tumor most often consists of either limb-salvage surgery, rotationplasty, or amputation. A surgical procedure called a thoracotomy (i.e., opening the chest cavity) also is used when adolescents have metastases to the lungs.

Total removal of both gross and microscopic tumors is required to prevent recurrence. Factors that determine the choice of amputation or salvage therapy are tumor location, tumor size, presence of distant metastases, skeletal development, and patient preference. Whether or not the affected bone is broken at the time of diagnosis also affects the choice of treatment.

In up to 20 percent of osteosarcoma cases, areas of tumor develop inches away from the primary tumor. These areas, called skip lesions, can cause local recurrence in stumps after amputation. Prior to advances in CT and MRI techniques and radionuclide scanning, some surgeons removed the entire affected bone, resulting in disability and loss of function. Now, however, a variety of methods are used to salvage limbs. Bones from cadavers (called allografts) or pieces of the patient's own bone (i.e., fibula or iliac crest) are used. Devices made from cobalt, chrome, or steel can be custom designed to replace the diseased bone. In some cases, the bone is removed and not replaced.

Radiation

Osteosarcoma usually does not respond well to radiation. Because of the risk of recurrence for tumors treated with radiation, it is used only in treating patients whose tumors cannot be completely removed surgically.

Chemotherapy

Chemotherapy is resumed after surgery has removed as much of the tumor as possible. A combination of some of the following drugs is used to treat osteosarcoma: doxorubicin (Adriamycin®), high-dose methotrexate, cisplatin (Platinol®), and cyclophosphamide (Cytoxan®). Ifosfamide (Ifex®), and/or etoposide, are sometimes used for children who relapse.

Late effects

This section briefly outlines some common and uncommon late effects from treatment. Remember that you may develop none, one, or several of these problems in the months or years after treatment ends.

Physical impairments. One of the universal late effects from treatment for osteosarcoma is coping with physical impairments from amputation or limb-salvage therapy. After limb-salvage therapy or fitting with a state-of-the-art prosthesis, many survivors are able to resume an active lifestyle, while others struggle to regain mobility. For more information, see Chapter 17, *Muscles and Bones*.

Heart problems. Heart problems can occur months or years after treatment with anthracyclines (i.e., doxorubicin, idarubicin, or daunorubicin), high-dose cyclophosphamide, or chest radiation. Symptoms include shortness of breath, fatigue, wheezing, anxiety, poor exercise tolerance, rapid heartbeat, and irregular heartbeat. The number of survivors who develop this late effect is small, but regular checkups are crucial. Survivors often have no symptoms, but problems may be found on cardiac tests such as echocardiograms, electrocardiograms (EKGs), and Holter monitors. For more information, see Chapter 12, *Heart and Blood Vessels*.

Hepatitis C. Infection with the hepatitis C virus can develop in survivors who had blood transfusions prior to July 1992. For more information, see Chapter 15, *Liver, Stomach, and Intestines*.

Hearing loss. Cisplatin can result in mild to profound hearing loss in some children and teens. For more information, see Chapter 10, *Eyes and Ears*.

Learning disabilities. Treatment with high-dose methotrexate may result in cognitive problems. Learning disabilities can develop months or years after treatment ends. Typically, problems develop in the areas of mathematics, spatial relationships, problem solving, organization, planning, attention span, concentration skills, and social skills. For more information, see Chapter 8, *Brain and Nerves*.

Fertility. Female fertility usually is not affected by treatment for osteosarcoma unless the girl has very high doses of cyclophosphamide (more than 7.5 grams per square meter [grams/m²]) or ifosfamide (more than 60 grams/m²). In the majority of cases, girls treated for osteosarcoma have normal growth, sexual development, and fertility. The chances of having a normal pregnancy and birth are the same as in the general population.

Cyclophosphamide can cause a rapid decrease in sperm count in male teens who have passed puberty. Normal sperm production and motility generally return after treatment. After osteosarcoma treatment, younger males usually experience a normal puberty. However, young men who received very high doses of cyclophosphamide—more than 7.5 grams/m²) should have testosterone levels and sperm count checked. For more information about growth and fertility, see Chapter 9, *Hormone-Producing Glands*.

Second cancers. A rare side effect from treatment of osteosarcoma is developing second cancers. For more information, see Chapter 19, *Second Cancers*.

Rare cancers

Very small numbers of children are diagnosed every year with one of the rare childhood cancers. Because so few doctors see these diseases, diagnosis may be difficult and treatment may not be standardized. The uncommon cancers covered in this section are chronic myelocytic leukemia, histiocytosis, liver tumors, and soft tissue sarcomas. Although these diseases are discussed here briefly, the late effects that might develop after cure are discussed in greater depth in the chapters about organ systems.

If your disease is not covered in this chapter, go through the tables at the end of the chapter and the Children's Oncology Group's follow-up guidelines (*www.survivorshipguidelines.org*), find the treatments you received, and read about the tests you should get to monitor your health.

Chronic myelocytic leukemia

Chronic myelocytic leukemia (also called chronic myelogenous leukemia or CML) accounts for less than 5 percent of all childhood leukemias. In CML, large numbers of cancerous mature granulocytes (a type of white blood cell) appear.

The two major forms of chronic myelocytic leukemia are adult CML, which occurs primarily in adolescents and adults, and juvenile myelomonocytic leukemia (also called juvenile CML), which occurs mostly in infants.

Adult CML

Adult CML is characterized by a large spleen and high white blood cell count (usually more than 100,000). In more than 90 percent of teens with adult CML, analysis of cells in the bone marrow shows a genetic abnormality called the Philadelphia chromosome. This chromosome contains a translocation (where genetic material has traded places) involving chromosomes 9 and 22, abbreviated t(9;22).

Chemotherapy. The goal of treatment for adult CML is to lower the white blood cell count and to reduce the size of the liver and spleen. The current treatment is imatinib mesylate (Gleevec®). Previously, hydroxyurea (Hydrea®) or busulfan (Myleran®) were used. In some cases, the biologic agent interferon alpha is given alone or in combination with hydroxyurea or cytarabine (ARA-C).

Radiation. Before chemotherapy was used to treat adult CML, radiation of the spleen was a common therapy. When clinical trials proved that it was inferior to chemotherapy in prolonging survival, it was used only to reduce the size of painful massive spleens in patients whose disease was resistant to chemotherapy.

Surgery. Removal of the spleen also was common practice in the past until clinical trials showed no improvement in prolonging the chronic phase or survival.

Stem cell transplantation. Although Gleevac® and interferon alpha slow the progress of adult CML, the best hope for cure is stem cell transplant. The highest cure rates occur when the patient is transplanted during the chronic phase with marrow or stem cells from an identical twin, HLA-matched family member, or HLA-matched non-family member. Descriptions of the types of stem cell transplants and their late effects are at the end of this chapter under "Stem cell transplantation."

Juvenile myelomonocytic leukemia

Juvenile myelomonocytic leukemia (also called juvenile CML) usually strikes children younger than age 5. Unlike the adult form of CML, juvenile CML does not have a chronic phase, and the cells usually do not contain the Philadelphia chromosome. This disease progresses rapidly.

Stem cell transplantation. As with adult CML, chemotherapy generally is not a successful treatment for juvenile CML, and stem cell transplantation is the best hope for a cure. However, chemotherapy is sometimes used while preparing for transplant. Descriptions of the types of stem cell transplants and their late effects are at the end of this chapter under "Stem cell transplantation."

Histiocytosis

Histiocytosis is a poorly understood and frequently misdiagnosed disease. Patients can have a wide array of symptoms ranging from skin conditions to bone lesions. Approximately 1,200 new cases are diagnosed in the United States each year, but the true incidence is unknown because so many different types of doctors treat various aspects of the disease. It is common for children with histiocytosis to be seen by dermatologists, endocrinologists, and orthopedists, as well as oncologists.

Histiocytosis is a disease in which histiocytes (a cell of bone marrow origin) multiply and accumulate in various organs or bones in the body. Symptoms mimic other childhood illnesses or conditions, so the only way to obtain a definitive diagnosis is the thorough examination of a sample of affected tissue under an electron microscope.

Organs commonly damaged by the multiplying histiocytes are skin, bone, ears, lymph nodes, glands, lung, eye, liver, spleen, and bone marrow. Less frequently involved body parts are kidneys, jaw, thymus, thyroid, and intestines. Many of the lesions spontaneously heal with time. Diabetes insipidus is also commonly found at diagnosis.

There are three types of histiocytosis:

- **Langerhans' cell histiocytosis.** The most common type of histiocytosis, in which Langerhans' cells are found in lesions.

- **Class II histiocytosis.** A very rare disorder in which Langerhans' cells are not found in lesions. This is almost always a fatal disease, although stem transplantation is used experimentally to treat it.

- **Class III malignant histiocytosis.** A very rare malignant disorder best identified by lymph node biopsy. The disorder was previously always fatal, but new treatments are extending remissions significantly.

There are key differences in these three disorders in terms of diagnosis, treatment, and prognosis.

Langerhans' cell histiocytosis is poorly understood, and hence, numerous treatment methods have been tried over the years. The disease has been treated aggressively as an infection and just as aggressively with chemotherapy as a malignancy. Stem cell transplants are sometimes recommended for children with severe, unresponsive disease. Low-dose radiation is sometimes used for bone involvement, with doses ranging from 700 to 1,000 cGy.

Class II histiocytosis is treated with stem cell transplantation. Descriptions of the types of stem cell transplants and their late effects are at the end of this chapter under "Stem cell transplantation."

Children with Class III malignant histiocytosis are given induction therapy consisting of vincristine (Oncovin®), prednisone, cyclophosphamide (Cytoxan®), and doxorubicin (Adriamycin®). Maintenance drugs used are vincristine, cyclophosphamide, and doxorubicin.

Most survivors of histiocytosis have no long-term side effects from their treatment. For those who had numerous relapses of the disease or were treated with a stem cell transplant, the chances are higher of developing problems later in life. The following are very rare late effects of treatment for histiocytosis.

Heart problems. Heart problems can occur months or years after treatment with high doses of anthracyclines (i.e., doxorubicin, idarubicin, or daunorubicin), high-dose cyclophosphamide, or chest radiation. Symptoms include shortness of breath, fatigue, wheezing, anxiety, poor exercise tolerance, rapid heartbeat, and irregular heartbeat. Survivors often have no symptoms, but problems may be found on cardiac tests such as echocardiograms, electrocardiograms (EKGs), and Holter monitors. For more information, see Chapter 12, *Heart and Blood Vessels.*

Hearing loss. Some children with Langerhans' cell histiocytosis develop hearing loss after years of chronic ear infections. For more information, see Chapter 10, *Eyes and Ears.*

Diabetes insipidus. If the disease infiltrated the pituitary gland, diabetes insipidus often develops.

Uncommon problems. Very rare late effects include bladder problems (i.e., hemorrhagic cystitis and bladder fibrosis) from cyclophosphamide, and damaged joints (from osteonecrosis—death of blood vessels that nourish bones) from high-dose steroids. For more information, see Chapter 14, *Kidneys, Bladder, and Genitals,* and Chapter 17, *Muscles and Bones.*

Liver tumors

Liver tumors comprise fewer than 5 percent of all childhood cancers. The two most common types of childhood liver cancer are hepatoblastoma and hepatocellular carcinoma. Eighty percent of childhood hepatoblastomas occur before age 3, whereas hepatocellular carcinoma has two common incidence peaks in children: from birth to age 4 and from ages 12 to 15.

Surgery. The primary goal of surgery is to remove as much of the tumor as possible. Generally, surgery occurs soon after diagnosis. In cases where the tumor is very large or if the disease has spread to other organs, chemotherapy sometimes is given before surgery.

Chemotherapy. Chemotherapy almost always is used to treat both types of liver cancer. Chemotherapy can be given systemically (i.e., injected into the bloodstream and reaching all parts of the body) or regionally (i.e., delivered directly to the liver).

For hepatoblastoma, the most commonly used drugs are cisplatin (Platinol®), vincristine (Oncovin®), and fluorouracil (5-FU). Other drugs, such as doxorubicin (Adriamycin®), ifosfamide (Ifex®), carboplatin, and etoposide (VP-16 or Vepesid®) have been used for more advanced stages of the disease.

Initial treatment for hepatocellular carcinoma usually includes cisplatin and doxorubicin.

The following are possible late effects of treatment for liver cancers.

Heart problems. Heart problems can occur months or years after treatment with high doses of anthracyclines (i.e., doxorubicin, idarubicin, or daunorubicin), high-dose cyclophosphamide, or chest radiation. Symptoms include shortness of breath, fatigue, wheezing, anxiety, poor exercise tolerance, rapid heartbeat, and irregular heartbeat. Survivors often have no symptoms, but problems may be found on cardiac tests such as echocardiograms, electrocardiograms (EKGs), and Holter monitors. For more information, see Chapter 12, *Heart and Blood Vessels*.

Hearing loss. Cisplatin can result in mild to profound hearing loss in some children. For more information, see Chapter 10, *Eyes and Ears*.

Second cancers. A rare side effect from treatment with etoposide is developing second cancers. For more information, see Chapter 19, *Second Cancers*.

Soft tissue sarcomas

Childhood soft tissue sarcoma is a disease in which cancer arises in the body's soft tissues. Soft tissues include muscles, tendons (which connect muscles to bones), fat, blood vessels, nerves, and synovia (tissues around joints). Forty-seven percent of all childhood soft tissue sarcomas have a histology (which is how the cells look under a microscope) that is different from rhabdomyosarcoma (discussed later in this chapter). These soft tissue sarcomas include the following:

- **Synovial sarcoma.** This is the most common non-rhabdomyosarcoma soft tissue sarcoma in childhood. Synovial sarcoma is found most often in older children and is very rarely diagnosed in children younger than age 10. The disease occurs most frequently in the lower extremities, most often in the thigh or knee area. The second most common sites are the upper extremities, followed by the head, neck, and trunk.

- **Fibrosarcoma.** This soft tissue sarcoma occurs most often in infants and children younger than age 5 and in children between ages 10 and 15. These tumors usually develop in the extremities, and the majority of children diagnosed have localized disease. Infants diagnosed with this disease tend to respond to treatment better than do older children.

- **Malignant peripheral nerve sheath tumor** (also known as neurofibrosarcoma or malignant schwannoma). This is an aggressive malignancy that accounts for approximately 5 to 10 percent of all non-rhabdomyosarcoma soft tissue sarcomas of childhood. The disease often occurs in association with neurofibromatosis. The most common sites of origin are the extremities.

- **Malignant fibrous histiocytoma.** This form of soft tissue sarcoma most frequently occurs in the lower extremities and the trunk area. Other sites include the upper limbs, scalp, and kidneys.

The following are extremely rare forms of childhood soft tissue sarcomas. Young children with these diseases are generally treated on protocols based on those used for childhood rhabdomyosarcoma. Teens are usually treated on protocols similar to those used for adults with soft tissue sarcomas.

- **Leiomyosarcoma.** Leiomyosarcoma, which arises from smooth muscle, most often occurs in the gastrointestinal tract, especially the stomach.

- **Liposarcoma.** Liposarcoma arises in fatty tissue and is found most frequently in early adolescence. The most common sites of origin are the legs or trunk.

- **Hemangiopericytoma.** Hemangiopericytoma is a tumor of the blood and lymph vessels that occurs most frequently in infants.

- **Alveolar soft part sarcoma.** This rare soft tissue sarcoma, found most often in older children, arises from skeletal muscles of the extremities, head, and neck.

Treatment for non-rhabdomyosarcoma soft tissue sarcomas usually is with surgery and sometimes radiation therapy. Chemotherapy may be used to shrink large tumors to make them operable.

Although medical science has made advances in treating soft tissue sarcomas while reducing the side effects and long-term impact to the child, amputation is sometimes necessary. Limb-sparing procedures have made this less common.

Surgery. Surgery is the cornerstone of treatment for soft tissue sarcomas. The surgeon attempts to completely remove the mass with wide margins (i.e., removing a portion of the surrounding tissue) to ensure that no microscopic disease remains. This is often followed by 4000 to 5500 cGy of radiation. Investigational use of brachytherapy (which is implanting radioactive seeds for continuous low-level administration of radiation) is ongoing for children with rare soft tissue sarcomas. Another newer therapy used in current studies is intraoperative electron radiation. Radiation is directed at the site during surgery when the tumor and the surrounding areas are exposed.

Because these malignancies are so rare in children, treatment for non-rhabdomyosarcoma soft tissue sarcomas is based on experience with adults. However, children with non-rhabdomyosarcoma soft tissue sarcomas usually have a better outcome than do adults with the same diseases.

Chemotherapy. The use of chemotherapy after surgery is controversial. Patients with tumors too large to remove or whose disease has spread may be treated with vincristine, dactinomycin, and cyclophosphamide.

Retinoblastoma

Retinoblastoma is a malignant tumor of the retina in the eye. Approximately 300 children and adolescents younger than age 20 are diagnosed in the United States each year. Retinoblastoma usually is diagnosed in very young children and may be present at birth. Although it can occur at any age, 95 percent of cases are diagnosed before age 5. Children with more than one tumor or a tumor in both eyes (usually the hereditary form) tend to be diagnosed at a younger age than those with only one tumor and one eye involved (usually the non-hereditary form).

Treatment

Successful treatment of retinoblastoma depends largely on the size of the tumor and the extent of the disease. The staging system most widely used is the Intraocular Retinoblastoma System, which is based on tumor size, location, and presence of disease within the layers of the retina (called seeding).

Chemotherapy

Historically, chemotherapy was thought to have limited usefulness in treating retinoblastoma. Recently, however, chemotherapy has become the front-line treatment for selected groups of patients. Intraocular chemotherapy shrinks the tumors, which are then treated with cryotherapy and/or laser therapy. Drugs used in various combinations are vincristine (Oncovin®), etoposide (VP-16 or Vepesid®), and carboplatin (Paraplatin®).

Surgery and other therapies

There are several types of procedures used to treat retinoblastoma: enucleation, cryotherapy, and laser therapy. Decisions about the most appropriate treatment are made on an individual basis.

Removal of the eye (called enucleation) is a simple operation that eliminates the need for repeated examinations under anesthesia required by more conservative therapies. This step is taken only when absolutely necessary. The enucleation procedure is done under general anesthesia. In addition to removing the eye, the surgeon removes a section of the optic nerve. An orbital implant is placed into the socket immediately after the eyeball is removed.

Cryotherapy, sometimes called cryosurgery, is used to treat small primary tumors or new tumors that develop. Cryotherapy uses extreme cold applied by a small probe placed directly on the tumor. It is now often used in combination with chemotherapy and can also be used after radiation therapy.

Laser therapy, which uses infrared wavelengths of light, is sometimes used to treat small tumors.

Radiation

Retinoblastoma is a radiosensitive tumor. Radiation is used to destroy local disease while attempting to maintain vision. The two methods of radiotherapy used to treat retinoblastoma are external beam radiation and radioactive plaques. Historically, children have received a total of 3500 to 4600 cGy. Newer methods of delivering radiation are being used to try to reduce adverse long-term effects. These methods include intensity-modulated radiation therapy, stereotactic radiation therapy, and proton-beam radiation therapy (also called charged-particle radiation therapy). Radioactive plaque therapy (called brachytherapy) has been used in children with small, early stage tumors and in those with recurrent disease who have previously been treated with radiation.

Late effects

This section briefly outlines some common and uncommon late effects from treatment. Remember that you may develop none, one, or several of these problems in the months or years after treatment ends.

Bone growth. The most noticeable side effect of treatment for retinoblastoma is bone growth abnormalities around the eye, which develop after radiation to the orbit. Young children who have one or both eyes removed before age 3 may have an altered facial appearance when they mature due to the slowing of the growth of the orbit. After enucleation, a prosthesis needs to be placed and replaced periodically to foster orbital growth.

Dry eyes. A less common problem is decreased tear production, causing dry eyes and blurred vision. Some children who receive external beam radiation develop mild to severe keratitis sicca (inflammation of the cornea).

Loss of vision. Radiation can cause damage to the retina, resulting in loss of vision. Doses of 4500 cGy or below rarely result in loss of vision, but 5000 to 6000 cGy can cause retinopathy, and 6500 cGy can damage the retina and optic nerve, causing blindness. If systemic chemotherapy also is given, the risk of damage increases. Radiation-induced cataracts often occur if a child gets more than 1000 to 2000 cGy. In addition, vitreous leakage can occur near the edge of the tumor scar. For more information about these possible late effects, see Chapter 10, *Eyes and Ears.*

Second cancers. Children with the genetic form of retinoblastoma have an increased rate of developing second cancers, especially sarcomas, lung cancer, skin cancers, and breast cancer. For more information, see Chapter 19, *Second Cancers.*

Risk of passing on to children. Survivors with the genetic form of retinoblastoma can pass the risk on to their children. Genetic counseling prior to pregnancy can help survivors sort out their options. For more information, see Chapter 3, *Relationships.*

Rhabdomyosarcoma

Rhabdomyosarcoma (RMS) is the most common childhood soft tissue sarcoma. Approximately 350 children are diagnosed with RMS in the United States each year. Two-thirds of these cases are diagnosed in children younger than age 5. The disease has a slightly higher incidence in males compared with females. Black children have a slightly higher incidence than white children.

Description

RMS is a malignant soft tissue tumor of primitive muscle cells called rhabdomyoblasts. Instead of maturing into muscle cells, the rhabdomyoblasts grow out of control. Because muscles are located throughout the body, the tumors can appear at numerous locations. The four sites where RMS is most commonly found are the head and neck, genitourinary tract, extremities, and chest and lungs.

Treatment

Treatment depends on the location of the tumor, whether it has spread, its histology (meaning how it looks under a microscope), and its molecular genetics. Prior to the 1950s, the only treatment for RMS was surgical removal of the tumor. Many tumors were not completely removable, and up to 18 percent of children had metastatic disease at diagnosis. The addition of radiation in the 1950s and chemotherapy in the 1960s dramatically improved survival rates for children and teens with RMS.

Surgery

All children and teens with RMS have surgery, either to remove all or part of the primary tumor, or to perform a biopsy to reach a diagnosis. Surgery is used as early as possible in the course of treatment and is the quickest method to reduce the amount of the disease. However, complete removal may not be possible, particularly if the mass is located near vital blood vessels, if it deeply invades surrounding normal tissue, or if there are functional or cosmetic reasons for avoiding such a procedure.

During surgery the doctor removes as much of the tumor as possible and then samples surrounding tissues that are later examined by a pathologist. The pathologist determines whether the entire tumor has been removed or if some cells remain behind.

Second-look surgical procedures are sometimes done after chemotherapy to remove any remaining residual disease and determine whether remission has been reached. This is especially important for choosing appropriate further treatment, such as the amount of radiation to be given. Approximately 10 percent of newly diagnosed children have tumors that can be completely removed. In most cases, residual disease is present. For this reason, chemotherapy is used in all treatment protocols, and radiation is used in most.

Chemotherapy

Chemotherapy is given to all children and teens with RMS to destroy any cancer not removed surgically. Giving several anticancer drugs in combination has markedly improved the survival rate for this disease. The most commonly used drugs include cyclophosphamide (Cytoxan®), vincristine (Oncovin®), ifosfamide (Ifex®), etoposide (VP-16 or Vepesid®), doxorubicin (Adriamycin®), and dactinomycin (Cosmegen®).

Radiation

Radiotherapy is an important tool used to treat children and teens with RMS. Generally, those with stages I and II disease do not receive radiation therapy if their tumors can be completely removed. However, the need for radiation also depends on the histology of the tumor. Current protocols give patients with residual disease 3000 to 5100 cGy of external beam radiation although, in the past, higher doses of radiation were given. New radiation methods such as intensity-modulated radiation therapy (IMRT), fractionated stereotactic radiation therapy, and proton beam radiation are sometimes used for patients with head and neck RMS.

Most often, radiation is given approximately 1 to 3 months after chemotherapy has begun. However, children with tumors in the skull, meninges, or spinal cord may start radiation therapy soon after diagnosis.

Investigational use of brachytherapy (i.e., implanting radioactive seeds for continuous low-level administration of radiation) is ongoing for children and teens with RMS, especially those with small tumors in critical areas such as the head, prostate, bladder, or vagina.

Late effects

This section briefly outlines some common and uncommon late effects from treatment. Remember that you may develop none, one, or several of these problems in the months or years after treatment ends.

Loss of tissue and scarring. One universal late effect from surgery for RMS is loss of tissue and a scar where the tumor was removed. In cases where the surgeon performed a radical lymph node dissection, lymphedema (i.e., backup of lymph in extremities) can result. For more information, see Chapter 16, *Immune System*.

Altered growth. The growing bodies of young children given high doses of radiation develop an altered appearance in the areas radiated, because growth is affected. Because RMS can appear in different areas of the body, refer to the chapters about those specific areas for detailed information about late effects. For instance, high doses of radiation to the orbit and surrounding tissues causes asymmetry in growth and development in the bones around the eye. One orbit will be smaller than the other. Cataracts and other side effects can also develop after radiation. For more information, see Chapter 10, *Eyes and Ears*.

Bladder and kidney problems. In the past, children with tumors in the genitourinary area had the bladder removed in the initial surgery. The resulting permanent ileal conduit (i.e., diversion of the flow of urine to a bag outside the body) could develop many complications over time. Now, the bladder is only removed if the cancer remains after chemotherapy and radiation.

Radiation of the abdomen and/or pelvis that exceeds 2300 cGy can cause chronic nephritis (inflammation of the kidney) and a host of related kidney complications including fatigue, anemia, high blood pressure, hyperuricemia (excess uric acid in the blood), and gout. These problems can develop months or years after radiation treatment. Radiation of the abdomen can also cause fibrosis that obstructs the ureters. For more information about these problems, see Chapter 14, *Kidneys, Bladder, and Genitals*.

Problems after lymph node removal. Radical removal of the lymph nodes in the area of the testes or prostate can result in retrograde ejaculation or bowel obstruction. Problems with ejaculation and decreased sperm production are common in males who had RMS in or near the genitals. For more information, see Chapter 9, *Hormone-Producing Glands*.

Ovarian failure. Radiation to the abdomen can cause ovarian failure in some female survivors. For more information, see Chapter 9, *Hormone-Producing Glands*.

Curvature of the spine. Abdominal radiation at higher doses can also cause curvature of the back. For more information, see Chapter 17, *Muscles and Bones*.

Learning disabilities. Cranial radiation and intrathecal chemotherapy used to treat children with parameningeal RMS (in the membranes surrounding the spinal cord and brain) can cause cognitive problems. The severity of the damage depends on the child's treatment, age, and sex, with younger children being more at risk than older children or teens. Learning disabilities can develop years after treatment ends. Typically, problems develop in the areas of mathematics, memory, spatial relationships, problem solving, planning, organization, attention span, concentration skills, and social skills. For more information, see Chapter 8, *Brain and Nerves*.

Heart problems. Heart problems can occur months or years after treatment with anthracyclines (i.e., doxorubicin, idarubicin, or daunorubicin), high-dose cyclophosphamide, or chest radiation. Symptoms include shortness of breath, fatigue, wheezing, anxiety, poor exercise tolerance, rapid heartbeat, and irregular heartbeat. Few survivors develop this late effect, but regular checkups are crucial. Survivors often have no symptoms, but problems may be found on cardiac tests such as echocardiograms, electrocardiograms (EKGs), and Holter monitors. For more information, see Chapter 12, *Heart and Blood Vessels*.

Hepatitis C. Infection with the hepatitis C virus can develop in survivors who had blood transfusions prior to July 1992. For more information, see Chapter 15, *Liver, Stomach, and Intestines*.

Uncommon late effects. Children and teens who receive radiation have a slight risk of developing a second cancer. Those treated with VP-16 have a small chance of developing a second leukemia within 3 to 5 years of treatment. For more information, see Chapter 19, *Second Cancers*.

Wilms tumor

Wilms tumor is a primary cancer of the kidney. It accounts for 5 to 6 percent of all childhood cancers in the United States—approximately 500 children are diagnosed each year. Wilms tumor occurs most commonly in children younger than age 5. Girls have a slightly higher incidence than boys. Blacks and whites have similar incidence rates, but Asians are much less likely to develop Wilms tumor. A small percentage of Wilms tumors are believed to be inherited. In cases where the disease is inherited, there is a higher incidence of bilateral disease (meaning in both kidneys).

Treatment

Choice of treatment depends on histology (i.e., how it looks under a microscope), extent of disease (called stage), size of the tumor, and age of the child.

Surgery

Children diagnosed with Wilms tumor usually have a surgical procedure called a nephrectomy (removal of a kidney) performed before any other therapy is started. Occasionally, if the diagnosis is questionable, a biopsy will be performed prior to the nephrectomy. After biopsy or surgery, the pathologist examines the nuclei of the cancer cells under a microscope. If the nuclei of some of the cells appear larger than normal or irregular in shape, it is called anaplasia. If there is a large amount of anaplasia scattered throughout the tumor, it is called diffuse anaplasia.

Tumor cells that are not anaplastic are called Wilms tumor of favorable histology. Ninety-five percent of children with Wilms tumor have favorable histology. Children with unfavorable histology require more intense treatment.

For the majority of children, the goals of surgery are to remove the tumor, prevent rupture of the tumor capsule, and provide tissue for examination and staging. During surgery, the kidney with the tumor is removed, the other kidney is examined (to diagnose the 5 percent of cases in which both kidneys have tumor cells), and lymph nodes in the region are biopsied.

Chemotherapy

All children diagnosed with Wilms tumor receive chemotherapy. There are several chemotherapy drugs that are effective against this type of cancer. The use of dactinomycin (Cosmegen®) and vincristine (Oncovin®) has dramatically increased survival rates. Children with early stage disease are often treated with just these two drugs. For those who are diagnosed at more advanced stages, doxorubicin (Adriamycin®) and cyclophosphamide (Cytoxan®) may be added. In North America, only those children with bilateral Wilms tumor receive chemotherapy prior to surgery.

Radiation

In the past, all children with Wilms tumor received radiation, some at very high doses. But now, because of the risk of long-term complications from radiation therapy, the decision to use it to treat a child with Wilms is based largely on the stage and histology of the tumor.

Late effects

Some children with stage I or II disease have few or no long-term effects. Children with higher risk disease, or those who relapse and require more intensive treatment, sometimes pay a higher price. The following information briefly outlines some common and uncommon late effects from treatment. Remember that you may develop none, a few, or several of these problems in the months or years after treatment ends.

Growth problems. A child whose trunk is irradiated may have curvature of the spine and soft tissue underdevelopment in the radiated areas (most common in those treated prior to 1970). When lower doses of radiation (1000 to 2500 cGy) are given to all or parts of the spine, up to 40 percent of survivors have reduced sitting heights (measured from the rump to the top of the head). This problem is more common in children who were younger than age 6 and in adolescents going through their growth spurt when irradiated. For more information, see Chapter 17, *Muscles and Bones.*

Heart problems. In some patients, heart problems can occur months or years after treatment with anthracyclines (i.e., doxorubicin, idarubicin, or daunorubicin), high-dose cyclophosphamide, or chest radiation. Symptoms include shortness of breath, fatigue, wheezing, anxiety, poor exercise tolerance, rapid heartbeat, and irregular heartbeat. Survivors often have no symptoms, but problems may be found on cardiac tests such as echocardiograms, electrocardiograms (EKGs), and Holter monitors. In a study of Wilms tumor survivors who were treated with doxorubicin in National Wilms' Tumor Studies 1, 2, 3, and 4 and who did not relapse, more than 4 percent developed heart problems.[4] Abdominal radiation can cause damage to major blood vessels, including the aorta and renal vessels. For more information, see Chapter 12, *Heart and Blood Vessels.*

Hepatitis C. Infection with the hepatitis C virus can develop in survivors who had blood transfusions prior to July 1992. For more information, see Chapter 15, *Liver, Stomach, and Intestines.*

Fertility and pregnancy. Girls who had abdominal radiation can experience ovarian failure. Survivors who do become pregnant have a risk of delivering low birthweight babies, of impaired development of the fetus due to maternal scoliosis (curvature of the spine), or of reduced blood supply from damaged vessels. Offspring are not at risk of developing Wilms if the mother had the non-inherited form in only one kidney. Any young woman who had Wilms tumor should get genetic counseling to fully understand her particular situation, and, if pregnant, should be cared for by an obstetrician who specializes in high-risk pregnancies. This gives the best chance for a full-term pregnancy and a healthy baby. Children fathered by males treated for Wilms are just as healthy as children of fathers with no cancer history. For more information, see Chapter 3, *Relationships* and Chapter 9, *Hormone-Producing Glands.*

Newer technologies can sometimes help infertile couples have a baby. Counseling and support for infertile couples allow them to explore their options and address their feelings about infertility.

Digestive problems. A very small number of survivors who were treated with flank or whole abdomen radiation develop chronic gastrointestinal disturbances. For more information, see Chapter 15, *Liver, Stomach, and Intestines*.

Second cancers. Second cancers develop in a very small number of Wilms survivors. The most common—bone, breast, thyroid, leukemias, and lymphomas—are usually found in irradiated areas. For more information, see Chapter 19, *Second Cancers*.

Stem cell transplantation

Stem cell transplantation (i.e., bone marrow, stem cells, or cord blood) is used to treat several types of childhood cancers. In these procedures, the child or teen is given high doses of chemotherapy and/or radiation to destroy all of the cancer in the body. During this process, the bone marrow is totally destroyed. Normal marrow or stem cells are then infused into the child's veins. The marrow or stem cells migrate to the cavities inside the bones where new, healthy blood cells are then produced.

The three types of transplants are:

- **Allogeneic.** Allogeneic transplants are those in which donor bone marrow, stem cells, or cord blood is transplanted into the patient. The cells usually come from a sibling with a matching marrow type or a matched unrelated donor. In some cases, parents are used as donors. The risk of complications increases if the donor is mismatched or unrelated.

- **Syngeneic.** Syngeneic bone marrow transplants (BMTS) are those in which the donor is the patient's identical twin. Many late complications are avoided because the marrow is an identical match.

- **Autologous.** During an autologous stem cell transplant, the patient's own stem cells are extracted and cryopreserved (a type of freezing). The patient then undergoes radiation and chemotherapy, or high-dose chemotherapy alone. The frozen cells are thawed and infused into the child or teen intravenously.

The three sources of blood cell used for transplant are:

- **Bone marrow.** In a BMT, the donor's bone marrow is extracted from the hip bones. This is done in the operating room with the use of two large bore needles.

- **Peripheral blood stem cells.** For a peripheral blood stem cell transplant, the patient's or donor's stem cells—cells from which all other cells evolve—are harvested in a procedure called apheresis. Blood is removed through a catheter or vein in the arm and circulated through a machine that extracts the stem cells. The remaining blood is then returned to the patient or donor.

• **Umbilical cord blood.** Umbilical cord blood is a rich source of stem cells. In the 1990s, researchers began conducting transplants using the umbilical cord blood obtained during the birth of a sibling or from preserved unrelated donor cord blood.

Prior to the transplant, the patient's bone marrow is destroyed using high-dose chemotherapy with or without radiation. This portion of treatment is called conditioning. The purpose of the high doses of chemotherapy and radiation is to kill all remaining cancer cells in the body, make room in the bones for the new bone marrow, and suppress the patient's immune system so it will accept the donor's marrow.

Conditioning regimens vary according to institution and protocol, and also depend on the medical condition and history of the child or teen. Typically, chemotherapy is given for 2 to 6 days, and radiation (if part of conditioning) is given in multiple small doses over several days. The drugs most commonly used during conditioning are cyclophosphamide (Cytoxan®), busulfan (Myleran®), etoposide (VP-16 or Vepesid®), thiotepa, and melphalan (Alkeran®).

The transplant itself consists of simply infusing the stem cells or marrow through a catheter or intravenously into the patient, just like a blood transfusion. The stem cells travel throughout the blood vessels, eventually filling the empty spaces in the long bones. Engraftment occurs when the new marrow begins to produce healthy white cells, red cells, and platelets—usually 1 to 4 weeks after transplantation.

Late effects

This section briefly outlines some common and uncommon late effects from treatment with stem cell transplantation. Remember that you may develop none, one, or several of these problems in the months or years after treatment ends.

Graft-versus-host disease. Graft-versus-host disease (GVHD) is a frequent complication of allogeneic stem cell transplants. It does not occur with autologous or syngeneic transplants. In GVHD, the bone marrow provided by the donor (the graft) attacks the tissues and organs of the BMT child (the host). Approximately 30 to 50 percent of children and teens who have a related HLA-matched transplant develop some degree of GVHD. The incidence and severity of GVHD are increased for those children and teens who receive unrelated or mismatched marrow.

There are two types of GVHD: acute and chronic. Children and teens can develop one type, both types, or neither one. Acute GVHD usually occurs at the time of engraftment or shortly thereafter. Donor cells identify the patient's cells as different and attack the patient's skin, liver, stomach, or intestines. Acute GVHD is treated with cyclosporine, tacrolimus (Prograf®), and steroids (i.e., prednisone, dexamethasone). Prolonged use of steroids to treat GVHD can cause osteonecrosis (death of the small blood vessels that feed bones). For detailed information about these late effects, see Chapter 15, *Liver, Stomach, and Intestines* and *Chapter 18, Skin, Breasts, and Hair.*

If chronic GVHD develops, it usually starts 100 or more days post-transplant. It primarily affects the skin (itchy rash, discoloration of the skin, tightening of the skin, hair loss with a dry flaky scalp, nail changes—dry and brittle), eyes (dry, light sensitive), mouth and esophagus (dry mouth, tooth decay, difficulty swallowing), intestines (diarrhea, cramping, weight loss), liver (jaundice), lungs (shortness of breath, wheezing, coughing), and joints (decreased mobility). Survivors with chronic GVHD can develop one, a few, or several of these problems. There are many medications, including tacrolimus (Prograf®), steroids, and mycophenolate (CellCept®), that can be used to treat chronic GVHD.

Cataracts. Numerous late effects can occur from total body irradiation (TBI) used during conditioning. Often, children and teens develop cataracts after transplant. If the TBI is given in one dose, the likelihood of developing cataracts is much higher than if TBI is given in smaller doses over several days (called fractionated). Currently, if radiation is used, it is given in fractionated doses. Decreased tear production is also common after transplant. For more information, see Chapter 10, *Eyes and Ears.*

Growth problems. Radiation can affect growth. Children who received prior cranial radiation, spinal radiation, or total body radiation should be monitored for learning disabilities, dental problems (e.g., facial bone and jaw growth, delayed development of permanent teeth, incomplete root development), and growth hormone deficiency resulting in delayed or decreased growth. Children and teens who receive TBI also may have a low thyroid function due to decreased production of thyroid hormone. For more information, see Chapter 9, *Hormone-Producing Glands.*

Problems with puberty. For the most part, children and teens who were given only cyclophosphamide during conditioning have normal sexual development. Children and teens who had TBI, however, may experience delayed puberty (the incidence is lower if the radiation was given in several small doses). All children and teens who received TBI should be followed closely by a pediatric endocrinologist who can prescribe hormones to assist in normal pubertal development. Girls are more likely than boys to need hormonal replacement; boys usually produce testosterone but not sperm.

Fertility. Children and teens who received TBI usually—but not always—become sterile; that is, after growing up, girls will not be able to become pregnant, and boys will not be able to father children. The ability to have a normal sex life is not affected. Some children treated with cyclophosphamide but no radiation have remained fertile, and to date, all offspring have been normal. For more information, see Chapter 9, *Hormone-Producing Glands*.

Hepatitis C. Infection with the hepatitis C virus can develop in survivors who had blood transfusions prior to July 1992. For more information, see Chapter 15, *Liver, Stomach, and Intestines*.

Second cancers. Children or teens who received a stem cell transplant have a small risk of developing a second cancer, particularly if TBI was used. The type of cancers most commonly seen post-transplant are leukemia, lymphoma, and bone and soft tissue sarcomas. For more information, see Chapter 19, *Second Cancers*.

TBI can also cause late effects to the lungs, heart, liver, and bowel. Any body system treated with radiation can be damaged, so follow-up needs to be done for the rest of one's life.

Recommended follow-up for survivors

Some tests are recommended to monitor your long-term health. By screening for problems that may occur, you can quickly identify and treat them. Most survivors of childhood cancer should have the following tests every year: complete blood count, liver function studies, urinalysis, and measurements of blood pressure, pulse, respirations, height, and weight. In addition, the following tables list some tests you should have based on the specific treatments you received. Refer to Table 6-1 for tests after chemotherapy, Table 6-2 for tests after radiation, and Table 6-3 for tests after surgery. Other treatments are listed in Table 6-4.

For comprehensive and up-to-date recommendations, refer to the long-term follow-up guidelines from the Children's Oncology Group at *www.survivorshipguidelines.org*. Recommendations are being regularly updated as new information is learned about late effects, so survivors and their healthcare providers should check these recommendations periodically.

Table 6-1. Tests After Chemotherapy

If Treatment Included	Recommended Follow-Up Testing
Bleomycin (Blenoxane®) Busulfan (Myleran®) Nitrosoureas (CCNU, BCNU)	• Chest x-ray, PFTs (breathing tests) baseline, then as needed.
Cisplatin (Platinol®) Carboplatin (Paraplatin®)	• Complete pure tone audiogram (hearing test) or brainstem auditory evoked response baseline and then at least yearly if hearing loss is detected. For survivors who also had cranial or ear irradiation, test yearly for at least 5 years. • Blood tests: BUN, Cr, Na, K, Cl, CO2, Ca, Mg, PO4 baseline and then periodically if indicated. • Creatinine clearance baseline, then every year if abnormal. • Fasting lipid profile baseline, then as needed.
Cyclophosphamide (Cytoxan®)	• Blood tests: LH, FSH, estradiol/testosterone baseline at age 13, then as needed.
Ifosfamide (Ifex®)	• Semen analysis. • Menstrual history (females every year after puberty). • Yearly discussion of any urinary problems. • Blood tests: LH, FSH, estrogen/testosterone baseline at age 13, then as needed. • Urinalysis every year. • Creatinine clearance baseline, then as needed. • Blood tests: BUN, Cr, Cl, CO2, Ca, Mg, PO4 baseline and periodically if indicated.
Nitrogen mustard (mechlorethamine or Mustargen®) Lomustine (CCNU) Carmustine (BCNU)	• Complete blood count every year. • Semen analysis (upon request). • Chest x-ray, PFTs (breathing tests) every 3 to 5 years (only if you received BCNU).
Daunorubicin (Cerubidine®) Doxorubicin (Adriamycin®) Epirubicin Idarubicin Mitoxantrone	• Electrocardiogram (EKG) and echocardiogram baseline, then every 1 to 5 years depending on risk (higher risk from higher cumulative dose, young age, being female, radiation to chest). • Holter monitor (24-hour EKG test) every 2 to 5 years depending on total dose. • Exercise testing. • If pregnant, see an obstetrician who specializes in high-risk care.
High-dose cytarabine (ARA-C)	• Neurologic examination. • Neuropsychological evaluation baseline, then as needed if educational or vocational problems emerge.
Asparaginase	• None, unless associated with acute problems.

Table 6-1. Tests After Chemotherapy (continued)

If Treatment Included	Recommended Follow-Up Testing

Methotrexate (systemic)
Intrathecal medications:
  Methotrexate
  ARA-C
  Hydrocortisone
	• Neuropsychological testing baseline, then every 2 years if any learning problems noted.
	• Educational assessment every year.
	• Bone density evaluation baseline, then as needed.

Mercaptopurine (6-MP or Purinethol®) Thioguanine (6-TG)	• Liver function tests baseline, then as needed.
Prednisone Dexamethasone (Decadron®)	• Evaluation for joint pain. • Bone density evaluation baseline, then as needed. • Growth evaluation. • Examination for cataracts every year.
Vincristine (Oncovin®)	• Neurologic exam yearly for 3 years, then as needed. • Examination for peripheral neuropathy yearly for 3 years, then as needed.
Etoposide (VP-16 or Vepesid®) Teniposide (VM-26)	• Neurologic examination. • Skin exam every year for 10 years. • Complete blood count every year for 10 years. • Counseling about second cancers.

Table 6-2. Tests After Radiation

Radiation Given	Recommended Follow-Up Testing
Bone	• X-rays every 5 years. • Evaluation of bone growth and overlying soft tissue in area irradiated every year.
Cranial Nasopharyngeal	• Educational assessment every year. • Neuropsychological testing baseline, then every 2 to 3 years. • Neurologic evaluation every year. • X-ray of full set of teeth (Panorex) at age 5. • Monitor for early or delayed puberty. • Growth curve every year (every 6 months between ages 10 to 12). • Bone age (x-ray of hand) at 9 years of age for a baseline, then every year until puberty (based on risk factors). • Blood tests: growth hormone, somatomedin C, IGFBP3, and others as indicated. • Complete eye examination by ophthalmologist every year that includes check for cataracts. • Blood tests: Free T4, TSH, fasting glucose, fasting lipid profile every year.

Table 6-2. Tests After Radiation (continued)

Radiation Given	Recommended Follow-Up Testing
Flank	• Observe for scoliosis (curvature of the spine) every year (every 6 months during puberty).
Chest or mantle	• Blood tests: Free T4, TSH every year. • Chest x-ray, PFTs (breathing tests) baseline, then as needed. • Fasting glucose and lipid profile every 3 to 5 years. • Breast self-exam every month. • Breast examination by healthcare provider every year. • Mammogram 8 years after radiation or by age 25 (whichever comes last), then every 2 years until age 40, then every year (females only). • Growth curve (sitting and standing heights) every year until fully grown. • Dental exam every year. • EKG and echocardiogram baseline, then every 1 to 5 years depending on risk (higher risk from higher cumulative dose, young age, being female, radiation to chest). • Exercise testing. • If pregnant, see an obstetrician who specializes in high-risk care. • Counseling about not smoking.
Whole lung	• Chest x-ray. • PFTs (breathing tests) every 3 to 5 years. • Breast self-examination every month. • Breast examination by healthcare provider every year. • Mammogram 8 years after radiation or by age 25 (whichever comes last), then every 2 years until age 40, then every year (females only). • Growth curve (sitting and standing) every year until fully grown. • EKG/echocardiogram/chest x-ray baseline, then every 1 to 5 years depending on risk (higher risk from higher cumulative dose, young age, being female, radiation to chest). • Holter monitor (24-hour EKG test) every 2 to 5 years depending on total dose. • Exercise testing. • Counseling about not smoking.
Spinal	• Evaluation for scoliosis (curvature of the spine), kyphosis (curvature of spine in hunchback shape). • Blood tests: Free T4, TSH every year. • Growth curve (sitting and standing heights) every year. • Blood tests: LH, FSH, estrogen (females baseline at age 12, then as needed). • Evaluate stage of puberty.

Table 6-2. Tests After Radiation (continued)

Radiation Given	Recommended Follow-Up Testing
Spinal *(continued)*	• EKG/echocardiogram/chest x-ray baseline, then every 2 to 5 years depending on risk (higher risk from higher cumulative dose, young age, being female, radiation to chest). • Exercise testing.
Testicular (males only)	• Testes exam every year by a healthcare provider. • Testicular self-exam every month. • Blood tests: LH, FSH, testosterone at age 14, then as needed. • Evaluate stage of puberty. • Sperm count (as requested)
Neck and jaw	• Dental exam every year. • Complete eye examination by ophthalmologist every year that includes check for cataracts.
Leg	• Monitor for leg-length discrepancy.
Orbit (eye)	• Complete eye examination by ophthalmologist every year. • X-ray of orbits every 3 to 5 years. • Blood tests: LH, FSH, estrogen/testosterone (baseline at age 12, then as needed). • Evaluate stage of puberty.
Whole body (TBI)	• Growth curve (sitting and standing heights) every year. • Bone age (x-ray of hand) as needed. • Urinalysis (check for blood, protein, sugar). • Puberty evaluation every year from ages 8 to 18. • Blood tests: LH, FSH (baseline at 12, then as needed). • Menstrual history (females) every year after puberty. • Blood tests: Free T4, TSH every year. • Complete eye examination by ophthalmologist every year that includes check for cataracts. • Skin checks and counseling on protecting skin from the sun.
Abdomen Pelvis Inverted Y	• Blood tests: LH, FSH, estrogen/testosterone (baseline at age 12, then as needed). • Evaluation for scoliosis (curvature of the spine) and kyphosis (curvature of spine in hunchback shape). • Blood culture if you have a fever. • ALT, AST, bilirubin at baseline, then as needed. • Colonoscopy every 5 years starting 10 years after the radiation or age 35, whichever occurs last. • Creatinine, BUN, Na, K, Ca, Cl, CO_2, Mg, PO_4 at baseline, then as needed. • Evaluate stage of puberty and obtain menstrual history. • Semen analysis (males). • Nutritional history.

Table 6-2. Tests After Radiation (continued)

Radiation Given	Recommended Follow-Up Testing
Abdomen Pelvis Inverted Y *(continued)*	• Stool test for blood every year. • Urinalysis every year. • If pregnant, see an obstetrician who specializes in high-risk pregnancies.
All areas	• Skin check of irradiated areas every year.

Table 6-3. Recommendations and Tests After Surgery

If Treatment Included	Recommendations and Follow-Up Testing
Adrenal gland removal	• Information about symptoms of adrenal insufficiency.
Abdominal surgery	• Serum magnesium every year.
Amputation	• Examination with attention to range of motion and muscle contractures. • Prosthesis check every 6 months until skeleton has stopped growing, then yearly. • Antibiotics prior to dental work if an allograft.
Enucleation (removal of the eye)	• Socket examination each year. • Evaluation by ophthalmologist every year.
Laparotomy	• Gastrointestinal and nutrition status evaluation.
Limb salvage	• Bone x-ray every year. • Evaluation by an orthopedic surgeon every 6 months until skeleton has stopped growing, then yearly. • Counseling about exercise restrictions.
Nephrectomy (removal of a kidney)	• Blood pressure every year. • Urinalysis every year (check for blood, protein, sugar). • Blood tests: BUN, Cr, Ca, Na, K, Cl, CO_2, Mg, PO_4 baseline and then as needed. • Counseling about kidney protection.
Neurosurgery	• Neuropsychological evaluation baseline, then as needed. • Evaluation by neurologist and rehabilitation specialist every year.
Splenectomy	• Penicillin daily (erythromycin if allergic to penicillin). • Antibiotics prior to dental work. • Pneumovax (recommendations on frequency vary). • Annual influenza vaccine. • Fever above 101° F requires a blood culture and evaluation for infection by a doctor.

Table 6-4. Other Tests

Issue	Recommended Follow-Up Testing
Transfusions	• Baseline HIV blood test. • Blood tests: If transfused prior to July 1992, have HBV (hepatitis B virus) and HCV (hepatitis C virus) tests.
Primary disease	Counseling and surveillance for second cancers if the primary disease was: • Hodgkin lymphoma. • Hereditary retinoblastoma. • Sarcoma. • Neuroblastoma. • ALL if treated with cranial radiation.
Health maintenance	• Low-fat diet. • Exercise. • Lifestyle counseling. • No smoking. • Moderate alcohol use.
Family history of cancer	• Counseling about risk of second cancers. • Genetic evaluation.

Chapter 7

Fatigue

The patient is cured when he can again
do the things he loves to do.

—Stanley A. Herrings

FATIGUE IS SOMETHING almost all children and teens experience while being treated for cancer. For a small percentage of survivors, however, the profound tiredness lasts long after treatment. People with fatigue have little energy and feel emotionally, physically, and mentally tired. Fatigue may have an identifiable physical cause, or it may remain an elusive—but life-altering—late effect of treatment. This chapter describes fatigue, its causes, and its treatment. It also includes the voices of many survivors who live with and cope with chronic fatigue.

Contributors to fatigue

During treatment, the effects of drugs, surgery, and radiation can sometimes combine to cause overwhelming fatigue. Survivors hope and expect that this frustrating condition will resolve when treatment ends. Most survivors are able to resume activities with normal energy levels. Others have occasional or constant exhaustion. Cancer-related fatigue is different than being tired from normal activities because it takes less activity to tire you out, it isn't completely relieved by sleep and rest, and it can last a long time. This unexpected and unwelcome late effect can cause physical, mental, emotional, and financial distress. At a time when you expect renewal, you find that you cannot make it through the day.

Research on cancer-related fatigue in childhood cancer survivors is fairly limited and findings have been mixed. Some studies have shown lower rates of fatigue among childhood cancer survivors when compared with survivors of cancer in adulthood, while others have found similar rates of fatigue. More research is needed to get a better understanding of how fatigue changes over time, what factors influence it, and what can be done to decrease it.

The first step in coping with fatigue is to understand that it can be a late effect of treatment. The next step is to give your healthcare provider a specific description of how the fatigue affects your life. According to clinical guidelines published in 2011, your healthcare provider should screen you for fatigue at regular intervals during and after cancer treatment, and then as needed.[1]

Usually, fatigue doesn't occur by itself. More often, it occurs along with other symptoms (called "symptom clusters"). Stress can make fatigue worse. Many factors can contribute to fatigue that persists long after treatment ends, including the following:

- Nutritional deficiencies
- Sleep disturbance
- Depression or anxiety
- Inactivity
- Chronic pain
- Certain medicines
- Obesity
- Alcohol/substance abuse
- Hormone imbalance (i.e., thyroid, testosterone, estrogen, growth hormone)
- Gastrointestinal problems
- Liver dysfunction
- Heart or lung disease
- Kidney disease
- Low red blood cell counts (called anemia)

Most often, the exact cause of persistent fatigue is unknown. Fatigue can improve over time, but it can take a long time. And while it lasts, fatigue can have a far-reaching impact on every aspect of life.

> I had Hodgkin's when I was 13 and again when I was 26. I have no chronic fatigue, although I lost my stamina after the radiation in my teens due to restricted lung capacity. I can't run more than a half mile no matter how good of shape I am in. It utterly exhausts me. I work harder than most people I know. But if I feel like taking a day off, I do. I stay healthy and take good care of myself.

I think I was unusual in that I didn't have fatigue when I was initially treated in the early 1970s. I finished my senior year at Berkeley during radiation treatment and did my first year of graduate school during chemo. Looking back on it now, I think I was a little bit nuts. But I felt I had to keep pushing. Fatigue did not become a problem for me until the chronic heart failure began in 1997. Now every day is a battle to find enough energy. I find it hard to believe that I once saw patients from 7 in the morning until 7 at night and then often went to a meeting afterwards.

But I also know that currently my fatigue is exacerbated by depression, and I can feel a certain heaviness set in that makes the fatigue even worse when I am coping with the depression. When I get a handle on the depression (I have had lots of psychotherapy, and I sometimes take an antidepressant), my fatigue becomes much more manageable.

I think there is a real place for psychotherapy after treatment. It isn't a sign of weakness to go in search of help, nor a sign of deep mental disturbance, but an admission that sometimes certain events are more than we can cope with. The hard part is finding a psychotherapist who can appreciate the nature of the trauma and make good interventions.

Signs and symptoms

Chronic fatigue can interfere with all of the activities of daily life. It can wax and wane or be constant. Following are some of the signs and symptoms of fatigue:

- Whole body tiredness, weariness, or exhaustion even after sleep

- Mental and emotional exhaustion

- Difficulty concentrating, remembering, or completing tasks

- Confused thinking

- Decreased ability to work, do regular activities, or start new projects

- Decreased interest in enjoyable activities

- Feelings of sadness, frustration, or irritability

- Decreased sexual desire

- Spending more time resting or sleeping

  Chronic fatigue is the worst late effect I've had to deal with after treatment for Hodgkin's. I've had it for 22 years. I used to be a very active

*person—give me a list of 100 things to do and I'd do 110. Now, I nap
2 hours every single afternoon. By 2 p.m., I shut down completely—I
can't move anymore, I can't think anymore. So I just go to bed. My husband can tell as soon as it starts because I start to mix up my words and
my speech slurs. But, you know, I try to appreciate all the things I can
do: I can see, hear, taste, walk. I try to focus on all the things I can do,
rather than fixate on the things I can't.*

· · · · ·

*I was diagnosed in August 1990. For 9 years I have felt fatigue. I just
thought that I was lazy. Over the years I have developed such a guilt
complex because I tire easily. I have seen my husband suffer and give up
so much because of me. Cancer treatment left me infertile. Sex drive is
right out the window also.*

*Friends cannot seem to understand my fatigue, and my employer is
beyond understanding me. I even work in a hospital. I have tried to work
full time but just cannot do it. I want to, but the body just plays out too
much. Bedtime is 8 p.m., just to make it through the next day. I have cut
my hours back to 3 days a week. Well, I need every other day just to
recoup from one. I feel like I am always trying to come up with some sort
of an excuse that they would understand, other than I am tired.*

Chronic fatigue is very hard on relationships with loved ones. You may not
have the energy to go out with your spouse to have dinner or visit friends.
Your interest in sex may disappear, or you may just be too tired by the evening even if you are interested. You may not have the energy to take your
children to the park or play in the backyard. Your friends may not understand that you can look great but have no energy. If your fatigue forces you
to work less or stop work entirely, your income may decrease. You may feel
guilty or lazy. All of these worries—big and small—can take a toll.

*It's hard explaining even to dear friends that I just don't function the way
I did pre-treatment. I'm still trying to find that balance between challenging myself and knowing my limitations. If anything, I drive myself
way too hard.*

*I'm a rather private person. I don't like telling people that I've had can-
cer and that cancer still has an effect on my life. People say things like,
"But you look so healthy. And you're done with treatment. Why don't you
just get over it?" Well, I'm sure if I could "just get over it" I would. But
it's not that easy.*

*I do get angry when people who know I've had cancer expect me to per-
form like any other 22 year old. I know they can't really imagine what I
feel like. But I'm not so sure I want to tell everyone what it does feel like.*

It's a bit of a bind when you look healthy and desire to work hard, but you just don't have the stamina that you used to.

Many children also suffer from fatigue long after treatment ends.

Many years after her treatment for neuroblastoma, Paige still has fatigue and a low energy level. She is very tired at the end of school and her activity of choice is always TV or Gameboy®. She plays soccer and basketball, but she doesn't have a lot of stamina and gets frustrated.

Survivorship healthcare professionals have observed that children with cognitive changes, in particular, seem to have more fatigue.

My daughter was treated on a high-risk ALL protocol that included 1800 cGy of cranial radiation and 17 doses of intrathecal methotrexate. She had the radiation when she was 3 years old. Among her many side effects is profound fatigue. Through elementary school and middle school, she would come home from school and go straight to bed for a few hours. We had to wake her up to eat dinner. It was worse in high school, so she had lots of testing done, and they found out that she was mildly growth hormone deficient and also had the poorly understood post-radiation fatigue. The doctor told her that her brain had to work so hard to process input from the world around her that it just got very tired very fast. After she went on growth hormone and also a drug called Provigil® (used for people with narcolepsy), she could stay awake long enough to eat and do homework. She still sleeps 10 or 11 hours a night, but she is able to stay awake all day. It's been 20 years since the radiation, and sadly, we think this late effect is a permanent one.

Screening and detection

A thorough physical and psychological evaluation is needed to identify possible causes of fatigue and determine what may be treatable. It helps to keep a record of your pattern of fatigue prior to going to your healthcare provider. For instance, you could note on your calendar how long you work each day, how many naps you take, how long they are, and how much you sleep each night. Many survivors force themselves to go to work but feel absolutely exhausted by the afternoon. This is an important piece of information to share with your healthcare provider.

Your evaluation should include the following:[2]

• Review of cancer history, treatment, and current status

• Complete physical examination

- Fatigue history
  - When it started, how long it has lasted, any changes
  - Actions or events that make the fatigue better or worse
  - Effect of fatigue on job, daily life, and relationships
- Assessment of contributing factors, such as:
  - Pain
  - Hormone levels (i.e., thyroid, testosterone, estrogen, growth hormone)
  - Current medications, including over-the-counter medicines and supplements
  - Emotions (e.g., depression and anxiety)
  - Sleep and napping habits
  - Level of physical activity
  - Nutrition history, including weight gain or loss and changes in appetite
  - Other health conditions that could affect fatigue

> I've never had debilitating fatigue, but in the 33 years since treatment, I've always struggled with having enough energy. When I worked a 40- or 50-hour week like everyone else, I had no energy to cook meals or clean house or do anything but collapse when I came home. I had to grieve when I finally realized it was from the treatment, because I could have managed it a whole lot differently. Now I do energy management. The things I really want to do, I make sure I do. I'm very up front with people. I tell them I have limits on my energy and will say, "This is a good time to do it," or "Can we do this together, then I'll sit and watch while you do that?" People are very understanding.

Medical management

Fatigue in long-term survivors of cancer can range from being a nuisance to being a disabling condition. For some survivors, the fatigue comes and goes. For others, energy and stamina are permanently reduced.

> I've never felt less than anyone else because I couldn't keep up. I've always viewed my life from the standpoint that I've been to hell and back and I'm doing mighty fine keeping the pace that I keep. I compare myself to me, not to others who are sick or healthy, or to the "past Carol"— only to the "present Carol." If I set my goals and meet them for myself, then I'm content.

When I need help, I ask for it. I learned a long time ago that asking for help allows another person to give of herself. I like to give, so I think it's nice to offer someone else that opportunity.

Your healthcare provider can consult the National Comprehensive Cancer Network (NCCN) Guidelines for Cancer-Related Fatigue for ways to manage fatigue, based on its possible causes and your individual situation and health needs. Medical management can include pharmacologic (i.e., medicines) or non-pharmacologic interventions, such as:

- Enhancing activity level with exercise, physical therapy, or occupational therapy.
- Consultation with a sleep expert to improve "sleep hygiene" (i.e., the things you do to get a good night's rest).
- Counseling and support (individual or group) to help with emotions and stress management.
- Consultation with a nutritionist about diet and supplements.
- Medicines for pain, emotional distress, and anemia, if needed.

Survivors with fatigue caused by heart damage sometimes benefit from medication and/or cardiac rehabilitation programs.

Sometimes there is no medical treatment for fatigue even when the cause is known. Many brain tumor survivors and some leukemia survivors treated with cranial radiation have fatigue from unknown causes. This exhaustion can affect a survivor's education and social life. Counseling for these survivors can include how to get accommodations in school through an Individualized Education Program or Individualized Transition Plan (see Chapter 4, *Navigating the System*). Some options are to go to school half days, allow more time to get from class to class, and participate in adaptive physical education.

I watched my son Bobby sink into a sedentary lifestyle after his bone marrow transplant, and it scared me. He was so tired after transplant that he just laid around at home. He would toss and turn all night long and then fall asleep just as he was supposed to be getting up for school. He would fall asleep in class, be unable to focus and learn, and then fall asleep on the drive home, crawl into bed for a few hours, get up to eat and do schoolwork at 10 p.m., then toss and turn again for half the night. Even if he didn't nap in the late afternoon, insomnia seemed to be a chronic problem, and he was always so tired.

We took him out of school to homeschool him for 11th and 12th grade, and he did beautifully. If he had a bad night, he slept until he woke on his own, then did his schoolwork at his own pace. If he had difficulty with a lesson, he reread it until he understood it. He still sat around the rest of the time, so I pushed him to go to the local health club. He then joined an aikido class taught at the health club and that was very helpful. He got out to exercise for 4½ hours per week. He started riding a bike to a job last spring. I began to notice increased good health, good color, toned muscles, and more energy than ever before.

Counseling for all survivors suffering from post-cancer fatigue can address several issues. Psychological distress that existed prior to cancer or resulted from cancer treatment may make fatigue worse. Resolution of these issues may improve your energy level. Therapists who specialize in this area can also work with you to devise an energy conservation plan. Supportive discussions about the effect the low energy has on your life may result in new ways to adapt to the condition. Counseling may also help lift the burdens of negative feelings such as thinking that you are lazy or selfish.

One of my ways of conserving energy is to just sit down. When I am doing chores and my energy level dips, I sit down for 15 minutes with my legs elevated. I allow my mind some quiet time also. I stop thinking about what is awaiting my attention. It will all still be waiting after my rest. This rest gives my body and my mind a chance to rejuvenate. I find it most helpful.

• • • • •

To save energy, I usually just sit down for a little bit. Or if it's bad, I take a 20-minute power nap. I also find bouncy music and playful kittens to be energizing.

As for weather, I find that sunshine makes me want to go outside and play, but once I'm out there I don't last very long. It feels like the sun drains me. With all the clothing I have to wear in winter I feel like I'm dragging a whole other person around with me as well, so I get tired then. But I always feel less guilty in the winter because no one wants to go out and do energetic things. Everyone's content with watching a movie or some other sit-down activity.

The following are other general suggestions for coping with chronic fatigue:

• Experiment with your activity and rest patterns and monitor your fatigue

• Avoid or modify activities that cause additional fatigue

- Conserve your energy
- Schedule activities for when you have the most energy
- Set priorities
- Minimize stressful situations as much as possible
- Rest
- Adopt good sleep habits
- Accept help when you need it
- Eat a balanced diet that is low in caffeine and junk food
- Engage in reasonable exercise approved by your healthcare provider
- Find activities to refresh your mind or distract yourself (e.g., walk, listen to music, garden, bird-watch, fish, cook, knit, paint, play with pets, watch a funny movie, get a massage)
- Practice meditation and relaxation exercises
- Focus on what you can do, not what you can't do

My daughter was a soccer player until she was diagnosed. Last weekend, watching the women's World Cup, she said she can't believe she ever could run for 90 minutes straight. She loved soccer, but cannot participate yet. Her first year in remission was most remarkable by the fatigue. It was a huge problem for her. She had to delay her entrance into college for a year to go through treatment and recovery. If it were not for the office of student disabilities at her university, she wouldn't have made it through the first year.

Good news, though, the second year went better. She is now able to rollerblade and can get up the stairs. I think she learned to budget her energy just like others budget their time. She can no longer dance all night, but she can dance and that's a good thing.

Chapter 8

Brain and Nerves

Although the world is full of suffering,
it is full also of the overcoming of it.

—Helen Keller

THE NERVOUS SYSTEM in the body has two main parts: the central nervous system and the peripheral nervous system. The central nervous system (CNS) is composed of the brain and the spinal cord. The peripheral nervous system is a network of nerves throughout the body. The CNS and peripheral nervous system work together to monitor, coordinate, and control all activities of the body. Changes in the functioning of the brain or nerves can profoundly affect both health and quality of life.

As the number of survivors who have received treatment affecting the nervous system increases, more is being learned about long-term effects on the CNS. These effects can impact survivors' education, social lives, relationships, and job performance.

This chapter discusses the treatments that can cause changes in the brain and nerves. It lists signs and symptoms, discusses how to screen for these effects, and looks at how they can be medically managed.

The brain

The brain is the body's main information processing center. This complex organ weighs approximately 3 pounds and is protected by membranes called meninges, a cushion of fluid, and the skull. The three main structural parts of the brain are the brain stem, the cerebellum, and the cerebrum. The brain stem connects the brain to the spinal cord. It coordinates most of the functions necessary for survival, such as breathing, heart rate, and sleep. The cerebellum controls muscles to allow smooth and coordinated movement. It also monitors posture and balance. The cerebrum controls all voluntary, or conscious, activities of the brain, including speech, language, hearing, memory, and learning.

Organ damage

The brain can be damaged by tumor growth or treatments such as radiation, surgery, and chemotherapy. The survivors most at risk for brain damage are children and teens treated for leukemia, brain tumors, and tumors of the head and neck such as rhabdomyosarcoma.

The tissues of the brain are very sensitive to radiation. The dose and location of radiation and the child's age, sex, and individual vulnerability all play a role in how much the radiation will affect brain function. Those at highest risk are children under the age of 2. Children under the age of 5 are at very high risk, and children ages 5 to 8 are at high risk. Girls show a greater sensitivity to radiation than do boys. However, any child whose brain is irradiated may develop long-term changes in brain function. Because the damage to healthy cells depends in part on the total dose of radiation, this discussion will first deal with children who received less than 2500 centigray (cGy) of whole brain radiation.

Radiation doses below 2500 cGy

Most children who are irradiated to avoid the spread of leukemia receive either 1800 cGy or 2400 cGy to the whole brain. Children who have stem cell transplants may also receive radiation to the brain. Depending on the year children received transplants, they most commonly received 1000 to 1200 cGy of total body irradiation (TBI), usually the smaller dose.

Children who received 1200 to 1800 cGy often develop learning difficulties that may be subtle. The changes are more pronounced in those who received 2400 cGy. Greater doses of chemotherapy into the brain from intrathecal medications or high-dose systemic methotrexate may increase the effects from the radiation. Very young children (younger than 5 and particularly those younger than 2) whose brains are growing and developing are more at risk than are older children and teens.[1,2] Changes in the ways children or teens think, remember, and learn are called cognitive late effects.

> My daughter has problems absorbing new concepts, especially math ideas. For example, we were doing multiplication—the factors of 12 (2 lots of 6, 6 lots of 2, 3 lots of 4, etc.). We used pencils for the lots and after playing with the piles of pencils for a while, I really thought she had got it. She could tell me all the factors of 12, and make the lots from the 12 pencils. Next morning I asked her, and she couldn't remember any factors of 12! Even with the pencils in front of her.

She has good and bad days. Some days it's like she is operating through a fog, everything is too difficult. She can't concentrate. She just wants to be left alone to draw pictures or whatever. Mental effort is too much.

She gets very frustrated (understandable!), and in class there just isn't the time to go over the same things day after day until she finally gets it. It is an insidious problem, because she is bright and sharp and well behaved in general, and doesn't look like she should have a learning difficulty.

Learning difficulties usually become evident gradually, beginning a year or two after radiation and continuing to evolve many years after 1800 to 2400 cGy of radiation to the brain. Typically, problems are noted in mathematics, spatial relationships, memory, problem solving, attention span, and concentration skills. These late effects can cause changes in learning style as well as social behavior. It is important that parents and educators remain vigilant for potential learning problems to allow for quick intervention.

My daughter received 1800 rads (cGy) of cranial radiation and intrathecal methotrexate when she was 17 months old. She is now 9 years old and in third grade. She has many learning challenges, including slower processing speed, attentional difficulties, and difficulty with short-term memory and multi-step processing. She benefits from additional help in school. In the past she has needed additional drilling in phonics, math fact repetition, and refocusing on multi-step directions, as well as additional time to complete testing. It is challenging for her to maintain her focus throughout the day.

After much observation, I am convinced that these kids have a quirky organizational system. My husband and I both realize that school is a struggle for her. We have sought help through the special education system, and our daughter is now classified as traumatically brain injured. Her self-esteem is high, and she is a very bright, verbal child with a lot of strengths. We are working diligently with all of her teachers and all of the resources available to ensure that she gets the best education possible.

· · · · ·

I had 2400 rads of radiation when I was 15. I don't think it changed my intellectual functioning at all. I finished high school, college, and attended graduate school. I'm now a physician's assistant.

The growth of the skull (cranium) of young children who receive 2400 cGy of cranial radiation may slow, leaving the child with a smaller head than he would otherwise have had. The areas on either side of the eyes may develop a slightly pinched look. This late effect develops in approximately 3 out of 10 children. Children who were given 1800 cGy of cranial radiation may also develop this late effect, although to a lesser degree. Children under the age of 5 when treated are most at risk.

Parents of children who had 2400 cGy of cranial radiation, and in some cases as low as 1800 cGy, sometimes report that the child's affect (i.e., emotions shown on the face) has changed. Rather than a face that reflects what she is thinking and feeling, her face appears expressionless. This can affect making and keeping friends, because facial expressions and other body language are a big part of effective communication. Other parents notice reduced curiosity and interest. Although not much research has been done on these late effects, they are included here because they occur in some survivors and can affect the way those survivors deal with the world.

I asked my son's therapist if she thought anti-depressives might help because I thought my son was depressed. The therapist evaluated him and said he wasn't depressed, but his affect was so flat it just seemed that way. She said when a person doesn't show emotions in their face or tone of voice, whoever is talking to them thinks they don't feel anything. She told me that they still feel as much, but their ways to express it have been altered.

• • • • •

I've never heard anyone talk about this, but my daughter's personality changed big time after her treatment for relapsed ALL (acute lymphoblastic leukemia) that included radiation. She was always a very exuberant and verbal child. She talked early and was just full of it. She used to laugh and joke all the time. Now she's quiet and never jokes. I don't think she understands jokes anymore due to cognitive problems from the radiation. It's very hard for me. I don't think she remembers who she used to be, but I do.

Slow processing speeds can impact overall decision making and the ability to make good judgment calls. The amount of information a survivor has available to make decisions may be lessened, because the process of considering options might be slow. Again, this is not a universal late effect, but it affects a significant percentage of survivors who received cranial radiation.[3]

My daughter is very vulnerable because she believes whatever anyone tells her. The kids with behavior problems seek her out because she will just go along with whatever mischief they dream up. Even when we discuss it later and she explains that she knows she wasn't supposed to do those things, she always says, "They really wanted me to go along, so I did." It's scary.

Children who received cranial radiation doses of 1800 or 2400 cGy are at risk for problems with hormone production, puberty, and growth. Children who were younger than age 8 when they received radiation are at highest risk. There is also a small risk that the thyroid might not produce enough thyroxin. This risk increases if spinal radiation was also received. It is important to remember that the risk continues throughout life, and in some children, the effects do not appear until a decade or two after treatment has ended. These issues are covered in depth in Chapter 9, *Hormone-Producing Glands.*

Children, especially girls, who received radiation to the brain at a young age are at risk for becoming overweight. The exact reason why some children become overweight after radiation is unclear. This is discussed in Chapter 17, *Muscles and Bones.*

A rare effect from radiation to the brain that occurs during treatment and may be progressive is leukoencephalopathy. Children who develop this disorder may have lasting problems with balance (ataxia), difficulty swallowing (dysphagia), or speech problems (dysarthria). Other symptoms are seizures, blindness, and coma. Leukoencephalopathy usually occurs in children or teens who relapsed and received cranial radiation plus high total doses of intravenous and/or intrathecal methotrexate.

Radiation doses above 2500 cGy

In the past, many children or teens with brain tumors received 3500 cGy to the whole brain, with a boost of up to 5540 cGy to the tumor bed (i.e., the place where the tumor originated). Others received high-dose radiation only to the tumor itself. Currently, lower doses of radiation are used. Specific disabilities may partly depend on which area of the brain received the highest dose of radiation. However, in general, the higher the dose and the younger the age, the more dramatic the effect on brain functioning.

Higher doses of radiation cause slower brain processing speeds and greater drops in IQ scores. The location of the tumor also influences the type and severity of learning disabilities that may develop. For example, children with temporal lobe tumors may have problems with memory. Learning may also be affected by medications used to treat seizures, or by surgical complications, hydrocephalus, vision problems, and hearing loss.

I'm 28 and was diagnosed with an astrocytoma when I was 15. This brain tumor was surgically removed, and I had radiation treatments for several months to follow. Some of the details are a little fuzzy still. I graduated high school with my class and enrolled in college. I started as a theater/dance major but was unable physically and mentally to keep up with the pace. So I changed my major to science. I graduated in 1994, and you couldn't get me out of there fast enough! I was experiencing what I now know to be long-term effects. It was very hard keeping up in class. I wasn't aware until after the fact that I had real symptoms and that there were laws to protect me. I just thought I wasn't smart enough to excel.

Children or teens with brain tumors who get very high-dose radiation to the brain can have multiple and life-altering late effects. Brain tumor survivors can develop seizure disorders, gait and balance problems, hand/eye coordination problems, personality changes, and learning disabilities. Radiation to the pituitary and hypothalamus can cause problems with growth, puberty, and fertility (see Chapter 9, *Hormone-Producing Glands*). Vision problems, cataracts, and diminished hearing can also develop after radiation (see Chapter 10, *Eyes and Ears*). All of the above late effects from high doses of radiation to the brain can range from mild to severe.

I'm 22 now and had an astrocytoma when I was 10. I had surgery, chemotherapy, and radiation to my head and spine. They ended up removing some of my vertebrae because I had so much tension from scoliosis and kyphosis. I get around in a wheelchair now. The radiation affected my ovaries and I'll never be able to have kids. I'm also pretty short (4'6") and skinny, but I try to eat nutritious food. I go to a healing center and exercise to try to keep a strong upper body. One of my legs is pretty bent, so the massage therapist works on that.

With the use of proton beam radiation, there is hope that the risks to healthy brain tissue will be minimized.

Chemotherapy

Chemotherapy used to treat leukemia and some sarcomas can also cause learning disabilities that are sometimes subtle. Intrathecal methotrexate and high-dose methotrexate with leucovorin rescue can cause learning disabilities, though usually much milder than those caused by radiation.[4] Therapy for acute lymphoblastic leukemia sometimes includes triple intrathecals (methotrexate, hydrocortisone, and ARA-C) and has been associated with learning disabilities similar to those seen with lower doses of radiation. Very young children (younger than age 5 and particularly younger than 2) whose brains are growing and developing are more at risk from chemotherapy to the brain than are older children and teens.

> My son was on a high-dose methotrexate protocol and developed learning disabilities. He was having problems with concentration, organization, and mathematics. At that time, medical personnel were not aware of the potential for learning problems as a result of treatment. He really didn't get any help until high school when the learning specialist on the staff tested him. She decided to treat him like a head injury patient. She taught him to concentrate for longer periods of time. His schedule was redesigned so that it was in 15-minute blocks. She taught him numerous tricks like word associations to improve his short-term memory. She was the first person who really got through to him, even though he has had tutors before. She was the first to say, "Yes, you have a problem, and this is what I can do to help." It worked. He graduated from a well-known university and is doing well in the investment field.

• • • • •

> My son was on a high-dose methotrexate protocol from age 3 to 6. He entered preschool while on therapy, and we enrolled him in a private kindergarten because of the small class size. He transitioned to public school in second grade with no problems. He is now 18, an A student who excels in math. He has had no after effects from his years of treatment.

Surgery

Surgery to the brain can cause a host of late effects. The body system and amount of damage depend on the part of the brain that was operated on, the amount of healthy tissue that was removed, and complications after surgery.

> My daughter Sarah had two surgeries to the posterior fossa near the brain stem. All side effects from the first surgery resolved. But after the second she had balance and vision problems and she also lost the ability to write with her right hand. She learned to write with her left hand, but her printing in earlier years was beautiful and the messy printing really bothered her. Being left-handed caused some output problems at school because she just wasn't as quick as before.

As with all the late effects described in this book, these cognitive late effects are not all-or-nothing phenomena. You may have none of these late effects, a few, or many. These lists of possible problems are not meant to fit you into a category, but rather to cover all of the possibilities so that problems, if they develop, can be identified and treated early to give the best possible outcomes.

Signs and symptoms

Brain damage from cranial radiation was first recognized in the late 1970s because survivors were having difficulty in school. Some young survivors were easily distracted and had trouble learning. This spawned many studies of neurocognitive changes from treatment.

Signs and symptoms of damage from radiation and/or chemotherapy include problems with the following:

- Handwriting

- Spelling

- Reading or reading comprehension

- Understanding math concepts, remembering math facts, comprehending math symbols, sequencing, and working with columns and graphs

- Remembering and copying shapes

- Using calculators or computers

- Learning to ride a bike or tie shoes

- Auditory or visual language processing: trouble with vocabulary, blending sounds, and syntax

- Attention deficits: becoming either inattentive, hyperactive, or both

- Short-term memory and information retrieval

- Social maturity and social skills

> I had cranial radiation when I was a child and have some problems remembering things. Occasionally I have trouble figuring out in a conversation what point the speaker is trying to make. But I'm an adult now and feel very socially competent. I've discovered who I am. So I don't take these little glitches too personally.

- Understanding facial expressions or gestures

- Understanding deceit, cunning, or manipulation

- Planning and organizational skills

- Showing emotions on the face

Cognitive problems usually develop within a year or two of radiation and progress over time. So if your child used to color within the lines and draw proportional figures but gradually loses these abilities, the radiation and/or chemotherapy are probably the culprits. The effect on individual children is quite variable. Some children have no late effects, some develop very subtle disabilities, and others develop life-altering problems.

> My daughter had 1800 cGy of radiation when she was 3 years old. During preschool and kindergarten, she had the most beautiful handwriting. She was also a great artist and could draw using perspective at an early age. By the time she was 7, however, her handwriting started to deteriorate and she had trouble writing in a straight line—her sentences tending to slope up. She reverted to drawing stick figures. She started pressing really hard on the paper when drawing or writing, and the process became very laborious. She now mostly uses a word processor for writing projects, and we are negotiating with the school for her to use a laptop (they call it assistive technology) in school. She has problems with math and has social difficulties because she can't really follow conversations well. Her neuropsychological scores range from the 5th to the 95th percentile.

• • • • •

> My daughter had 1800 rads of cranial radiation when she was almost 5 years old. The possible side effects listed on the consent form included a drop in IQ. We were concerned, but our doctor said, "There are no options now; if the late effects develop, you'll deal with them then." Three years later, she was tested for the gifted and talented program in our school district. I bawled when the letter came in asking for permission to place her in the gifted school. Clutching the letter in my hand, I drove to the clinic to hug the doctor one more time.

You should suspect learning difficulties if any of the following learning changes occur:

- Your child was an A student prior to cancer, and she is now working just as hard and getting Cs.

- Your child takes 3 hours to do homework that used to take 1 hour.

- Your child reads a story and then has trouble explaining the plot.

- Your child frequently comes home frustrated from school, saying he just doesn't understand things as well as the other kids.

- Your child's teacher complains that she "just doesn't pay attention" or "just needs to work harder."

- Your child says he doesn't like school.

If any of the above situations are occurring, take action to begin the evaluation process before your child's self-esteem plummets. It is often hard to take this first step because some children affected by radiation and/or chemotherapy can often reason well and think clearly and may be above average academically in several areas. They may fall behind their classmates, however, on tasks that require fast processing skills, short-term memory, sequential operations, and organizational ability (especially visual). Once identified, these differences can be addressed in school through extra help with memory enhancement, eliminating timed tests, improving organizational skills, and providing extra help in mathematics, spelling, reading, writing, and speech. Early intervention can make a huge difference.

When my daughter stopped reading aloud in second grade, we thought it was because her younger sister had surpassed her in reading ability. But the neuropsychologist told us that it was because she couldn't hold that many balls in the air at once. Reading aloud requires juggling several skills at the same time: read the words, hold them in your brain, form the words, use your mouth. She couldn't do that many things simultaneously. However, silently, she can read and comprehend at the fifth grade level. When we got the report back, I showed her and told her it was really good news. She said, "Why?" And I said, "Because you don't have to read aloud. The majority of the time, adults read silently, and you're great at that. So just forget reading aloud. You don't have to do it anymore." She got a big smile on her face.

• • • • •

I was diagnosed with leukemia in 1976 when I was 5 years old. I had 2400 rads of cranial radiation and while still in grade school was told I had a perceptually impaired learning disability. I had difficulty copying from the board. I have trouble following a line straight across and then going to the next line down. When I read, I use a piece of paper under each line, then move to the next. On the board, it just all got jumbled up in my mind.

These things were a big problem in grade school, but less and less as I continued my education. I now have a master's degree in social work. It was a big help learning about my legal rights. I took my SATs timed and only completed half of the items. When I took the GREs (tests to enter graduate school) untimed, it was so much better. They allotted me 4 hours, and I only took 3. I was relaxed, not worried about the time, and thus able to concentrate more. I did quite well. I am still a poor speller, but that's what spell check is for! I also get words mixed up, for instance, recently I wrote "not for prophet" instead of "not for profit."

It is also important to remember that higher cognitive functioning often remains intact; it is just getting the information in ("processing") that is impaired. Children who were gifted usually remain so; children with average abilities retain them. Their performance may be slower; they may require extra instruction in memory enhancement and organizational skills, but they can still achieve to their potential. There are thousands of survivors in their late teens and 20s who are successfully attending high school or college, or are pursuing professional careers.

> For me, the most difficult part of each semester of graduate school has been exam time. The normal stresses of the competitive academic program are compounded by my feelings of being different and even some ostracism for getting certain testing accommodations that aren't available to other students. A few students have thought that I get an unfair advantage or even questioned my acceptance into the program if I can't keep up with the rigors of time-pressured tests and crowded testing environments. At times, all my emotions about having cancer resurface when I have had to talk about my learning disability with other students. I have opted to take advantage of confidential services as much as possible; however, some students notice that I'm not in the same exam room with them. I feel like I have lost some friends after telling them about my learning disability, yet those difficult experiences make me truly grateful for the friends who have understood.

Addressing these issues with the schools can be tough because these disabilities are very different from those the schools are most familiar with. It usually takes a lot of time and effort to get the best and most appropriate education for survivors with cognitive problems. Older survivors need to learn how to advocate for themselves when they go to college or enter the workforce. These issues are covered in detail in Chapter 4, *Navigating the System*.

> My Katie (then 2½) received radiation two times a day for 3 days in 1993 prior to a bone marrow transplant for juvenile chronic myelogenous leukemia. My husband and I were told that as a result, Katie would be sterile, be forever at risk for secondary cancers, lose some IQ, develop cataracts, not reach her original expected height, and have a whole host of shorter-term problems.

> I remember sitting in the waiting room thinking, they're zapping away my baby's babies. They're zapping away her laughter, her insight, her joy, her very being.

> That was 6 years ago, and today Katie is alive and my joy. What did the radiation do, at least what I can tell right now? She has problems with

reading and with math. She sometimes has problems making logical jumps from one thought to another. For reading and math, we work with the school and have her on an intensive program. So far, she is reading at grade level and is slightly below grade level for math.

She is shorter than her classmates and has had the cataract in her right eye removed. We live with these late effects, and to tell you the truth, they're not all that bad. At least we knew about them, were prepared, and knew how to approach the school system. I really feel for parents of learning-disabled children who struggle for years before they find there is help available.

But all this long gobbledygook aside, I want to let you know what radiation didn't do. It didn't take the soul and spirit of my child. She is a lovely, lively, happy child. I don't know if she'll ever work in a research lab, but she certainly has all the expectations for a full life just like the majority of her peers. She tells me she wants to be a vet who specializes in horses. I have no reason to think that can't happen. She is inquisitive, humorous, affectionate, and very social. I think she'll make a great vet. She might need some extra help in chemistry classes, but heck, so did I.

Additional signs and symptoms associated with radiation to the brain (for brain tumors, relapsed leukemia, or bone marrow transplant following relapse) are:

• Problems with balance and coordination.

> *The damage from Matt's brain tumor affected his balance, coordination, and walking. By the time he was 3, he had outgrown the double stroller we used to tote him and all of his medical gear in. We went right to a pediatric wheelchair, even though he is a part-time user. It is great for festivals, a walk outside when the neighborhood kids want to push, travel by bus to/from school, etc. I can't even tell you how the steering and maneuvering compares to a stroller! He uses his walker or a forearm cane for short distance walking. We do use a wagon outdoors under direct supervision, which he loves, and an occasional push on a trike. We're trying to find a tricycle that he can pedal.*

• Impaired growth.

• Altered fertility with higher doses of radiation.

• Early or delayed puberty.

• Problems making and keeping friends.

• Second cancers.

My son is 8 years old and has been a medulloblastoma survivor for half his life. He has many late effects from the chemo, radiation, and surgery: hearing aids, glasses, Pullups® at night, inability to walk alone, very poor balance, and slow speech. He lost all abilities after surgery. He was unable to walk, move purposefully, or eat for several months. He is working hard and making slow but steady progress. He told me one day that he just wanted to run like the other kids. I get teary-eyed hearing that. I am so very grateful for the technology that has saved his life, but he doesn't understand what happened. I remember a lot of events and dates now as "before the tumor" or "after the tumor." He is such a trouper, though. He does not see himself as handicapped. He is usually a happy guy, always cracking a joke, and seldom complains.

Children who had radiation to the head may also experience permanent hair loss or thinning hair, dental problems, hearing loss, and cataracts. These late effects and the ones listed above are covered in other chapters in this book.

I had neuroblastoma when I was 9 months old and leukemia when I was 3 years old, more than 30 years ago. I've had surgery, radiation to the flank and cranium (I don't know the doses), and chemotherapy. I'm more than a foot shorter than my brothers, have had glasses since I was 3, have cataracts in both eyes, and am infertile. My hair is thin all over my head and my muscle tone is weak. My baby molars didn't fall out until I was 30. I've paid a big price for my survival, but I've also had a pretty good life. My emotional well-being is good, and I've achieved many of my goals.

Seizure disorders are another lasting effect that can develop in the brain after surgery, radiation, or chemotherapy. They occur most commonly during treatment, although they sometimes begin many years after therapy. Seizures are caused by electrical disruptions in the brain. There are many types, ranging from mild partial seizures, in which the child does not lose consciousness, to generalized seizures involving convulsions and loss of consciousness. Signs and symptoms of seizures include the following:

- Staring into space
- Not hearing people talking
- Glassy eyes
- Auras (i.e., an abnormal smell, taste, abdominal sensation, or emotion that precedes a seizure)
- Stiff body
- Smacking lips and mumbled words

- Convulsions

- Jerking or twitching in parts of the body

Ways to screen for and treat all of the above late effects are covered in the next part of this chapter.

Screening and detection

Any child at risk for cognitive problems should have neuropsychological testing done as soon as possible after diagnosis. This can happen after treatment starts, when the child starts feeling better, or after treatment ends. The first test is called a baseline.

Neuropsychological tests are done by Ph.D. psychologists who specialize in evaluating how children learn and think. These tests usually take 4 to 6 hours, and may be done over 2 days for younger children or those who are easily fatigued. All of that time is spent with the child, and the parents are interviewed separately. The psychologist gives a series of general tests appropriate for the child's age level, and then another series of more and more specific subtests based on the results of the general ones. Pediatric psychologists usually make the testing fun for children, and children need to know this ahead of time so they don't worry.

The baseline testing is used as a yardstick to measure future changes in brain functioning. Many institutions do baseline tests, then repeat them every 2 to 3 years until adulthood. Parents and older survivors use the information from these tests to advocate for the most appropriate education. Getting and paying for neuropsychological tests and advocating for the best education are covered in Chapter 4, *Navigating the System*.

> *I was treated in the 1970s and had cranial radiation and lots of intrathecal methotrexate. I have difficulty remembering how to spell, and there is a lot of information I simply don't seem to be able to retain, like addition and multiplication facts. I also have some other memory problems like forgetting directions to familiar places. I forget what exit to take and frequently get lost. I keep notes in my glove box with written directions to help me find my way around. I didn't initially realize it was treatment-related until another survivor friend and I were driving around one day. She had 2400 rads of cranial radiation when she was 2. And she was making the same mistakes navigating as I do. And she got just as stressed about it. She and I are a bad combination in a car!*

Survivors at risk for long-term effects from treatment to the brain need extensive, periodic evaluations throughout their lives. These should include an educational analysis every year while in school, yearly dental exams, yearly evaluations of puberty and growth, yearly eye and hearing examinations, education about second cancers, and a discussion about any problems that have developed. See the tables at the end of Chapter 6, *Diseases*, for lists of recommended follow-up tests based on specific treatments.

Our son, now age 10½, was recently diagnosed with what is called a nonverbal learning disability. It is amazing since he is the best speller, best reader, and best at math in his class. We found out because we are in a long-term effects study at Stanford. He went through a week of tests and when we had the conference, I was shocked by their findings because he has always done so well in school. He is even in the gifted program.

His particular condition will usually show up in junior high or high school when they do more conceptual thinking. After speaking to the bone marrow transplant (BMT) department last week, they confirmed that this is a common side effect of all of the spinal chemo he had (he relapsed in his CNS twice) and the radiation related to the BMT. The psychiatrists were very supportive and gave lots of information for the school district and teachers. It was still a shock.

Medical management

Because treatment that affects the brain can cause a wide constellation of medical late effects, medical management includes a thorough evaluation and referral to appropriate specialists. An important component of medical management is a clear discussion of the risks for specific late effects to the brain and nerves. These should occur at each follow-up visit, as some of the late effects do not arise until years after treatment and are, in some cases, progressive.

My daughter Melissa was diagnosed with low-risk ALL when she was 3 years old. She relapsed in the CNS 18 months into treatment. She was then given 2400 rads (cGy) of cranial radiation as well as spinal radiation. Her CNS problems really started when she had a seizure that lasted 90 minutes. We have used every seizure drug available, with limited success. They are partial complex with some generalization. She tends to get them at night when she's tired. We need to see the neurologist frequently.

Medical care should include referrals not only to medical specialists, but also to professionals who can help address any psychological, social, or educational issues that arise. Many institutions have educational liaisons who help parents and survivors understand the laws governing appropriate education. Sometimes these specialists travel to the school to attend

Individualized Education Program (IEP) meetings. Some institutions have transition specialists who work with survivors as they shift from pediatric medical care to adult care. These specialists can also help survivors with educational and vocational planning.

In the early 1970s, at age 3, I had 2400 rads of cranial radiation. I always had to struggle and work harder in school than anyone else to get good grades. When I took the LSATs to get into law school, I was very disappointed in my performance. I went back to the hospital where I was treated and was stunned to discover that my learning difficulties were caused by my treatment for leukemia. I had my first educational assessment and it showed strong aptitudes in vocabulary, comprehension, and verbal reasoning. But I had poor short-term sequential memory and processing speeds. I hired an educational consultant, worked on my areas of weakness, and applied to take the LSATs under untimed conditions. My scores were much improved, and I will graduate from law school this year.

Recent research has examined the role of cognitive remediation in helping survivors overcome learning problems caused by treatment. This therapy teaches methods to improve memory, attention, and math skills. Children learn strategies that help them keep on task and lessen attention drift. They also learn ways to organize both their thoughts and work habits and practice ways to retain information.

Although children and teens may develop attention problems after treatment, these are not the type usually diagnosed as attention deficit hyperactivity disorder (ADHD). Some researchers, however, are using medications effective for that disorder to treat survivors with attention problems, and these children are showing improved attentional skills. Parents and medical professionals need to do a careful risk/benefit analysis for each child to determine if using these medications is appropriate.

Medical management of seizure disorders starts with a thorough evaluation from a pediatric or adult neurologist. Many medications are available to treat seizure disorders, and sometimes the survivor will need trials with different drugs to find out which ones control the seizures the best with the least number of side effects. Parents should ask the treating physician about added effects from these medications on the child's already impaired thought processes.

If these methods do not help and the seizures interfere with daily life, surgery may be recommended. An excellent resource for understanding seizures and treatment options is *Seizures and Epilepsy in Childhood: A Guide for Parents, Third Edition*, by John Freeman, M.D.; Eileen Vining, M.D.; and Diana Pillas.

> *My son has partial complex seizures. At the beginning, he had occasional staring spells. We then witnessed a big seizure, and he was immediately put on the first of many medications. We have tried every medicine known to man as single therapy. Last year we tried double therapy, but it didn't eliminate the seizures. Depending on which medication he is on, the seizures have been shorter or longer, milder or more frequent, but never eliminated. The emotional behavior side effects from the drugs have been hard to cope with. He gets very argumentative and has trouble controlling his impulses. Most seizure meds also make him sleepy, which causes more problems with school. He was on a continuous EEG (electroencephalography) for several days at a hospital to evaluate whether he was a candidate for surgery, and he was not.*

Some clinics have support groups for long-term survivors where they can share experiences with their peers. Some follow-up clinics link survivors going off to college or into the workplace with mentors who are several years ahead of them in the process. Mentors can provide a lifeline of advice, support, and friendship. Medical management should address all aspects of life: social, educational, vocational, and medical.

Because no one can know it all, survivors, their families, and their physicians must become lifelong learners about the newest research and treatments. Although this is a challenge, it also provides hope that some late effects that cannot be treated today may be able to be addressed in the future.

Nerves

Peripheral nerves gather information and send it to the spinal cord and brain. The central nervous system (CNS) processes the information and sends instructions to the body. For instance, if you touch a hot stove, a sensory receptor in your hand senses the heat and a nerve carries that information to the CNS. The CNS then sends instructions through nerves to the muscles of your arm and hand to pull your finger away from the stove.

The CNS receives billions of signals about conditions inside and outside the body and sends responses that allow coordinated and smooth functioning of all body parts and organs. Damage to nerves from radiation or surgery can disrupt or block these signals.

Organ damage

Children are remarkably resilient, and after treatment for cancer ends, many resume normal activities at age-appropriate levels. But there are some children, particularly those who received cranial radiation, who have chronic problems with strength and coordination. Others who had chemotherapy or radiation have persistent problems with sensation or motion. This section covers damage to the nerves themselves.

> I had astrocytoma and had lots of radiation, surgery, and chemo. I also had a spinal hemorrhage. I got kyphosis afterwards and when they operated on that they had to take out part of my spine. The bones were very brittle and they did a spinal fusion. I am now in a wheelchair. I can feel my lower body, but I can't walk.

Chemotherapy, particularly vincristine, often causes acute peripheral neuropathies. Usually these are characterized by foot drop (when the front of the foot does not lift while walking), problems with balance, winging out of lower legs when running, and poor coordination. For some survivors, these symptoms persist for months or years. Survivors have noted changes in both muscle strength and sensation.

> I was treated for ALL 25 years ago. I got a lot of peripheral neuropathy on treatment. The sensation in my feet and my muscle coordination are still off. I was never as athletic after treatment as I was before.
>
> • • • • •
>
> Judd finished his treatment at age 6 and had some muscular weakness. He tried organized sports, but preferred individual sports like skiing. Over several years, he gradually regained his strength and coordination so that his athletic ability is average.
>
> • • • • •
>
> My daughter was off the scale on her reactions to vincristine. During the first part of her treatment for high-risk leukemia, she couldn't walk, lift her head, even open her eyes. It has been 7 years, and despite lots of therapy, she still walks flat-footed, has generalized weakness, and is a couple of years behind her peers in gross motor functions.
>
> • • • • •
>
> The massive doses of vincristine used to treat my son's rhabdomyosarcoma exacerbated what were already existing sensory integration issues and motor problems. At diagnosis (age almost 5), he was not drawing recognizable pictures yet or able to write his name legibly, much less tie shoes or do other more complex activities with small motor skills. He

was lagging in gross motor skills as well, but definitely dropped back a lot in balance and coordination during chemo, experiencing substantial foot, ankle, and wrist weakness and neuropathy in the hands and feet. He started kindergarten at age 5, unable to handle a pencil, unzip his lunchbox, zip his coat, or get safely up and down the stairs to his classroom by himself. It took fighting tooth and nail to get him in-school occupational therapy and physical therapy services because he was reading at the fifth-grade level and therefore not "learning disabled."

At 8 he still has foot-slapping and is having major problems in motor planning. We wonder if the extreme muscle weakness/poor muscle tone is just from the chemo exposure or would he have been where he is now anyway? Our guess, of course, is that the chemo had an additive effect on an existing problem. We find our oncologist is a little defensive on the subject (I guess doctors have some guilt about what treatments do to kids, too), so we don't discuss the motor and muscular issues up in clinic. It's hard—of course we know there was no way to avoid the chemo, but that doesn't alter what we're dealing with here and now. We wish they would share more hard information with us on the length and severity of these late effects and just what areas they are actually known to affect, so we'd have known what to be looking for a long time ago.

Children who relapse and have higher total doses of chemotherapy are much more at risk for persistent nerve problems than children or teens who are treated once and cured.

My son was treated for leukemia and relapsed twice, then had a bone marrow transplant. He's had cranial radiation, spinal radiation, lots of vincristine, and lots of intrathecal methotrexate. He has partial nerve damage to the muscles running down his legs, and also in his feet. The doctors do not feel this will improve. His only recourse at this time is major physical activity, gaining strength in muscles that he can. This would include weight lifting machines and long distance running. We have not started this yet. He is not too thrilled about it, and he is old enough to make up his own mind. He is very much a team player, and does not enjoy solitary activity, so I would need to get a personal trainer for him.

· · · · ·

My 7-year-old daughter was born with neuroblastoma, relapsed at 3 months, then developed a brain tumor at age 5. She has neurofibromatosis so she's at risk for multiple tumors. She's had over 5 years of chemotherapy, including lots of vincristine. She had massive acute neuropathies, but the long-term effect is paralyzed tendons in her left ankle. I wanted to make sure it was neuropathy and not some other treatable problem, so

I took her to an ankle and foot orthopedic specialist in Manhattan for a second opinion. He gave her a very thorough exam and said it was a very localized neuropathy that affects two tendons in one ankle. It causes her to walk on the outside of her foot and makes her unstable. She now wears a brace that helps her foot align properly.

• • • • •

The nerve damage isn't clear-cut. Tim had severe foot drop from the vincristine while on the relapse therapy. He had some foot drop on regular therapy, but not bad and it did resolve. During relapse, he was also very weak and in bed most of the time. After Tim's treatment ended, the heel cord stayed tight. We were told it was probably a combination of nerve damage from the vincristine and a lack of exercise and having his feet in a prone position for so long. He got braces and wore them whenever he was at school. He also walked a lot more. We hoped that would be enough to straighten/ lengthen it again. Unfortunately, his feet collapsed more and more. The braces were always rubbing and uncomfortable because of the position of the foot.

This past spring, we saw an orthopedic doctor. He determined that the braces would not work without further intervention first. We had the choice of surgery to lengthen the heel cords, or a series of casts. We decided on the surgery. His feet are in much better position now, but still not "normal." The left foot, especially, will only go so far. He will likely need a brace on the left foot permanently, and at least a shoe orthotic on the right.

Surgery anywhere in the body can cut nerves and thus affect function or sensation. For example, both spinal cord and urinary tract surgeries can leave the survivor incontinent (i.e., unable to control urination or bowel movements). Survivors of limb-salvage surgery sometimes have areas in the limb that have no sensation to touch.

Pressure on nerves from a prosthesis, wheelchair, or crutches can also affect nerve functioning.

One big problem with late effects is that sometimes it's hard to know what's caused by cancer and what's not. For instance, I've used crutches for 25 years. The doctors told me that this might affect the nerves in my hands and arms. And I have noticed less sensation in my hands. My fingers are just not as sensitive as they used to be. But it's been 21 years, so maybe it's because I'm getting older. I don't know if this is natural because I have nothing to compare it to.

Survivors of Hodgkin lymphoma (formerly called Hodgkin's disease) treated on older protocols, including high-dose radiation, can experience neuropathies that affect sensation and function. The neuropathies can also result from vincristine in the combination drug therapy called MOPP and from vinblastine in ABVD, another combination of medicines. They occur during treatment and may subside with time or persist.

I had 4500 rads of mantle radiation 30 years ago. I don't have any pain in my legs from the neuropathy. I do have pain in the middle and lower back on my left side, which is probably where the nerves are being affected. Besides loss of strength in my thighs and hips, the upper legs feel like wood. Not really numb, just kind of heavy and stiff. I have a small foot drop but do not need a brace yet. I've fallen only a couple of times—don't know how many falls it will take before I look for some kind of aid.

What I struggle with mostly is how much energy it consumes to move around. Walking is no longer an automatic, unconscious process. I have to stay aware of where I'm walking—a simple sidestep or bump from my dogs and I lose it. My right leg over-extends as a way of compensating and that makes my stability worse. So I'm always reminding myself to flex that right knee. It just takes a lot of energy to move about and it's pretty clumsy at best.

My neurologist has told me there is no treatment—just perhaps braces, walkers, wheelchairs, etc., to help adapt to the limitations, but no magic pill or therapy that will reverse it. I'm grateful that there isn't much pain associated with it so far—have enough of that to deal with in my neck and shoulders right now from the fibrosis and atrophy. When my hubby massages my back, I also find that my walking is easier for a short while. Maybe getting the muscles softer and circulation improved allows more nerve conduction. Don't know. I do grieve the loss of my leg functions. It's just a sadness, no anger.

• • • • •

I had lots of problems when I was on ABVD. It just freaked me out. It was like my legs were asleep from the hips down, and it hurt very, very badly. I couldn't stand up for longer than 10 minutes at a time. It was one of the creepiest side effects. Now I have late problems as well— peripheral neuropathy of unknown origin, but obviously possibly related to treatment—and am on chronic medication to manage the excruciating foot pain that it causes. Fortunately, my doctor worked out a winning combination with me and has been great about helping me cope with it.

I was diagnosed with neuroblastoma when I was 5 months old. I had 3 years of chemotherapy, including vincristine. I have no late effects to my nerves at all.

I had 7 weeks of radiation to treat Hodgkin's in the early 80s. I developed permanent neuropathy in my fingertips. It freaked me out because I was a clarinetist. At first it felt tingly. Now if I rub my fingertips it just feels dead. It's a nasty side effect, but the best side effect is my survival.

Rarely, survivors report numbness, tingling, and electrical sensations in their arms and/or legs, which worsen when bending or twisting the head or neck. These sensations usually occur within months of high-dose radiation that includes the spinal cord, but can appear years afterwards. These symptoms usually resolve on their own within months.

A very rare late effect after radiation to the brain and intrathecal chemotherapy is atrophy or death of the optic nerve, which can cause blindness. Another very rare complication of radiation to the head and neck is vocal cord palsy.

Pressure from tumors directly on nerves can also affect motion and function.

My daughter Terri was diagnosed with an astrocytoma in her spinal cord 5 years ago. The pressure from the tumor has damaged nerves and her left arm hangs by her side most of the time. The left arm sits most comfortably when twisted with the palm facing backward. Her left arm is shorter and smaller than the right and I don't think it is growing very much at all. There is no expectation that she will ever get movement back again. In 1994, Terri's left shoulder began twitching. This was diagnosed as spinal myoclonus and may be due to either scoliosis or the tumor itself. The shoulder continuously twitches every 3 seconds. Despite this, Terri is very happy and healthy and enjoys school.

Signs and symptoms

Signs and symptoms of nerve damage include the following:

- Twitching face
- Decreased strength in hands and feet
- Poor coordination
- Pain

- Dulled or absent sensation
- Paralysis
- Decreased vision
- Changes in the voice

> We had Justin tested through the school district, and the district is giving him his physical therapy. He's weak in the hips and walks with his feet turned out. He's resistant to taking physical risks; for instance, he sits down and slides off things rather than jumping off. He just loves to go to physical therapy.

• • • • •

> My son had a brain tumor and developed posterior fossa syndrome afterwards. He couldn't speak or swallow and lost control of many of his bodily functions (he was back in diapers). The left side of his face is paralyzed and his left eye turns in. That eye also doesn't close all of the way, so we use Lacri-Lube® at night and eye drops during the day. When he smiles, the left side of this face stays the same, but the right side of his face smiles.

Screening and detection

A thorough follow-up visit should include a full neurological examination and a discussion about physical activities. Any indication that there may be damage to the nerves should result in a referral to a neurologist for further testing. Vision changes should be evaluated by an ophthalmologist.

> When I brought my daughter to the endocrinologist 3 years after her treatment for leukemia ended, he asked her to hop up on the table and she couldn't. He looked at me and said, "Get this child into physical therapy. She should be able to do that easily." She's had physical and occupational therapy for 4 years now, and is much improved. Her legs remain straight rather than flailing around when she runs and her balance is much improved. She is still about 2 years behind her peers in gross motor function, though, and I don't know if she'll ever really catch up.

Medical management

Survivors with nerve damage from treatment may benefit from a referral to physical therapy for help with coordination and strength problems. Occupational therapy (OT) is often helpful if hand/eye coordination and visual-spatial problems persist after treatment.

My son's leukemia relapsed twice and he had a bone marrow transplant. The vincristine did a number on his hands/arms. His muscle damage is very obvious in his hands. He cannot hold a pencil well, even to this day. His handwriting is terrible. He still has pains running up his arms if he has to write very much, and his hands fall asleep and he has to shake them out. Shooting a basketball is almost impossible. To gain the power to shoot, he throws way offside, causing him to fall. His general weakness in his arms is permanent, but we hope, with weight training, there might be some improvement. He has compensated by becoming very keyboard-oriented. He does all of his school work on the computer, which was recommended by the neuropsych department.

• • • • •

OT was very helpful for Gina. She began it at the hospital and continued when she entered school. She had OT for 5 years or so. The therapist helped her learn to write, and OT improved her spatial awareness and hand/eye coordination (piano lessons helped with this too). She still cannot snap her fingers, but this year at camp she climbed to the top of the climbing tower (quite a feat for anyone), and when she went to YMCA® camp last week she was thrilled to complete the high ropes course.

I don't believe she would be where she is today without OT. Intervention is necessary and important, and the earlier the better.

Chapter 9
Hormone-Producing Glands

The future enters into us, in order to transform
itself in us, long before it happens.

— Rainer-Maria Rilke
Letters to a Young Poet

SOME GLANDS PRODUCE SUBSTANCES called hormones, a term derived from the Greek word *hormaein*, which means "to excite." Hormones are released in tiny amounts, but they travel throughout the body to orchestrate complicated processes such as growth, puberty, reaction to stress, temperature regulation, and urine output. Disruptions in the balance of these chemical messengers can profoundly affect both health and quality of life. All of the hormone-producing glands working together make up the body's endocrine system.

The glands discussed in this chapter—hypothalamus, pituitary, thyroid, testes, ovaries, and adrenal—can be affected by treatment for childhood cancer. Other glands—parathyroid, pancreas, and pineal—are not discussed, as their functions usually remain untouched by treatment.

Hypothalamic-pituitary axis

The hypothalamus and the pituitary gland are located deep in the brain and are connected by a stalk. The hypothalamus and pituitary work together to control all the other glands in the endocrine system. The hypothalamus—often called the master gland—produces substances that instruct the pituitary to release or stop releasing hormones.

Before describing the effects of treatment on the hypothalamus and the pituitary, it is helpful to understand what substances each organ produces and their function in the body. The following chart outlines this information:

Hypothalamus Hormone	Pituitary Hormone	Function
Thyrotropin-releasing hormone (TRH)	Thyroid-stimulating hormone (TSH, also called thyrotropin)	Stimulates thyroid growth and secretion
Growth hormone-releasing hormone (GHRH)	Growth hormone (GH)	Increases body growth, muscle strength, energy, cognitive development
Gonadotropin-releasing hormone (GnRH)	Follicle-stimulating hormone (FSH)	Females: stimulates growth of ovarian follicles and female hormones Males: stimulates sperm production
Gonadotropin-releasing hormone (GnRH)	Luteinizing hormone (LH)	Females: stimulates ovulation and female hormones Males: stimulates testosterone production
Corticotropin-releasing hormone (CRH)	Adrenocorticotrophic hormone (ACTH)	Stimulates adrenal growth and secretions that help the body respond to emotions (especially stress)
None	Antidiuretic hormone (ADH or vasopressin)	Reduces the volume of urine
Prolactin-releasing factor Prolactin release-inhibiting factor	Prolactin	Regulates breast development and milk production in females

The hypothalamus-pituitary axis (HPA) works somewhat like a thermostat. It is programmed to secrete specific hormones under certain conditions and continues to do so until receiving a message to shut off secretions. For example, assume that the thermostat in your home is set at 70°. When the room temperature drops below 70°, the thermostat turns on the heater. The heater will continue to run until the room reaches a preset value within the thermostat (for example, 73°), and then the thermostat turns off the heater.

An example of this feedback loop system in the body is when puberty begins. When it's time for a girl to begin developing, the hypothalamus releases GnRH (gonadotropin-releasing hormone), which stimulates the pituitary to release FSH (follicle-stimulating hormone) and LH (luteinizing hormone). These hormones start the development of the ovaries. When the ovaries begin to mature and release hormones (estrogen and progesterone), the loop is complete and puberty proceeds normally. If, however, the prepubescent girl had high-dose abdominal radiation, the LH and FSH are released, but the damaged ovaries do not respond. The HPA keeps pouring out LH and FSH to start puberty, but the loop is never connected and the system never turns on. In this scenario, the girl would have high FSH and LH, but no estrogen. She would not begin puberty.

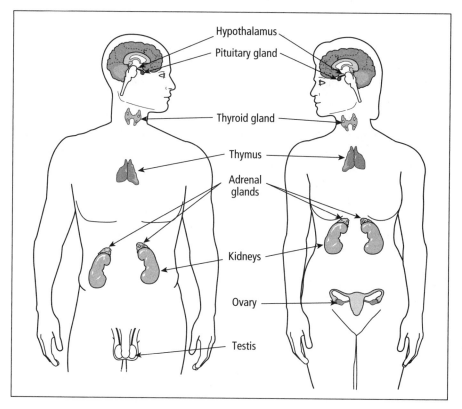

Figure 9-1. The endocrine system

Organ damage

The hypothalamus and the pituitary gland are not normally damaged by chemotherapy; however, abnormalities are commonly seen after radiation to the brain, face, or neck. The pituitary gland can tolerate up to 4000 centigray (cGy) and continue to function well. The hypothalamus is more delicate and can be affected by doses as low as 1800 to 2000 cGy. The amount of damage depends on total dose, method used to deliver radiation, and age of the child when irradiated.

Growth hormone deficiency is the most common problem after radiation to the HPA. It is often not immediately apparent and tends to worsen over time. Younger age at treatment and being female are additional risk factors for short adult height.

> Ethan was diagnosed with a brain tumor at age 5 and got radiation and chemotherapy over a 14-month period. Right at the end of treatment, his pediatrician noted that he had not grown nor had he gained any weight over the previous year. Because radiation carried the risk of hormonal damage, she suggested an endocrine work up, which revealed deficiencies of both thyroid and growth hormone. After 6 months of thyroid hormone replacement, the situation was unchanged, and growth hormone (daily shots) was initiated. The results were astounding. After the first month of growth hormone, Ethan had his pre-cancer energy back. He was impish in a way he hadn't been in 2 years. His appetite ramped up and he grew. The one problem we had was that he later had signs of premature puberty. He needed to have additional shots of Lupron® (once a month, but intramuscular) to halt that process. Growth hormone was a big success for Ethan. At 17, he is a bit shorter than his siblings, but not by much, and most importantly, he doesn't feel short. He recently went to adult maintenance doses of growth hormone (still once a day, but a smaller amount) and he does it all himself.

The survivors most affected by damage to the HPA are those who were treated for brain tumors. Almost all children treated with more than 3000 cGy to the brain experience growth disruptions. In contrast, children with leukemia who received 1800 to 2400 cGy of cranial radiation have less frequent, milder problems with growth.

> I had astrocytoma when I was 10. The radiation affected me and I can't have children. I have to take a pill to have a period. I'm in my 20s and am 4'6".

· · · · ·

> My treatment for leukemia (diagnosed at age 11) and three relapses lasted almost 14 years. I was on four different protocols and had a bone marrow transplant. I had 2400 cGy of radiation plus whole body radiation prior to my transplant. I've had no problems with growth—I'm 6'1". I have no endocrine problems. Cognitively I'm fine. I have all my hair. I've had such a great outcome.

· · · · ·

> My daughter had 2400 rads of cranial radiation and also spinal radiation to treat her relapsed acute lymphoblastic leukemia. Until then, she

was at the high end of the growth scale, but she stopped growing. When we started growth hormone, she grew an inch in the first 2 months. She's now 10 years old and is 4'4".

Survivors whose growth is most likely to be affected are:

• Survivors of childhood brain tumors. Surgery in the area near the HPA and high doses of radiation can both cause severe growth slowdowns.

• Children treated for leukemia with whole brain radiation. The younger the age when irradiated, the more pronounced the effect on height.

• Children who had spinal radiation (see Chapter 17, *Muscles and Bones*).

• Children who were treated with total body radiation prior to a stem cell transplant (this term includes bone marrow transplants). A single high dose of radiation causes more problems than radiation given in smaller doses.

• Children (especially girls) who enter puberty before age 8 (called precocious puberty).

• Children (especially girls) who have an early puberty (ages 8 to 11) but not a precocious one can have somewhat reduced final heights.

Our son Chris was a big boy until his treatment for medulloblastoma. His height froze for a year while he was being treated. He had surgery to remove the tumor and both cranial and spinal radiation. He's now on the shorter end of average for kids in his grade.

• • • • •

My son had high-risk leukemia, relapsed twice in the CNS (central nervous system), and had a bone marrow transplant (BMT). He had 2400 cGy of radiation to his brain and spinal cord, then total body radiation and Cytoxan® prior to transplant. He has not grown much since the BMT. He is entering seventh grade, and is 4'10". His friends have all continued to grow, so this is starting to bother him. He has not really started puberty yet, either. He still has the little boy voice. He has been followed by an endocrinologist, who said he will decide what to do this January if puberty hasn't started yet. He was always at the 95th percentile of height before cancer, but he definitely is not anymore.

An early growth spurt coupled with early sexual maturation can also result in short stature. This happens because the bones stop growing when sexual maturity is reached. When this happens at a young age, the child loses 2 or 3 years of additional growth.

My daughter had 1800 cGy of cranial radiation starting the week she turned 4. She began puberty at 8 and was done at 10. She hasn't grown since. She is 4'11" and wears a size 3½ shoe.

Children or teens who received high-dose radiation (more than 3500 cGy) to the area of the hypothalamus and pituitary often develop a variety of hormonal abnormalities. They are at risk for growth hormone deficiencies; early sexual development; deficiencies in production of LH, FSH, adreno-corticotrophic hormone (ACTH), and thyroid-stimulating hormone (TSH); and may produce too much prolactin. These problems may develop years after treatment, so these survivors need long-term endocrine follow-up. Although this chapter describes each of these problems separately, survivors often have combinations of endocrine problems.

My daughter has hormone deficiencies due to radiation to the pituitary. She had rhabdomyosarcoma in the nasopharynx and was treated with 5400 rads of radiation. The pituitary had to be included in the radiation fields because the tumor was right next to it. She is growth hormone, thyroid, and estrogen deficient. The estrogen and thyroid are replaced by daily medication. We opted not to use growth hormone since she was about 5'3" when she became deficient. Her cortisol is fine.

There are numerous other problems from damage to the HPA that do not directly involve growth. These rare problems are listed here:

• Hyperprolactinemia (too much prolactin) can occur in children who receive more than 3000 cGy to the HPA. In females, prolactin is involved in breast development when there is adequate estrogen, progesterone, and growth hormone. Teens or women with too much prolactin stop having periods. Men who produce too much prolactin may have a lower sexual drive.

• Panhypopituitary dysfunction is a complication in children with brain tumors who get more than 5500 cGy to the HPA. In these cases, the production and secretion of all substances produced by the HPA stop and hormone replacement is necessary.

Signs and symptoms

Signs and symptoms of damage to the HPA can take many forms. Common late effects are decreased growth, early or late puberty, and low levels of LH and FSH hormones.

Decreased growth. Decreased growth is a common problem for all children and teens on therapy for cancer. Many children experience catch-up growth after treatment ends. A few survivors continue to have slowed growth long after therapy ends. Signs and symptoms of impaired growth are:

• Growing less than 5 cm (2 inches) a year.

• Significant changes in the growth percentiles (e.g., a child who used to be in the 90th percentile who is now in the 50th percentile).

• Below normal height for pubertal status.

• Below normal sitting height.

• Growth hormone deficiency.

• Slow bone growth. This can be missed if height and weight are not plotted on a growth graph periodically and followed over time.

Early (precocious) puberty. Precocious puberty can occur in children who were treated with cranial radiation. Signs and symptoms of precocious puberty are:

• Physical signs of puberty in girls (e.g., breast development, underarm hair, body odor) before the age of 8.

> *My daughter is 7 years old, 49" tall, and weighs 80 lbs. She had 2 weeks of cranial radiation to treat her leukemia. I can't remember the rads she was given. She doesn't have body odor yet, but lots of breast development (her 12-year-old sister asked if it could be transplanted). She also has some pubic hair. We have been told some of this could be from damage to the hypothalamus.*

• Physical signs of puberty in boys (e.g., testicular enlargement, development of the penis, underarm hair, facial hair) before the age of 9.

• Growth hormone deficiency.

Although parents are often relieved to see growth during puberty, their child may end up very short if puberty does not start at a normal time and last the usual number of years.

Late puberty. Puberty can also be delayed by treatment for childhood cancer. Normally, puberty begins by age 13 in girls and 14 in boys. However, if hormones produced by the pituitary (LH and FSH) are disrupted or decreased by treatment, girls and boys may not start puberty at the normal time. Signs and symptoms of delayed puberty are:

• No signs of sexual maturation in girls (e.g., breast development, underarm hair, body odor) by age 13.

My daughter is 17, and had one of the first bone marrow transplants for AML (acute myelogenous leukemia). She never really went into puberty. She developed no body hair, breasts, or any of the other things associated with the teen years. When they tested her blood, they found levels of hormones similar to a woman in menopause. She's since had breast augmentation surgery and takes birth control pills to try to replace the hormones she's missing.

- No signs of sexual maturation in boys (e.g., development of the penis, underarm hair, deepening voice) by age 15.

- Children being shorter than their peers because they haven't had a pubertal growth spurt.

Abnormal LH or FSH hormone levels in females. Signs and symptoms of low LH or FSH in females during or after puberty are:

- Puberty stopping.

- Menstruation stopping.

- Changes in duration, frequency, or character of menstruation.

- Signs of low estrogen, such as hot flashes, vaginal dryness, low libido (sex drive), sleep disturbances, pain during intercourse, or infertility.

I was treated for ALL (acute lymphoblastic leukemia) as a child and started my period when I was 12½. I had normal periods for 6 months, then relapsed when I was 13. During treatment, it fluctuated—I'd go several months without a period, then I'd have one. That was 20 years ago, and I still have irregular periods, though I have had children. Birth control pills help regulate my periods now.

Abnormal LH or FSH hormone levels in males. Signs and symptoms of low LH or FSH in males during or after puberty are:

- Puberty stopping.

- Soft, small testicles.

- Low or absent sperm count.

- Changes in libido or sexual performance.

Screening and detection

Any child or teen who had radiation to the brain should be carefully screened for growth failure. A healthcare provider should measure standing height and plot it on a growth chart (i.e., graph that shows if the child is growing normally for his age) every 6 months. Sitting heights should also be obtained for any survivor who had radiation to the spine (i.e., total body radiation, mantle, spinal). The heights should be analyzed in light of the child's pre-cancer growth, current bone age (determined from a hand x-ray), stage of puberty, and height of parents.

I had a bone marrow transplant when I was 7 and because of the side effects of some treatment, I ended up having a very early period. I was so happy at the time, and we assumed it was a good sign that things were going well. However, as it turns out, starting my menstrual period at such a young age caused me to be much shorter than I would have been. I was one of the tallest kids in my class until grade eight. Then they all kept growing and I stayed the same height.

Any child who, after treatment, is growing slowly (i.e., less than 2 inches a year) or is in the fifth percentile or below for height should have the following tests:

• Bone age (measures the maturation of bones in the hand).

• Thyroid function tests.

• Somatomedin-C (IGF1) and IGFBP3 (blood tests that measure the amount of hormone available to support normal growth).

• Blood work to check on the functioning of other major organs. For example, if the kidneys are not working well, a child will not grow optimally.

All children with growth concerns should be referred to a pediatric endocrinologist.

I had an ependymoma when I was 8 years old. I'm now the second to shortest kid in my class. When I was 12, my endocrinologist put me on Lupron® to prevent an early puberty and to get as much growth as I can. It's a shot every 28 days. It doesn't bother me because it is for a good cause. I go to my regular pediatrician to get it and he's a good shot giver. Now we are discussing whether to go on growth hormone.

All children should be evaluated for puberty status after radiation to the HPA, regardless of age. Any child who appears to be entering precocious puberty should have a bone age (x-ray of the hand) and GnRH testing done. Most facilities also test growth hormones in any child who appears to be entering precocious puberty because the two problems—slowed growth and early puberty—tend to occur together. Children entering precocious puberty should be referred to a pediatric endocrinologist with experience treating survivors of childhood cancer.

*My son was treated with radiation for astrocytoma. We just found out
that his GH (growth hormone) is really low. The highest number he had
was 4.9 out of all four blood draws. We also got the "wonderful" news
his testosterone level was 463, which is equivalent to an adult male! And
he's only 9 years old. So now we go back to the children's hospital to get
growth hormone and Lupron® to stop the poor child's puberty. We haven't
explained to Justin yet that this means one shot a day for the GH and
one shot every 28 days for the Lupron®.*

Some teens do not begin puberty at the normal age. This can be caused
by organ failure (see sections about ovaries and testes) or lowered LH and
FSH production due to HPA damage from radiation. These adolescents
should have a comprehensive evaluation by a pediatric endocrinologist
that includes bone age, LH and FSH levels, testosterone or estradiol (estrogen) levels, and thyroid function tests for those who had high levels of
radiation (more than 3000 cGy) to the HPA. For survivors who had more
than 5000 cGy to the HPA, tests of cortisol and prolactin levels also are
recommended.

Medical management

Healthcare providers of survivors at risk for problems stemming from HPA
damage should discuss the signs and symptoms with parents (or older survivors) and give a thorough yearly evaluation. The following are the current
methods used by most follow-up clinics to treat HPA problems:

- **GH deficiency.** Replacement GH is given in a daily shot.

- **Low LH and FSH.** Females who produce no LH or FSH are usually treated with estrogen and synthetic progesterone (progestin). Adolescents and
  women with partial deficiencies may require only monthly progestin therapy to cause a period. These medications should be prescribed only by a
  pediatric endocrinologist experienced in treating survivors of childhood
  cancer or by an obstetrician with expertise in reproductive endocrinology.
  Males with low LH are given sustained-release testosterone (through an
  injection into the muscle every 2 to 4 weeks, a daily patch on the skin, or
  in a cream).

- **Precocious puberty.** The drug Lupron® is given through a monthly
  injection into the muscle to stop puberty until the time it should begin.
  Replacement GH and GHRH are given if the child also has low GH. A
  psychologist or other mental health professional may be helpful in dealing with the emotional effects of beginning puberty too early.

- **Hyperprolactinemia (too much prolactin).** This condition is treated with bromocriptine or a related medication.

Children who are growth hormone deficient should be evaluated again once they have achieved their adult height to determine if they require adult growth hormone replacement. Growth hormone affects many things other than growth, such as fat-to-muscle ratio, bone density, mood, cognitive function, and heart health. The criteria for receiving growth hormone in adulthood are stringent. Many children who are given growth hormone during childhood do not need growth hormone into adulthood, but many do (although they need a smaller dose). There have been concerns about the long-term safety of growth hormone. To date, studies support the safety of growth hormone and ongoing studies continue to monitor for any negative long-term effects.

Thyroid

The thyroid is a small, butterfly-shaped gland located in front of the trachea in the neck. An exquisitely sensitive gland, it enlarges and becomes more active during puberty, pregnancy, or times of great stress. It also alters its size and shape during women's menstrual cycles.

The three hormones secreted by the thyroid are triiodothyronine (T3), thyroxine (T4), and calcitonin. T3 and T4, which contain iodine, have far-reaching effects on almost all tissues in the body and are intimately involved in physical growth, metabolism, and mental development. Calcitonin helps regulate the amount of calcium in the body. If T3 and T4 levels are low or nonexistent, growth hormone secretion is decreased, and what is released is not effective.

The thyroid's functioning can be disrupted by radiation to the gland itself or to its regulator—the HPA. The pituitary gland produces TSH that prompts the thyroid to produce the exact amount of hormones needed by the body.

Organ damage

The thyroid is generally not affected by chemotherapy. If damage occurs, radiation is usually the culprit. Children or teens who had total body radiation, mantle radiation for Hodgkin lymphoma, or radiation to the head and/or neck are at the highest risk for a malfunctioning thyroid. Several types of thyroid problems can develop after radiation.

Compensated hypothyroidism. High TSH and normal T4 may occur if the thyroid is working too hard. There are usually no symptoms. An irradiated and/or overstimulated gland is at increased risk for developing tumors, both benign and malignant. Survivors with compensated hypothyroidism are sometimes given supplemental thyroid hormone to allow the gland to rest.

> My Hodgkin's disease was treated with chemotherapy and mantle radiation in 1989. My total cGy ranged from 2500 to 2800, with areas of involvement getting the highest boost.

> Naturally, we were warned at the start that I could have thyroid dysfunction from treatment. My hematologist monitored this periodically after treatment via the standard T4/T3/TSH blood work, which was fine until March 1993. My doctor said that my TSH was a little high, but my T4 was normal, and explained that I would need to start thyroxine if my T4 came back low the next time. It didn't, but my TSH was still high, so we just kept monitoring annually since I wasn't really having any symptoms. I have had off-and-on episodes of feeling cold, and I also find it interesting that my major weight gain occurred just before those tests went awry.

> When I began to see a new doctor, he discussed the situation with me and said that he felt I should start thyroxine replacement even if my T4 remained normal, since there is some evidence that prolonged elevation of TSH may increase the risk of thyroid cancer. I've been on 0.1 mg of Synthroid® once daily since March 1997. We monitor my blood work twice a year, and he thinks I may have to go up on dosage—most people, he says, eventually do need more. His feeling was that I'd probably feel a lot better on it, and I do have more energy now.

Most often, compensated thyroid dysfunction is found on routine screening of at-risk survivors. An elevation in the TSH is the first sign of thyroid gland dysfunction.

Primary hypothyroidism. Survivors who received more than 1500 cGy of radiation to the neck or more than 750 cGy total body irradiation (TBI) are at risk for primary hypothyroidism (increased TSH and low T4). Survivors of Hodgkin lymphoma, non-Hodgkin lymphoma, head and neck tumors, and those who had TBI prior to a stem cell transplant may develop this problem. Hypothyroidism sometimes occurs in patients treated with craniospinal radiation for leukemia.

> Twenty years after high-dose mantle radiation for Hodgkin's, my thyroid went haywire. I lost 20 pounds, and my doctor did blood work and found

an underactive thyroid. I took the supplement and had no problem until 7 years later when he found nodules in the thyroid. When they removed the thyroid, it was very atrophied from the radiation.

Hypothyroidism is very common in Hodgkin lymphoma survivors who received mantle radiation. Treatment at a young age may also increase the likelihood of developing a thyroid problem.

I had a BMT 12 years ago with 1800 rads (cGy) of cranial radiation during the procedure. Fortunately, I've never had any thyroid problems.

• • • • •

My daughter had 1800 cGy of cranial radiation when she was 4 years old. She developed hypothyroidism when she was 9 and has been on Synthroid® ever since then.

Thyroid dysfunction can occur soon after radiation, but more typically starts 3 to 5 years after treatment.

Thyroid-stimulating hormone deficiency. This late effect, characterized by low TSH and T4 levels, is very uncommon but can occur after radiation to the head or after a stem cell transplant.

Hyperthyroidism. Hyperthyroidism (low TSH and elevated T4) occurs when too much thyroxine is produced, causing the body to use energy faster than it should. It is not well understood, but has been found in very small numbers of survivors who were treated with neck radiation.

Thyroid cancer. Radiation to the neck can result in thyroid cancer later in life, so all survivors at risk need lifelong evaluation of thyroid function.

I had 4400 rads of mantle radiation in 1968. In 1978 I developed a goiter. When they removed it they thought it was a cyst, but the pathologist found malignant cells in it. I didn't have to do anything for it since it was caught so early. I did go on thyroid replacement.

• • • • •

I recently had my thyroid removed. The surgeon showed me the pathology report. It said stuff like "atrophy, fibrosis, multi-nodular goiter" and "consistent with irradiation." In the final analysis the thyroid could have stayed in because there was no cancer, but there was no way to tell if there was cancer without removing it because it was in such bad shape. Frankly, I am glad it is gone.

Signs and symptoms

Hypothyroidism. Signs and symptoms of an underactive thyroid (hypothyroidism) include the following:

- Fatigue or lethargy
- Hoarseness
- Difficulty concentrating
- Depression or mood changes
- Constipation
- Weakness
- Intolerance to cold
- Swelling around the eyes
- Poor growth
- Delayed puberty
- Puffy face and hands
- Weight gain
- Dry or rough skin
- Brittle hair
- Joint or muscle aches
- Slow heart rate
- Low blood pressure
- High cholesterol
- Decreased tolerance for exercise

Hyperthyroidism. The signs and symptoms of an overactive thyroid (hyperthyroidism) include the following:

- Nervousness or anxiety
- Difficulty concentrating
- Fatigue
- Muscle weakness or tremor
- Rapid or irregular heartbeat
- Excessive perspiration
- Heat intolerance

- Diarrhea
- Weight loss
- Menstrual irregularities
- Protruding eyes
- Tenderness in the neck
- Decreased tolerance for exercise

Screening and detection

Free T4 and TSH levels should be checked every year after radiation to the head, chest, or neck, and anytime symptoms develop. Women who take oral contraceptive pills should also have their thyroid levels checked periodically. These are simple blood tests. At some facilities, radioactive iodine uptake by the thyroid is measured. At every yearly follow-up appointment, a survivor's thyroid should be palpated (felt by hand) and growth of children and young teens should be plotted on a chart. If a healthcare provider can feel a thyroid nodule (bump), an ultrasound of the thyroid will be done to evaluate it. Some institutions now use ultrasounds for screening.

Thyroid problems can occur years or decades after treatment for cancer, so a yearly check is necessary for the rest of your life. If any abnormalities are detected during an examination, referral and follow-up by an endocrinologist or surgeon are necessary.

Medical management

Survivors' healthcare providers should talk to them about the signs and symptoms of thyroid problems so they will be recognized early. Although thyroid problems are common in survivors who had radiation to the head and neck, treatment is generally easy and effective. Treatments for thyroid problems include:

- **Compensated hypothyroidism (high TSH, normal T4).** Daily pill of thryroxine to suppress excessive gland activity.
- **Primary hypothyroidism (high TSH, low T4).** Replacement with the hormone thyroxine (daily pill).
- **Thyroid-stimulating hormone deficiency (low TSH, low T4).** Daily thyroxine.
- **Hyperthyroidism (low TSH, high T4).** Radioactive iodine to destroy the thyroid, then daily replacement with thyroxine.

- **Thyroid nodules.** Patients with nodules detected by ultrasound should have a thyroid scan and evaluation by both an endocrinologist and a surgeon. If the scan shows nodules, a biopsy should be performed.

- **Thyroid cancer.** A thyroglobulin level (blood test) should be done before the thyroid is removed. If the tumor secretes the thyroglobulin hormone, this simple blood test can be used in the future to screen for recurrence of the cancer. Patients with thyroid cancer usually have the thyroid removed (called a thyroidectomy) and get radioactive iodine afterwards. After surgery, thyroxine replacement is necessary.

Female survivors who are at risk for thyroid problems and are planning to become pregnant should have a blood test done to evaluate their thyroid function. Both the American Association of Clinical Endocrinologists and the American College of Endocrinology recommend that all women planning to become pregnant be screened before they conceive, because mothers with thyroid disease have a higher risk of having children with neurological defects.

Testes

The testes are the male reproductive organs. These oval glands are each approximately 2 inches long when fully mature. They are enclosed in a sac called the scrotum. Each testicle contains hundreds of densely coiled tubes (called seminiferous tubules) that contain spermatogonia—cells that produce sperm. The creation of sperm depends on the presence of adequate FSH (follicle-stimulating hormone) and healthy germ cells.

Leydig cells, found throughout the testicles, produce the hormone testosterone. Leydig cell function is prompted by LH (luteinizing hormone). These two cell lines—spermatogonia and Leydig cells—react very differently to treatment for cancer.

Organ damage

The testes can be damaged by radiation, chemotherapy, or surgery. The following information is about "primary failure," when treatment affects the testes themselves.

Radiation: Spermatogonia

Spermatogonia are very sensitive to radiation. One hundred to 500 cGy of radiation to the testes can cause a temporary drop or stoppage of sperm production, and more than 600 cGy usually results in permanent sterility.

When sperm production is permanently affected, reduced testicular size and softer testicles result. Survivors likely to have received these doses are:

- Boys treated for testicular leukemia.
- Recipients of stem cell transplants whose conditioning included radiation.
- Boys or teens with Hodgkin lymphoma treated with "inverted-Y" radiation.
- Boys or teens with soft tissue sarcomas in the thigh, groin, or abdomen.

If damage to sperm-producing cells occurs before puberty, the first clue that there is a problem occurs when the testes do not grow to a normal size during puberty. These boys develop secondary sexual characteristics (e.g., facial hair, deepening voice), but the testes remain small and soft. If the teen is rendered infertile by treatment after puberty, his testicles may become softer and smaller over time.

Radiation: Leydig Cells

Compared to spermatogonia, testosterone-producing Leydig cells are very resistant to radiation. Whereas male sperm production is affected quickly by small amounts of radiation, it takes approximately 2000 or more cGy to the testes before Leydig cells start to become damaged. The younger the patient, the more severe the effect of the radiation on the Leydig cells.

Cranial or craniospinal radiation, given to children with ALL or brain tumors (other than those near the pituitary), rarely causes damage to testosterone production.

Chemotherapy

Chemotherapy can be devastating to the production of sperm, although sperm production may resume months to years after chemotherapy ends. The drugs that most affect sperm are the alkylators:

- Mechlorethamine and procarbazine (contained in MOPP—mechlorethamine, vincristine, procarbazine, and prednisone)
- Cyclophosphamide (contained in COPP—cyclophosphamide, vincristine, procarbazine, and prednisone)
- Ifosfamide
- Chlorambucil
- Nitrosoureas
- Melphalan

The higher the doses of these drugs, the more damage may occur to the sperm-producing cells.

> My stage IVB Hodgkin's was treated with five and a half cycles of ABVD [adriamycin, bleomycin, vinblastine, dacarbazine] and radiation. We banked sperm, but my disease was pretty far advanced. We didn't have time to put a lot of wigglies in the freezer, and they were not of very good quality. A few weeks after completing radiation in February 1997, my sperm count was 13 million—fair to middlin', as we would say in the South, where I'm from—with very good motility. I can still hear the dignified, enthusiastic East Indian accent of the lab technician telling me that "they are swimming most vigorously." I was told I should have no problem fathering a child.

Chemotherapy used to treat boys with leukemia does not usually affect sperm production unless high doses of cyclophosphamide were given. Vinblastine, bleomycin, and etoposide used to treat other cancers can temporarily affect sperm production, but the majority of survivors, over time, recover the ability to produce sperm.

> I had industrial doses of cyclophosphamide many years ago and was told that I would not be able to father children. It was the most devastating part of the whole experience. But I kept thinking in the back of my mind that it would all work out. And it did. My wife and I now have an 18-month-old son and another baby on the way.

It was thought for many years that testosterone-producing Leydig cells were immune to damage from chemotherapy, but this has proven not to be the case. High doses (nine courses or more) of MOPP or COPP can cause irreversible damage to the Leydig cells. These high doses are generally only seen in survivors who relapsed and received large amounts of chemotherapy drugs.

> I had Hodgkin's twice and had a total of eight cycles of MOPP and two of ABVD. I had mantle radiation too. I had a semen analysis and found out that I was infertile. After I got married, I lost all interest in sex. I thought it was because I didn't want to talk about my cancer history, and my wife seemed to always want to talk about it. When the nurse practitioner asked me about our sex life, I told her that I just wasn't interested anymore. She had a check done on my testosterone, and it was only 50 (normal is 350 to 1,000). When I started taking testosterone, my libido increased. I was so glad that we talked about it, and my nurse's frankness took away the taboo. It is hard to talk about sexual problems, but it really changed my life.

Patients treated during adolescence can have low testosterone and high LH. There can also be a lowering of libido despite a normal testosterone level. This means that for a survivor who received and is experiencing any abnormalities in puberty or sexual functioning, a thorough evaluation may help determine the cause and identify solutions.

> My 18-year-old son is not very active 5 years after his bone marrow transplant, perhaps because he has very low testosterone levels. His doctor recommended waiting on hormone shots until he had need of an energized sex drive. She suggested we might not want to do it in his late teens/early 20s, sort of "Let sleeping dogs lie."

In this situation, an endocrinologist should talk with the young man about his testosterone level and how it affects his life. Replacement testosterone does not just govern sex drive; it affects energy, stamina, and secondary sexual characteristics, and it contributes to an overall sense of well-being. It is also important to psychological and sexual development. Many teens and men with low-functioning Leydig cells feel much better when taking supplemental testosterone.

The preceding information discussed primary failure—damage to the glands themselves. Spermatogonia and Leydig cell functioning can be affected by damage to the HPA as well; this is called "secondary failure." A dose of 4500 cGy to the HPA in the brain can shut down both Leydig cells and sperm production. If there is nothing wrong with the testes but they have been shut down by the brain, they can be stimulated with hormones to produce sperm. It's vital to determine whether a survivor has primary or secondary failure so he can get the best treatment.

> I have been taking testosterone for about 10 years—first a shot every 2 weeks and now the patch. I feel much better when taking the patch. I feel stronger and my physical well-being is much better. With one patch my hormone level is in the low normal range. If I use two my level is almost in the middle of the range.

Surgery can also affect sexual functioning in males. If a survivor had an abdominal lymph node dissection, side effects can include impotence or inability to ejaculate. For more information, see Chapter 14, *Kidneys, Bladder, and Genitals*. Surgery for a brain tumor involving the hypothalamus or pituitary also can disrupt the functioning of the testes.

Survivors may be concerned about the health of any children they father. The research is reassuring in this regard. The children of male survivors are just as healthy as those of the general population (the one exception are children born to a parent who carries the gene for an eye tumor called retinoblastoma). For more information, see Chapter 3, *Relationships*.

Signs and symptoms

Signs and symptoms of damage to the testes depend on age during treatment. If testosterone-producing Leydig cells are damaged before puberty, boys usually won't go into puberty. If the Leydig cells are damaged after puberty, survivors may lose interest in sex and may become impotent.

If the sperm-producing cells are damaged before puberty, the testes won't grow as large as they normally would have. Survivors will have testosterone, so will look like a normal male and can function sexually like a normal male, but the testes will be smaller and softer. If sperm-producing cells are damaged after puberty, sexual functioning will be unaffected, but the survivor may not produce sperm. Therefore, function is normal, but the survivor may be infertile.

Primary testicular failure. Signs and symptoms of primary testicular failure (i.e., damage directly to the testicles) include the following:

- Absence of or change in libido (sex drive) if Leydig cells are affected
- Low or absent sperm counts
- Increased breast size

Secondary testicular failure. Signs and symptoms of secondary testicular failure (damage to the HPA) include the following:

- Lack of secondary sex characteristics (e.g., facial and pubic hair) and decreased testicular size
- Decreased libido
- Impotence
- Low testosterone levels

Screening and detection

Survivors should receive a thorough annual evaluation if they received chemotherapy or radiation that might have damaged their testes. Also, any boy showing signs of puberty before age 9 or who has not begun puberty by age 14 needs to be examined by an endocrinologist. This examination may include the following:

- A thorough history, including height, weight, and age when puberty occurred in all members of the family. The history should rule out other causes of precocious or delayed puberty, including hypothyroidism, medications such as steroids for bodybuilding, illegal drug use, chronic disease, or malnutrition.

- A careful physical evaluation, including evaluation of facial hair, underarm hair, pubic hair, length of penis, and size of testes.
- Analysis of a semen sample and a discussion about ejaculations, erections, and libido.
- Growth plotted on a chart to evaluate growth progression.
- LH, FSH, and testosterone levels.
- Prolactin level if radiation was given to the HPA.
- Discussion about fertility and libido.

Recovery of sperm production sometimes occurs 10 or more years after treatment. These tests should be repeated yearly for men who have a low sperm count.

Medical management

Male survivors who do not produce sperm as a result of direct damage to the testes (called primary failure) must simply wait to see if sperm production recovers over time. They should have periodic sperm counts and evaluations of testosterone production, as testosterone replacement may improve a sense of well-being.

> My second bout with Hodgkin's appeared in my groin. I had radiation to the groin and chemotherapy. My wife and I were warned that I would be infertile, so I went to a sperm bank before treatment started. It's been 2 years since I was treated, and I have periodic sperm counts, but still produce no sperm. The doctors don't expect me to ever produce sperm again.

Even if teens have no sperm production after treatment ends, it can return. Healthcare providers should explain if new advancements in reproductive technology, such as intracytoplasmic sperm injection, might be an option for survivors who want to father a child. Survivors should not assume that they are infertile; they should use birth control unless they are trying to become a parent.

In addition, if the testes have been shut down by radiation or surgery to the brain, survivors may begin to produce sperm if they received LH and FSH supplementation.

Teens or adults with primary Leydig cell damage need replacement testosterone. A testosterone patch or injection into the muscle every 2 to 4 weeks are the most common methods of supplementation for males with low testosterone. The treatment begins at the time of normal puberty and starts with doses of 25 to 50 mg per month of testosterone enanthate (not methyltestosterone). Dosage is increased by 50 mg every 6 months until the survivor is receiving 200 to 300 mg per month. This treatment helps the development of the genitals. In addition, the growth of prepubertal boys with low testosterone levels may be enhanced by injections of growth hormone (if they are growth hormone deficient). Boys with Leydig cell damage should be treated by a pediatric endocrinologist with experience treating survivors of childhood cancer.

High-dose radiation (more than 5500 cGy) to the HPA can cause hyperprolactinemia. Treatment with bromocriptine can sometimes resolve the symptoms, which include decreased libido, impotence, and low testosterone.

Children or teens with pelvic tumors (e.g., rhabdomyosarcoma, Ewing sarcoma) who receive high doses of abdominal radiation may have nerve damage that affects sexual functioning. Even with hormone replacement, these survivors sometimes continue to have sexual problems. Working closely with a pediatric endocrinologist and urologist will help survivors achieve the best possible outcome given their treatment.

Medical management also includes counseling to help cope with the possibility of late effects on sexuality and fertility. For infertile males, counseling is helpful to explore other ways to become a parent (such as using donor sperm or adoption). Also, education about the difference between infertility (the inability to father a child biologically) and impotence (the inability to have or maintain erections) is tremendously important. The majority of male survivors of childhood cancer are able to have satisfying sexual relationships.

Ovaries

Ovaries are the main reproductive organs of the female. They are approximately 1½ inches in length when fully developed after puberty and are located in the abdomen on either side of the uterus. The major functions of the ovaries are development of eggs (ova) and production and release of sex hormones. Normal ovarian function is crucial for optimal growth, puberty, and fertility.

The ovaries of younger girls are more resistant to ovarian damage than those of older teens. However, each ovary contains a finite number of eggs, so any damage to them is irreparable. The good news is that the ovaries are very treatment resistant, and it takes a considerable amount of radiation or chemotherapy to damage them.

Organ damage

The ovaries' functioning can be disrupted by radiation to the glands themselves or to their regulator—the HPA. Damage to the ovaries is called "primary failure" and damage to the HPA is called "secondary failure."

Radiation to ovaries

Female children or teens who had radiation to the abdomen for Wilms tumor, Ewing sarcoma, or lymphoma (and some older protocols for leukemia), or had TBI, are at the highest risk for primary ovarian failure.

The effect of radiation on the ovaries is dependent on age and dosage. In older adolescents, the ovaries may be damaged at doses of 500 to 800 cGy. During puberty, radiation doses of 800 to 1000 cGy can cause the ovaries to shut down. Some prepubertal girls, however, can get 1000 to1200 cGy and still retain ovarian function. Once an ovary fails, it totally stops producing eggs and hormones. It is an "all-or-nothing" gland.

> My daughter's growth hormone was low before her BMT at age 13, and now it's really low. She's 5 feet tall, and we don't think she'll grow any more. Her 11-year-old sister is now taller than she is. She had some breast development and a period prior to the transplant, but her ovaries have totally failed. She was also an emotional basket case after the transplant. The pituitary was sending out hormones to the ovaries, but they weren't working. So the pituitary just kept sending out more and more hormones. She was put on low-estrogen birth control pills, and within a couple of months her breasts started to develop. They put her on higher-dose pills and she started having periods. She also takes Synthroid® for her thyroid.

Older girls who stop having their periods after doses of up to 1000 cGy may resume their normal cycles months to years after treatment ends.

TBI prior to stem cell transplant can also cause ovarian failure. Young girls may not start puberty, and teens past puberty may stop having periods. Some female transplant survivors never develop secondary sexual characteristics (e.g., breasts, pubic hair) or start menstruating.

The preceding information concerns primary failure—damage to the glands themselves. Female survivors who had high-dose radiation to the pituitary or hypothalamus (for treatment of brain tumors or rhabdomyosarcoma) are at risk for secondary ovarian failure—reduction in hormones regulating the ovaries. The hypothalamus secretes GnRH, which stimulates the pituitary gland to release FSH and LH. FSH regulates ovarian follicular growth and LH regulates ovulation. Young girls who received cranial radiation for leukemia have a slightly increased risk for precocious or early puberty (see earlier section about the hypothalamic-pituitary axis).

Chemotherapy

Primary failure of the ovaries has been associated with chemotherapy, but it usually takes very high doses to cause damage. For instance, girls who haven't gone through puberty can take up to 15 to 20 grams of cyclophosphamide (Cytoxan®) and may still retain function, although they are at risk for premature ovarian failure in the future. After six cycles of MOPP, girls' ovaries usually still function well. High doses of busulfan combined with cytoxan as a pretransplant regime often causes ovarian damage.

Sometimes older survivors of childhood cancer experience an early menopause (in other words, menopause begins in the 20s or 30s instead of the 40s or 50s). As this risk can affect when and if survivors are able to have children, it's important to discuss this with your physician.

> I was treated with six cycles of ABVD (no radiation) over a 9-month period for Hodgkin's in 1977. I went into menopause at age 36. I started getting itchy and sex became very painful. I first went on Premarin® and Provera® and had very bad mood swings and painful breasts. I know lots of women who this works well for, so it's a matter of finding the right supplement for you. We experimented with different doses and cycles, but it still wasn't working well for me. When I changed to Estrace®, symptoms decreased vastly. One of the nice side effects is that I have very smooth skin and almost no wrinkles. I'm 46 years old and look good. And sex is enjoyable again.

Girls treated for leukemia before or after puberty generally retain good ovarian function. However, a small percentage of girls treated in the 1970s and early 1980s with craniospinal radiation have damaged ovaries if the ovaries were in the radiation field. The majority of girls treated for ovarian germ cell tumors remain fertile if they have one intact ovary and their uterus.

A great concern of many female survivors is their ability to have healthy children if they become pregnant. The research is reassuring in this regard. The children of the vast majority of female survivors are just as healthy as those of the general population. For more information, see Chapter 3, *Relationships*.

Signs and symptoms

The signs and symptoms of ovarian problems depend on age. If ovaries fail before puberty, female survivors won't start puberty. They may grow pubic hair, prompted by the adrenal glands, but they won't develop breasts or begin menstruation.

Survivors who were treated after puberty may stop having periods, get hot flashes, and have decreased interest in sex.

Girls with precocious puberty begin to develop breasts and pubic hair before the age of 8. In addition to possible psychosocial problems, precocious puberty causes the growth of long bones to slow or stop. Girls whose precocious puberty is not stopped can be very short.

Screening and detection

Survivors who received chemotherapy or radiation that might have damaged the ovaries should get a thorough annual evaluation. Also, any girl showing signs of puberty before age 8 or who has not begun puberty by age 14 needs an examination by a pediatric endocrinologist. A full evaluation of ovarian function includes the following:

- A thorough history, including information about puberty (or lack thereof), menstruation (e.g., date of first period, date periods stopped), menstrual irregularities, pregnancies, difficulties becoming pregnant, libido, heights of parents, age at which mother and sisters began menstruating, and symptoms of hypothyroidism (e.g., dry skin, constipation, sensitivity to cold).

- A complete physical, including height, weight, stage of puberty, and uterine size.

- FSH, LH, and estradiol levels beginning at puberty.

- If a survivor does not have a period by age 14 and has few or no secondary sexual characteristics (e.g., breast growth, pubic or underarm hair), referral to a pediatric endocrinologist is necessary.

- If a survivor used to have periods, but they have stopped for more than 6 months, or if she have hot flashes or breast discharge, referral to an endocrinologist is necessary.

Teenagers who have never had a period or whose periods have stopped should also have the following tests:

- Bone age (x-ray of hand)

- Ultrasound of ovaries

- Blood tests: Free T4, TSH, DHEAS, testosterone, and prolactin

The levels of LH, FSH, and estradiol tell the story. If it's a central problem—from the brain—the FSH, LH, and estradiol will all be low because the system was never turned on. If the ovaries are failing, FSH and LH will be high, and estradiol will be low.

Medical management

The medical management of girls whose ovaries have shut down is somewhat controversial. Consequently, it is extremely important that survivors be followed by a pediatric endocrinologist experienced in treating survivors of childhood cancer. An internist, family practice healthcare provider, or pediatrician may be able to provide care after a pediatric endocrinologist has thoroughly evaluated the situation and recommended treatment.

Some healthcare providers treat prepubertal girls experiencing ovarian failure with estrogen first, then add progesterone after a year. Growth hormone is suggested if the girl is growth-hormone deficient. When the girl is fully mature (with complete breast development, pubic and underarm hair), she is maintained on birth control pills.

Girls experiencing a precocious puberty are given medication to stop puberty so they will continue to grow normally. When the drug is discontinued, a normal puberty begins. Survivors at risk for premature ovarian failure may want to consider oocyte (egg) or embryo freezing if they may want to have a child in the future. In addition, post-pubertal girls who need a stem cell transplant can also undergo a procedure to procure oocytes for future use.

For information about fertility and pregnancy, see Chapter 3, *Relationships*, and the website of Fertile Hope at *www.fertilehope.org*.

Adrenal glands

There are two adrenal glands, one on top of each kidney. Each gland is roughly triangular in shape and approximately 1½ inches long and a ½ inch wide. The outer portion of the gland (cortex) secretes aldosterone, cortisol, and androgens (sex hormones). Aldosterone regulates the excretion of sodium (salt) and potassium in urine. Cortisol (hydrocortisone) has several important jobs, including marshaling the body's reactions to stress and to inflammatory and allergic reactions. The adrenals are stimulated and controlled by adrenocorticotropin, produced by the pituitary gland.

Organ damage

Children or teens who had a kidney removed (e.g., treatment for Wilms tumor or kidney cancer) or an adrenal gland removed (e.g., for a neuroblastoma that started in an adrenal gland) usually function quite well with only one remaining gland. Abdominal radiation almost never damages the adrenal glands. Brain irradiation, however, can occasionally disrupt the functioning of the adrenal glands if the HPA was affected (seen only in rare cases when more than 5000 cGy of radiation was directed at the pituitary).

Signs and symptoms

The signs and symptoms of adrenal insufficiency are weight loss, lethargy, low stamina, low blood pressure, irritability, depression, craving for salty foods, darkening of areas of the skin, weakness, and vomiting. These symptoms can appear gradually or suddenly worsen during periods of stress—for example, during an illness or after an accident. The acute onset of symptoms is called an Addisonian crisis or acute adrenal insufficiency.

Symptoms of an Addisonian crisis include pain in the lower back, abdomen, or legs; severe vomiting and diarrhea; dehydration; low blood pressure; and loss of consciousness. Left untreated, it can be fatal.

A temporary form of adrenal insufficiency may occur when a person who has been receiving a glucocorticoid hormone (such as prednisone) for a long time suddenly stops taking the medication.

Screening and detection

Problems with the adrenal glands are rare after treatment for childhood cancer. However, cortisol levels should be checked in the following situations:

- If one adrenal gland was removed and the other gland received high doses of radiation

- If the pituitary received more than 5000 cGy of radiation

Healthcare providers should check cortisol levels in both the morning and evening. If cortisol is low, referral to an endocrinologist is necessary for further testing.

Medical management

Treatment for cortisol deficiencies is replacement hydrocortisone given once in the morning or in two equal doses. Higher doses are needed if you are ill or undergoing anesthesia.

Metabolic syndrome

There is a growing body of evidence that survivors of childhood cancer are at increased risk for metabolic syndrome, which consists of a group of symptoms including obesity, insulin resistance, high cholesterol levels, and high blood pressure. This syndrome can lead to type 2 diabetes and cardiovascular disease. Some types of treatment predispose children to metabolic syndrome, and an endocrinologist is best able to diagnose this late effect. Treatment will vary based on which symptoms the child or young adult exhibits.

Chapter 10

Eyes and Ears

*The best and most beautiful things in the
world cannot be seen, nor even touched.
They must be felt in the heart.*

—Helen Keller

EYES AND EARS CAN BE DAMAGED by treatment for some types of childhood cancers. Each eye is constructed of several layers of tissue that each react differently to cancer treatment. Some parts of the eye are resistant to damage, but other parts are extremely sensitive to cancer treatment. Hearing can be affected by chemotherapy—most notably the family of drugs that includes cisplatin—and radiation. Frequent ear infections and certain intravenous antibiotics can also damage hearing. This chapter covers the various late effects involving eyes and ears, the risk of developing them, and how to manage them if they occur.

Eyes

The eye is the organ of sight. This nearly spherical body has numerous layers. At the front is the transparent cornea; through the cornea the colored iris is visible. The space between the cornea and the iris is the anterior chamber, which is filled with a clear fluid called aqueous humor. In the center of the iris is a space called the pupil that contracts or expands to control the amount of light entering the eye. Directly behind the pupil is the lens of the eye. The cavity behind the lens is filled with a gel-like substance called the vitreous humor. The thin layer that lines this cavity is the retina, which detects the light signals that enter the eye. The optic nerve transmits light information from the retina to the brain. Figure 10-1 shows the anatomy of the eye.

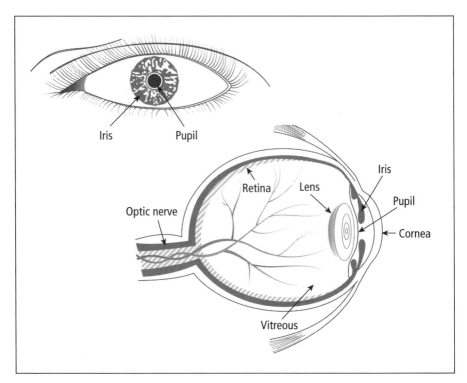

Figure 10-1. Anatomy of the eye

Organ damage

The eye can be damaged by radiation, treatment with steroids, or surgery. Vision can also be harmed if the optic nerve is damaged anywhere between the eye and the brain, which can happen from radiation, a tumor pressing on the optic nerve, or a tumor in the brain causing high fluid pressure around the brain and optic nerves. In addition, tumors in the brainstem (where the brain meets the spinal cord) can cause problems with eye movement or double vision.

When a cancer is in the eye, as in retinoblastoma, the affected eye might have to be surgically removed (called enucleation); this occurs less often now than in the past because of newer radiation techniques and chemotherapy protocols. Small and medium-sized retinoblastomas are often treated with some combination of chemotherapy, cryotherapy (freezing treatment), and photocoagulation (laser treatment). Large or advanced tumors may require enucleation.

Thirty years ago I was diagnosed with retinoblastoma when I was 18 months old. They thought it was the non-hereditary form because it was one tumor in just one eye. The eye was surgically removed, and I had no chemotherapy or radiation. I have no late effects other than wearing a prosthesis and having vision in only one eye.

The eye is exposed to low-dose radiation during total body irradiation (TBI) prior to some types of stem cell transplants. High-dose radiation is used to treat retinoblastoma, rhabdomyosarcoma, and other tumors around the eye. The eye may also be exposed to radiation given to treat brain tumors or leukemia.

Some common problems of the eye after treatment for childhood cancer are as follows:

- Hypoplasia (slowed growth of the bones around the eye)
- Cataracts
- Dry eye
- Shrinkage of the lacrimal duct, which drains tears from the eye
- Loss of vision

Ten years ago my newborn daughter was diagnosed with retinoblastoma in both eyes. She had one eye removed and both eyes radiated with 2200 cGy (centigray). Two years later the tumors returned in her remaining eye. The tumors regrew only 3 weeks after chemotherapy ended, so she had more chemotherapy. When that course had to be cut short due to side effects, they decided to remove the remaining eye. She has some learning problems from the radiation and wears two prosthetic eyes.

A common late effect is slowed growth of the orbits (eye sockets), which are the bony structures in the skull that protect the eyes. Each orbit is made up of seven bones, all of which can be damaged by radiation. This late effect is most noticeable in survivors who were treated at a very young age with more than 4000 cGy in the areas of the growing bones. Survivors with severe hypoplasia sometimes benefit from reconstructive surgery after the bones in the face are fully grown.

Joseph had 12 cycles of chemotherapy and 5000 cGy of hyperfractionated orbital radiation (twice daily for 6 weeks). With this treatment regimen, almost all of his above-the-neck side effects will be due to the radiation, not the chemotherapy drugs. Many of the side effects of radiation on the body are, of course, delayed for months or even years. He will suffer "bony hypoplasia," which means that the bony structures that absorbed radiation (in this case, his right temple and in and around the right orbit) will not grow any more, so his face will look increasingly asymmetrical as he grows up. The doctors are optimistic that it won't be too noticeable since he was turning 5 when treatments were done.

Cataracts—when the lens of the eye becomes opaque—are a frequent late effect of radiation treatment. Cataracts can cause vision loss, but they can often be treated with surgery. Higher doses of radiation cause more damage and shorten the time before cataracts appear. Cataracts appear earlier and become more severe if the child was treated at a young age. In addition, single, larger doses of radiation cause cataract formation more often than the same total dose given in several smaller fractions. Long-term steroid use (including prednisone and dexamethasone) or busulfan chemotherapy can also cause cataracts.

Naomi has had cataracts for the past 6 years as a result of high-dose prednisone and TBI from her BMT (bone marrow transplant). The cataracts are quite different from what we think of in terms of the elderly— they are not visible on the outside of the lens and in fact don't impair her vision. She has maintained 20/20 vision in spite of the cataracts, and there is no indication that that will change. The one thing that she does find is that the contrast of light to dark is affected. She can easily read the ophthalmologist's chart when it has black letters on a white background. The same chart done in tones of gray is very difficult for her to read. Also, white chalk writing on the blackboard is more difficult to read at times. Light really bothers her, either the bright summer sun or the reflection of the sun off the snow. The light hits the cataracts and disperses the light in the eye. So Naomi really needs to wear very good quality sunglasses with good UV (ultraviolet light) protection when out in bright sunlight.

Graft-versus-host disease and/or radiation can cause mild to severely dry eyes. Symptoms include irritation, burning, pain, blurred vision, sensitivity to light, and the feeling that a foreign body is in the eye. Dry eyes can be eased by using artificial tears.

Like most children who are a couple of years out of treatment, Joseph's scans and doctor visits are now more related to dealing with the long-term effects of the rhabdomyosarcoma cure than the disease itself. He has a big cataract on his right eye from the radiation, and his vision in both eyes is rapidly getting worse. He still needs eye drops every 2 hours all day because of damage from the radiation, and he has terrible problems with light sensitivity. But he always manages to compensate and doesn't let anything get in the way of his reading or play or computer games.

Loss of vision can involve central vision (the detailed vision used for reading), or the peripheral visual fields (side vision). Loss of peripheral vision can result from damage to the retina or optic nerve, or damage to the visual areas of the brain from brain surgery.

> I had an ependymoma (brain tumor) 6 years ago when I was 8 years old. I have visual field cuts. I don't see the whole picture that other people see. My peripheral vision is limited, as well as my lower field. This causes me a lot of problems. For example, I can't walk to school by myself right now because I don't notice cars moving on my left side as well as other unpredictable occurrences in city streets. I have to try to remind myself to keep turning my head. I can't follow any visual cues such as pointing, but instead rely on verbal instructions. I'm starting high school this year, so I've been going to the school with my mobility instructor to walk around and memorize the layout. The vision I do have is good, but it's only a fraction of what other people see.

Less common late effects to the eye or eye socket from radiation can include:

- Permanent loss of the eyelashes.

- Hemorrhaging of small damaged blood vessels in the retina (telangiectasias), typically occurring 3 to 5 years after treatment with more than 3000 cGy.

- Adhesions and scarring that limit the ability of the lids to fully close, making the eyes drier.

- Inflammation of the cornea (called keratitis), with sensitivity to light and pain at the surface of the eye.

- Ulcers, holes, or scarring of the cornea after treatment with more than 4000 cGy.

- Glaucoma (increased pressure within the eye), which can also be caused by steroid use.

- Secondary cancers.

Any of the late effects described in this section should be treated by an ophthalmologist skilled in treating survivors of childhood cancer.

> At the time he received the 5000 cGy to his eye, we were told Joseph would probably lose some vision in the treated eye, but they said the effect might be anywhere in the range from barely noticeable to completely blind. It's been 2 years and so far Joseph's vision tests at 20/20. But when I asked the ophthalmologist at the last visit if that meant we were out of the woods, he grimaced and shook his head. He's still

expecting something to show up and says we're not far out enough yet to know what the extent will be. Darn it.

Surgery, stroke, and some medications can also cause problems with the eyes and vision. If there is damage to the part of the brain that controls the muscles that move the eyes, this can result in an eye that does not move normally, and the two eyes not being lined up with one another. If this happens at an early age, the brain may start to ignore one eye, and the eye can lose vision as a result (called amblyopia). Amblyopia may need to be treated with patching therapy (patching the good eye to improve vision in the eye that is not being used). Surgery may help improve the alignment of the eyes, but it can't always restore a full range of movement.

> *Our son had an epidural hematoma (bleeding into the brain) after his surgery to remove a medulloblastoma. One side effect from this was that the left side of his face is partially paralyzed, and his left eye turns in toward his nose. One ophthalmologist told us that surgery can put it back in the right position, but it would forever remain fixed in that one place. After a year of therapy, he can now move the eye up and down and to the right. He can move it a bit toward the left, and his vision has improved.*

• • • • •

> *One of our daughter's seizure medicines caused vision disturbances. She developed tunnel vision and had trouble seeing. We changed the drug and it went away. She's at risk for cataracts from her cranial radiation, so we go to the eye doctor every year.*

Signs and symptoms

When children are old enough to talk, and certainly by school age, visual disturbances are usually detected and treated. However, if changes are gradual, a child may get used to them, and identification of visual late effects can be delayed. The following are signs and symptoms of late effects to the eye:[1]

• Blurry vision

• Double vision

• Blind spots or a decrease in visual field (range of vision)

• Increased sensitivity to light

• Difficulty with night vision

• Floaters across the field of vision that change or light up

• Pain in the eye

- Decreased tearing or excessive tearing/watering of eyes
- Persistent dry, scratchy eyes or eyelids

Screening and detection

You should be seen regularly by an ophthalmologist with experience treating survivors of childhood cancer if you:

- Had total body radiation.
- Received high-dose radiation to one or both of the eyes or nearby structures.
- Received radiation for a brain tumor or leukemia that included an eye in the radiation field.
- Used steroids for a prolonged period.

The ophthalmologist should perform a thorough evaluation that includes evaluation of vision, a test for glaucoma, checking for cataracts, and examination of the retina.

> *My 10-year-old daughter is 6 years out from her retinoblastoma relapse. We see the oncologist and ophthalmologist every 6 months for a checkup. Because she has a 30 percent chance of developing a secondary tumor, she has careful examinations and occasional CT (computed tomography) scans. When she started having headaches, she had an MRI (magnetic resonance imaging). Our doctor is great. When something worries us, she checks it out thoroughly. My daughter has a prosthesis for her eye and needs to go back every 6 months to get it resized and built up.*

Survivors not at high risk for eye damage will usually have a brief eye examination as part of their yearly follow-up examination. This should include a visual examination of the eyes and a vision test using a Snellen letter chart, or a picture chart for children who cannot read letters. Even children as young as age 3 can identify simple pictures on charts specially designed for preschoolers. Any abnormalities should result in a referral to an ophthalmologist.

> *Joseph has not had cataract surgery, but it is expected that he will develop one or more cataracts in the next year or so because of the 5000 cGy directed at the rhabdomyosarcoma in his orbit. We see a pediatric ophthalmologist frequently to stay on top of the late effects, and so far so good. Right after diagnosis the doctors explained the probability of cataracts and the surgery that is done to remove them if they are in the line of vision.*

For additional information about vision tests that you should have based on your specific treatment, you and your healthcare provider can refer to the Children's Oncology Group's survivorship guidelines at *www. survivorshipguidelines.org.*

Medical management

If you have any visual changes, you should be followed by an ophthalmologist skilled in treating survivors of childhood cancer. If you have cataracts or glaucoma, you may need glasses, medications, and/or surgery. Survivors who had one or both eyes removed will need a series of well-fitted prostheses as they grow, and education about caring for the prostheses.

A survivor's healthcare team should also provide referrals to resources to assist with adjustments related to limited vision. Special arrangements should be made with schools to provide preferential seating, eyewear protection, and other necessary accommodations. Long-term follow-up clinics can provide detailed information about educational regulations and opportunities for young people with visual impairments. For more information about education, see Chapter 4, *Navigating the System.*

> *My daughter has cataracts in both eyes due to the total body radiation from bone marrow transplant. Katherine is given dilating drops every morning so she can "see" around the cataracts. Because the dilating drops paralyze the focusing mechanism, Katherine wears bifocals. One lens is for normal vision and the other for reading.*

> • • • • •

> *My daughter was having a lot of problems in kindergarten seeing the board and doing her work. Even though we had been to the ophthalmologist 4 months before, we went back. Her eyesight had deteriorated considerably and was now 20/400 in the one eye, while the other was still 20/30. When we discussed the surgery, the doctor told us that if the capsule had been damaged by the radiation, a replacement lens could not be inserted, and he would not know until they got in and looked. Luckily, the capsule was fine and the new lens works great. Her eye now is 20/80.*

Artificial tears and ointments are used to protect the cornea and preserve vision in survivors with chronic dry eyes. A severe problem with dry eyes can sometimes be fixed by closing the tear draining ducts with either plugs or surgery (called punctal ligation). It also helps to avoid anything that contributes to dry eyes such as wind, fans, smoke, low humidity, or air conditioning.

After our son's surgery for medulloblastoma, the left side of his face was partially paralyzed. His left eye remains partially open all the time. When he first came home, we put drops in his eye every 3 hours and eye lubricant at night. Now we just watch it and use drops if his eye gets red. When the house is dry in the winter, we need to use more.

Survivors who develop corneal ulcerations as complications of dry eyes may need to be treated with antibiotic eye drops.

The major side effect we were warned of that has been a constant problem since treatment has been the radiation damage to the lacrimal gland in his right eye. He needs constant lubrication in that eye because it provides very little moisture by itself. It took us a long time to come up with the best way to keep his eye consistently moist, and in the meantime he had some major problems with corneal abrasions (causing painful light sensitivity) from the eyelid dragging over that dry little eye. Now he gets eyedrops every 2 to 3 hours during the day and a gooey eye ointment every night before bed. Missed drops mean eye damage, so he can't do sleepovers or extended play times with any kid whose parents aren't willing to give him his "drops and goop." How this system is going to work when he's too big to be in my care or the care of the school nurse all the time, I don't know, but I'm not borrowing worries for now. One alternative the doctors have suggested we could seek in the next couple of years may be surgery to "plug" the ducts which drain the eye, so that what little moisture the eye has won't just drain away so quickly.

Radiation-induced cataracts are progressive. Exposing these cataracts to extra sunlight may speed the progression. Sunlight can also aggravate glare symptoms from cataracts. Wearing sunglasses with UV protection when outside may help children and teens with cataracts.

I've had lots of radiation (left flank for neuroblastoma and cranial for leukemia) and years of chemotherapy. I have very bad vision as a result and have worn glasses since the age of 3. I also have small cataracts in both eyes, but they have never caused any problems. My eyes are also incredibly sensitive to sunlight.

Ears

The ear, the organ of hearing, is made up of three main parts: external, middle, and inner ear. The external ear includes the outer portion (auricle) and the external auditory canal. The middle ear is a cavity separated from the external ear by the eardrum, and it contains three small bones. The inner ear contains the cochlea (which is responsible for hearing), the vestibule (which senses position in space and motion), and the semicircular canals (which control equilibrium). Figure 10-2 shows the anatomy of the ear.

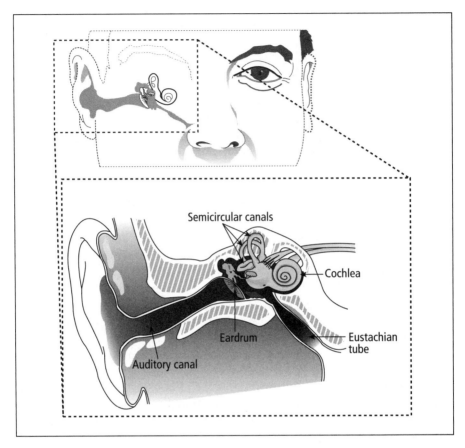

Figure 10-2. Anatomy of the ear

Organ damage

Ears and hearing can be damaged by chemotherapy, high-dose radiation, and some antibiotics.

Chemotherapy

Some anticancer drugs, primarily cisplatin, can cause substantial hearing loss in the high- to ultra-high-frequency range—6,000 to 12,000 Hertz (Hz). If more damage occurs, the lower frequencies also can be affected. Carboplatin is also associated with hearing loss but to a much lesser degree. Radiation to the head can intensify the hearing loss from cisplatin.

My daughter Sarah had an ependymoma treated with radiation when she was 4 and chemotherapy when it returned at age 6. She had a baseline audiology test before the chemotherapy and then another after the second chemotherapy. Because of the change in her hearing, the cisplatin was removed from the remaining two cycles of chemotherapy called for in her protocol. The doctors think that some of the chemotherapy side effects—including the hearing loss—were a result of the chemotherapy compounding damage already done by the radiation. She has high-frequency loss and her low frequencies are at the low end of "normal."

The damage generally occurs in both ears and is irreversible. Sometimes ringing in the ears (tinnitus) or a sensation of drifting in space or having objects drift around you (vertigo) can also occur. Children most at risk for chemotherapy-caused hearing loss are those treated for brain tumors, germ cell tumors, osteosarcoma, and neuroblastoma.

My daughter has mild-to-moderate high-frequency hearing loss after treatment for osteosarcoma. The hearing tests were, she says, the very worst part of cancer treatment because she knew she should be able to hear certain sounds and couldn't. Now, as a college freshman 6 years off treatment, she just got hearing aids. Adjusting to them is difficult, but she wants them and will persevere. She also has constant tinnitus, but she has adjusted to it.

Radiation

Survivors who had head and neck tumors treated with higher doses of radiation and/or older radiation techniques (from the 1950s and 1960s) often develop hearing loss. The most common diseases treated with high-dose radiation that can affect the ears are as follows:

- Nasopharyngeal carcinomas

- Parameningeal sarcomas

- Brain stem gliomas

- Medulloblastomas

- Ependymomas

Ethan's treatment for medulloblastoma, which included cisplatin, caused high-end hearing loss, which means that in rooms with a lot of people he can't hear at all. So at parties, he would kind of zone out because he really couldn't hear what people were saying to him, but in the classroom he was okay. But then he started to have hearing loss that was related to the radiation, and he lost hearing in the voice recognition range. He was only catching about 60–70% of what people were saying. Because of the kind of hearing loss it was, hearing aids were only of limited use, and because he was still growing, they had huge molds that really irritated him. So he didn't wear them.

The good news is that he's learned to lip read. The bad news is that as a 17-year-old high school student he is less adept at letting people know he needs to lip read, so he still misses big chunks of conversation. Ethan is very compliant with all the things that he needs to do related to learning—he sits in the front of the room, he has someone who reads tests to him because he can't read well enough, and all sorts of things that make him "different." But the hearing loss is something he doesn't really get yet. I know adults that had hearing loss as children who assure me that at some point this light bulb will go off for him and he will want to do what he can to compensate for it.

Children treated with less than 2400 cGy of cranial radiation (e.g., for leukemia or prior to stem cell transplantation) rarely develop any late effects in the ears.

Outer ear infections, which are common after high-dose radiation, can impair hearing by drying out and thickening the external ear canal and eardrum. Chronic middle ear infections (otitis media) can also be caused by radiation due to damage to the eustachian tube, which is responsible for drainage of the middle ear. When the eustachian tube cannot drain properly, middle ear infections can become chronic.

One effect that we were not warned of in advance has been a major problem. Joseph's sinuses, and particularly his eustachian tubes, were damaged enough by the 5000 cGy of radiation to the orbit that he has a real problem with sinus infections and ear infections. The sinus infections were worse during the year of chemotherapy but are still an ongoing problem 2 years later. The ear infections are definitely getting worse as the damage to the tubes is apparently making itself known, in conjunction with his existing allergies. His hearing has been so reduced by the fluid buildup lately that he's on Claritin®, and his pediatrician and the ENT (ear, nose, and throat specialist) are talking ear tube surgery.

The glands that produce earwax (cerumen glands) may produce less wax, and what is produced sometimes gets crusty and impacted. While the earwax is impacted, hearing is decreased and trapped moisture can increase the risk for ear infections. This late effect can also occur in survivors who developed graft-versus-host disease after stem cell transplantation. Impacted earwax can be removed by your healthcare provider. Using cotton-tipped applicators or other objects in the ear canal is strongly discouraged because they can actually push impacted earwax further into the ear canal.

Clare was tested post-treatment and she just had a very minor loss in the high-frequency range, probably from gentamicin (an intravenous antibiotic). However, she has had a different type of hearing loss the last few months, in the low-frequency range and more extensive. We have been to the follow-up clinic several times and they decided it was the huge earwax build-up as a result of the radiation.

An extremely unusual late effect of radiation to the ear is inflammation of the cartilage (chondritis), which can lead to cartilage damage and infection. This can occur after radiation doses of more than 7800 cGy given for brain stem gliomas.

The risk factors for permanent hearing loss in children or teens treated for cancer are as follows:

- Treatment with cisplatin, and to a lesser extent, carboplatin
- High doses of radiation to the head and/or neck
- Younger age at time of treatment
- Surgery involving the ear, brain, or auditory nerve
- Treatment with certain antibiotics such as gentamicin and amikacin (generally used for serious infections or fever when blood counts are low)
- Chronic ear infection
- Treatment with diuretics (drugs that help the body get rid of excess water)
- Poor kidney function

Signs and symptoms

Hearing loss should be suspected if your child:

- Does not startle or respond to loud noises.
- Does not respond to your voice consistently.
- Has a hard time understanding or following directions after age 3.
- Does not have clear speech.
- Fails to develop sounds or words that are appropriate for her age.
- Uses gestures instead of words.

Signs and symptoms of hearing loss typically associated with chemotherapy may be less obvious but should be suspected if your child:

- Confuses like-sounding words.

- Drops sounds off words or reports not hearing sounds such as th, f, sh, s, t, k, g, ch, and v.

- Reports he can hear but not understand words and speech.

- Has difficulty hearing in noisy situations or environments.

School-aged children who have lost some hearing may withdraw socially or have trouble in school. They may also describe ringing in their ears or dizziness.

> *My daughter Erin, who was treated for osteosarcoma, lost a fair amount of her hearing due to cisplatin. She doesn't think it's bad enough for hearing aids although they probably would help her a bit. She said when she went to the Young Adults Conference at Camp Mak-A-Dream, everyone who had trouble hearing would tap their ears and say "Cisplatin" as a reminder to speak up!*

Screening and detection

After treatment ends, appointments at the follow-up clinic should include an ear examination to look for infection, wax buildup, and eardrum perforation or scarring. Survivors should also have their hearing tested periodically following completion of treatment, because chemotherapy can have an impact on hearing up to 5 years after completion of the last round. Healthcare providers of survivors who had head or brain radiation may recommend periodic hearing tests because hearing problems can also sometimes develop several years after radiation. Anyone with abnormal test results should be referred to an audiologist or otolaryngologist (ear, nose, and throat doctor) for a thorough evaluation to determination whether assistive technology would be helpful.

> *I had cisplatin to treat my osteosarcoma. I lost some of my high-frequency hearing, but not enough to get hearing aids. It's worse in one ear than the other, because when I'm lying on one side I can hear my college roommate if she's talking, but I can't if I'm lying on the other side. I still get ringing in my ears that lasts for a few seconds then goes away.*

The most widely used method to test the hearing of children with cancer is pure tone audiometry. These tests should be administered by an experienced pediatric audiologist. Extended high-frequency audiometry may be used to test for hearing loss in the high-frequency range (4,000 to 20,000 Hz). This is especially important for younger children with limited language because many consonants ("th", "f", "p", "s") are in this range. If a child cannot hear these consonants it may be very hard for her to acquire clear speech, so early intervention can make an important difference.

Degrees of hearing loss, measured in decibels (dB), are:

- Mild (25–40 dB): Difficulty hearing distant speech, soft voices, or voices in a noisy place.
- Moderate (45–60 dB): Difficulty hearing speech in a quiet place.
- Severe (65–90 dB): Cannot hear loud voices or sounds.
- Profound (more than 90 dB): May hear only very loud sounds, and must rely more on vision than hearing to understand communication if they are not wearing hearing aids or have a cochlear implant.

Children at risk for hearing loss should also be tested for speech and language disorders. Assessments such as the Rossetti Infant Toddler Language Scale (used with children from birth to 36 months), the Preschool Language Scale 5th edition (used on children from birth to age 7), and the Goldman-Fristoe Test of Articulation 2nd edition (used on children ages 2 to 21) are used to identify speech and language disorders and evaluate the effectiveness of hearing aids, auditory training, and speech therapy programs.

Medical management

Medical management includes treating middle or external ear infections, and in some cases, placing tubes in the ears. Survivors with tinnitus (ringing in the ears) may benefit from intervention and should be evaluated by an audiologist or otolaryngologist. State-of-the-art hearing aids are needed for those with permanent hearing impairment. Newer digital technology can minimize background noise and maximize speech sounds, unlike hearing aids of the past. Proper fitting and follow-up testing are crucial. It is also important to develop a routine for maintaining the aids, cleaning the ear molds, and replacing the batteries. Ear molds will need to be replaced periodically; an indication that they should be checked is "feedback" or high-pitched noise coming from the hearing aids. Fostering language development with speech reading and signing is vital for those with profound hearing loss. Using the closed captioning while watching television can also be helpful. Coping with the emotional and psychological effects of hearing loss in children and teens is an essential component of care.

> Sarah wears hearing aids now and it hasn't been a problem. I give full credit to my husband. In the week before she got them, he regularly told her that there was a way to make her hearing better and wouldn't that be great. Sarah's hearing literally went overnight and the hearing aids

brought her hearing back overnight, so she knows what a difference they make. The technician at the hearing clinic let her pick the color of the ear molds. She picked bright pink. Also, in a growing child, the molds have to be replaced quite frequently (we were told probably 2 to 3 times a year).

Educators sometimes need the support and direction of medical caregivers. For instance, an FM system (a special type of assistive listening device) can be used by hearing-impaired children in school to amplify the teacher's voice. The teacher wears a microphone that transmits her voice via radio waves to a receiver that can be attached to the child's hearing aids, in a speaker mounted in the classroom, or to a personal speaker on the child's desk. Your child's healthcare provider should give you detailed information about educational regulations for young people with hearing loss. For more information about education, see Chapter 4, *Navigating the System.*

The American Academy of Audiology offers information about hearing loss on its consumer website at *www.howsyourhearing.org*. Links to various websites related to hearing loss in children can be found at *www.cdc.gov/ncbddd/ hearingloss/links.html*. In addition, the Children's Oncology Group's survivorship guidelines include an informational resource about hearing loss at *www.survivorshipguidelines.org*.

Chapter 11

Head and Neck

I never knew so young a body
with so old a head.

—Shakespeare
The Merchant of Venice

THE HEAD AND NECK can be affected both by tumors that originate in those areas and the treatment used to destroy the tumors. Even treatment for cancers elsewhere in the body can affect the vital structures and functioning of the head and neck. Because many of the tissues and structures located in the head and neck are growing rapidly during childhood and adolescence, they are very susceptible to damage from treatment for cancer.

This chapter covers damage to bones, teeth, glands, and other tissues in the head and neck. Signs and symptoms are listed, and methods to detect late effects in the head and neck are discussed. Finally, medical management of these late effects is outlined.

Organ damage

The parts of the head and neck that most often suffer long-term damage from treatment for childhood cancer are the bones, soft tissues, esophagus, mucous membranes, teeth, salivary glands, and taste buds. For information about the parts of the head and neck not covered in this chapter, see Chapter 10, *Eyes and Ears*, Chapter 8, *Brain and Nerves*, and Chapter 9, *Hormone-Producing Glands*. Some survivors who were treated for tumors in the head and neck do not develop any late effects.

> *My son was treated for Burkitt's lymphoma when he was 2 years old. He had a tumor in one of his tonsils that grew so large he had trouble breathing when he slept lying on his back. They removed the tumor surgically, and treated him for 64 days with Adriamycin®, Cytoxan®, methotrexate, and vincristine. He has absolutely no trouble breathing, swallowing, or talking.*

Bone growth

Bone growth in the skull, face, and jaw can be slowed or stopped by radiation. In the past, when children were given 2400 centigray (cGy) of cranial radiation to prevent leukemia relapse in the central nervous system, the growth of the entire cranium (i.e., bones of the head) would sometimes slow.[1] Cranial radiation can inhibit normal growth and expansion of the skull. This growth disruption is less likely to be found in children given 1800 cGy or less of cranial radiation when they are older than 5 years old.

> I was treated almost 30 years ago for leukemia. I had cranial radiation, but don't know how much they gave me. It did result in a smaller head, but since all of my growth was stunted, it's not so noticeable.

Direct doses of radiation to the jaw of a young child can cause underdevelopment of the mandible (jawbone). Children with parotid tumors or rhabdomyosarcoma in the head or neck receive radiation in this area.

Young children who were given high doses of radiation to the bony orbit of the eye to treat retinoblastoma or rhabdomyosarcoma near the eye often have an altered appearance, because the radiation causes the socket to grow less than the untreated socket. If the radiation is given to only one eye, the face appears more asymmetrical as the child grows.[1]

> I had both eyes removed in 1956 to treat retinoblastoma. I never wore prostheses—just sunglasses. My mom took care of the sockets when I was young, but they are not open now. Not shut tight—just not wide open either. The sockets have never changed size, so I guess they stopped growing when I had the radiation.

Soft tissues

Children or teens treated for rhabdomyosarcoma, nasopharyngeal carcinoma, or sarcomas of the head and neck can have soft tissue damage as well as underlying bone damage in the irradiated areas. Soft tissues can also be affected by scarring and blood vessel damage in the irradiated tissues. Such injuries can slow healing in the area and weaken bones by disrupting blood supply.[2]

Children or adolescents with Hodgkin lymphoma (formerly called Hodgkin's disease) who received mantle radiation are also at risk for underdevelopment of the structures in the areas irradiated, typically resulting in slender necks, narrow chins, and shortened distance between the shoulders.

I had a wonderful visit with a friend who is also a long-term Hodgkin's survivor and we discovered another late effect. It is so strange how these things crop up inadvertently. We were both headed for the same chair and discovered that we both like to have a place to rest our heads. Our necks are thin from atrophied muscles. I just always thought my neck was the only thin place on my body. It never occurred to me that this was a late effect. But she has the same thin neck, a little more pronounced than mine.

Carotid artery disease and an increased risk of stroke have been associated with radiation therapy to the neck in adults. Studies to determine whether survivors of childhood cancer who received radiation therapy to the neck are at risk for developing carotid artery disease are currently being conducted (see Chapter 12, *Heart and Blood Vessels*).

Sinuses

Most children and teens treated with chemotherapy and/or radiation suffer from acute damage to the mucous membranes in the nose and mouth. Many have severe ulcerations or mouth sores that are painful and cause great difficulty with eating and drinking. For the majority of survivors, these sores heal, leaving no lingering difficulties. However, for a small group, mucous membrane changes persist. Scarring in the nasal passages can interfere with normal mucus production and drainage, resulting in chronic sinus infections. Survivors can develop a constant post-nasal drip or a thick, continuous drainage from the nose.

These effects tend to be dose related. The people most likely to suffer from painful sinus infections are those who received high-dose radiation to the mouth and sinuses for rhabdomyosarcoma, Ewing sarcoma, osteosarcoma of the jaw, or Burkitt's lymphoma of the jaw. Children or teens who were given more than 4000 cGy to these areas are most likely to have these problems.

Clare had a chronic sinus condition caused by treatment for nasopharyngeal rhabdomyosarcoma. She had 5400 cGy of radiation. She got a sinus infection every other month and they were debilitating, lasting 2 weeks or so during which she felt terrible and didn't function well. Her doctors postponed surgery for 3 years hoping that it would improve, but it didn't. By then, Clare really wanted the surgery. She just had the surgery 2 weeks ago. After the procedure the surgeon came out to talk to us and he was beaming—a good sign. He said everything went just as he had hoped. They found a lot of obstruction, which they removed, and opened up four holes in her sinuses to promote drainage. Everything was biopsied and all was clear, which we expected, but it was still nice to hear.

• • • • •

Three years ago Joseph was diagnosed with orbital rhabdomyosarcoma. He spent a little more than a year on chemo, had 6 weeks of twice-daily radiotherapy, and three surgeries. His sinuses still show damage from the huge radiation doses, but it doesn't keep him from singing in the Madison Boychoir or enjoying other activities. It just means he needs to stick faithfully to his allergy medicines to avoid another endless round of sinus infections and awful headaches.

Teeth

The development and appearance of teeth can be affected by both radiation and chemotherapy. Radiation is more likely to cause problems when given in high doses to young children. Teeth that have not fully developed and have not yet erupted are also at risk. The damage to these tooth buds can be significant.

I had chemotherapy at 9 months of age to treat neuroblastoma, and cranial radiation and chemotherapy to treat leukemia at age 3. None of my permanent molars came in. I'm 34 and I still have most of my baby molars. A few have fallen out over the years and it's starting to cause me some problems.

• • • • •

Selah has been off treatment for almost 6 years. She received 10 doses of cranial irradiation when she was almost 5. Her 12-year-old molars are malformed due to radiation. We've seen them on the x-rays for years and knew they looked "funny." Now that they're up, they are different.

She also had cavities in them as soon as they erupted. Attaching braces was only possible by using glue because the orthodontist couldn't get a band around those molars. One option down the road will be to remove those and pull the wisdom teeth into place. As I told the orthodontist, "If this is the worst we have to deal with as a long-term side effect, I think we can handle it!"

• • • • •

I'm 27 and had 2400 rads of cranial radiation when I was 5. I've had no problems with my teeth. I didn't even get a cavity until I was 25. I didn't need braces either.

Abnormalities of the teeth that can develop from radiation or chemotherapy include the following:

- Absent teeth

- Abnormally small teeth (called microdontia)

- Short or thin roots

- Small crowns

- Poor bite (called malocclusion)

- Poor enamel

- Incomplete calcification

- Frequent cavities

- Enlarged pulp chambers

- Baby teeth that don't fall out at the usual time during a child's development

> I had radiation for retinoblastoma when I was 2½. When I was 8 years old, I noticed my permanent front teeth were pretty loose. I told my mom and they did a panoramic x-ray and found that I had abnormally small roots on all of my top teeth. They said they could last 2 years or 20 years. Well, I'm 23 now and still have them. I'm careful, though. I don't eat apples or corn on the cob. Just one more thing to deal with.

> • • • • •

> Coley was treated from ages 2 to 3 for hepatoblastoma (a type of liver cancer). She had four rounds of chemo (cisplatin, vincristine, and 5-fluorouracil) prior to surgery and two rounds of chemotherapy after surgery. I saw a spot on her back molar and was hoping that I was seeing things or that it was food stuck in her teeth. After all she had been through, I did not want teeth problems to enter the picture. But, the tooth started to hurt and she became a fanatic about brushing her teeth, hoping that if she cleaned them enough the pain would go away.

> I took her to a pediatric dentist who was just great. He looked in her mouth and said she had several cavities. Some of them he was not worried about because the teeth they were in were due to fall out soon and were not giving her pain, but she had two molars that might not be able to be saved. He also pointed out on the x-rays that the adult teeth under the gums were not the proper size and shape—some were at an angle. He told us that we had major dental work in our future.

Mouth

Saliva is a mix of secretions from the parotid gland (near the ear), sublingual gland (under the tongue), and submandibular gland (under the lower jaw) that lubricates the mouth and aids in taste and digestion. Diminished production of saliva (called xerostomia) affects overall well-being in many ways. A dry mouth can result in food not tasting good, teeth riddled with cavities, bad breath, and bone decay. Even kissing may lose its attraction.

> My daughter had problems with saliva production after chemotherapy and radiation for Hodgkin's. The braces she had were taken off sooner than planned and she had to use little tubes of dental stuff to lubricate her mouth. For a while after radiation, when she sang, she squeaked because of the dry mouth. The doctors told us that after a while the salivary glands would start secreting saliva again, but that she should have plenty of fluids. To this day (10 years later), she is always thirsty and keeps her fridge stocked with every type of drink imaginable.

The dose of radiation to the saliva-producing glands and the percentage of the glands that are radiated affect the amount of saliva produced. Children treated for head or neck soft tissue sarcomas are most at risk. Most glands regain the ability to secrete if the total dose of radiation to the area was less than 4000 cGy.[3] Graft-versus-host disease of the salivary glands can also affect saliva production.

Survivors with persistent problems with dry mouth can find information and support from Sjögren's Syndrome Foundation at (800) 4-SJOGREN or www.sjogrens.org.

> Just prior to my daughter's first radiotherapy session (extended mantle field for Hodgkin's), her radiation oncologist referred her to an oncology dentist for a thorough checkup and consultation. This oncology dentist made a mold of her mouth and had fluoride trays prepared. My daughter was instructed to religiously use a fluoride product (such as GelKam®) in the trays every night. The routine involves squeezing the gel into the trays, then placing them on her teeth for a specified amount of time. After that she removes them and is careful not to eat or drink anything for the rest of the night.
>
> She has religiously followed the fluoride regimen prescribed by her oncology dentist and is having very good success with her teeth. Just yesterday she visited the oncology dentist for her annual checkup. The dentist was very pleased with her diligent efforts. The point here is that

my daughter was forewarned about the devastating effects of radiation on her teeth. Because of this she has been able to prevent the damage that often occurs in survivors after mantle radiation.

• • • • •

I don't know if my dry mouth is a Hodgkin's thing or if it is being caused by my myriad of medications or one of my autoimmune problems. I have had it for 5 years or more. It didn't start until at least 20 years after treatment. I have never gotten used to it, but I am better at coping, except when I choke while eating. I keep a bottle of water with me at all times. I keep a full glass next to my bed. I chew gum more often. My doctor recommended lemon drops (sugar-free). I find that if I drink plenty of water, the dry mouth feels a little better. It is a horrible feeling walking around all day with the same Sahara mouth normal people just wake up with and brush away. The only time I am not thirsty is when I have water in my mouth.

Taste

Changes in taste continue to plague some survivors long after treatment ends. Radiation can cause long-term taste problems because it can destroy the microscopic structures of the taste buds, as well as cause dry mouth by damaging the salivary glands. Lack of saliva affects the taste buds' ability to accurately identify particular tastes. Many survivors crave foods high in salt and sugar, leading to problems with nutrition and dental health.

My daughter is 12 years out from her treatment for ALL (acute lymphoblastic leukemia). She was on a high-risk protocol that included cranial radiation. Her taste for most foods never returned. Prior to cancer, she ate everything with equal gusto. Now she refuses all meat but unseasoned chicken, and she hates most vegetables and fruits. She eats just a few foods, and I give her multivitamins to try to make up what she lacks in variety. She craves sweets, fats, and salt.

• • • • •

Since treatment for Hodgkin's 10 years ago, I find that I enjoy chocolate less and fruit flavors and sugary foods more. This has both positive and negative ramifications. On the positive side, I'd rather have orange sherbet than a Hershey's® bar; on the negative side, I'm a sugar junkie and really love sweets. I've never discussed it with anyone because I'm afraid they'd say I'm using my treatment as an excuse for bad habits. But a few years ago I read the Survivors of Childhood Cancer *book and felt reassured to learn that some survivors with decreased salivary flow post-mantle-radiation (that's me) do report increased cravings for sugary foods or require increased amounts of sugary tastes to satisfy them. It was only a small mention, but somehow I felt like jumping up and down and shouting, "See? See? I'm not crazy!"*

Esophagus

The esophagus is the tube that carries food and liquids from the mouth to the stomach. In Hodgkin lymphoma survivors treated with mantle radiation and others treated with direct radiation to the chest, neck, and spine, stomach acid can flow up into the esophagus, causing a burning sensation and tissue irritation. Over time, the esophagus can swell, causing an inflammation called esophagitis. This condition can be painful and can reduce the desire to eat. Barrett's esophagus (which is changes in the cells of the esophagus) can occur in association with reflux in those whose gastrointestinal tracts were irradiated.

Severe esophagitis can lead to bleeding from the inflamed portion of the esophagus or the formation of scar tissue. This narrowing of the esophagus—called esophageal stricture—is often accompanied by choking and delayed stomach emptying. The combination of these two problems can result in discomfort and weight loss.

In addition, some survivors have trouble swallowing because of damage from a tumor, prolonged vomiting from chemotherapy that damaged the esophagus, or complications from surgery or a tumor in the part of the brain that controls swallowing.

> *I had Hodgkin's disease stage IIA in 1968 and was treated with high-dose radiation. I started having food blockages about 8 years after treatment. At first it was very infrequent, but it soon became a constant problem. I also had a great deal of reflux. The reflux caused a stricture of scar tissue to develop at the lower end of the esophagus, which had to be stretched often. At its worst I got stretched every month. There is some risk in the dilations, especially if your esophageal tissue is thin or compromised in some way. Often my doctors would view the procedure under a fluoroscope to make sure nothing ruptured.*

> *In 1988, I moved and changed doctors. My new doctor taught me to do self-dilation, which was easy enough to do. I used spray anesthetic and inserted a flexible, weighted, rubber tube. I did it once a week. And as the medical research got better, new medications such as Prilosec® have 100 percent managed the reflux. With the reflux gone, the stricture also vanished. I also have motility problems in the esophagus, probably caused by damage to the vagus nerve.*

Vocal cords

Radiation to the neck can cause damage to the vocal cords and changes in the voice. The voice can become high and thin after 3000 cGy or more of radiation to the neck. Hoarseness sometimes occurs at doses greater than 4500 cGy to a radiation field that includes the vocal cords.

Signs and symptoms

Signs and symptoms of damage to the bones in the head and neck are as follows:

- Bone underdevelopment
- Altered or asymmetric appearance

Signs and symptoms of damage to the mouth or throat are as follows:

- Missing teeth
- Crooked teeth
- Cavities
- Small teeth
- Short teeth roots
- Enamel problems
- Dry mouth caused by decreased salivary flow
- Altered taste
- Bad breath

Signs and symptoms of sinus problems are as follows:

- Chronic post-nasal drip
- Chronic discharge from nostrils, especially on the irradiated side
- Pain in cheekbones or above eyebrows
- Headaches
- Bad breath

Symptoms of esophageal reflux are as follows:

- Difficulty and/or painful swallowing (especially dry foods)
- Burning discomfort beneath breastbone (called acid indigestion or heartburn)

- Burning feeling in the throat
- Feeling of food coming back up in the throat
- Bitter or sour taste in the mouth
- Weight loss
- Belching
- Hoarseness
- Breathing problems, such as asthma, coughing, wheezing, or vocal cord inflammation

Screening and detection

Screening for problems in the head and neck starts with a careful physical examination of the sinuses, nostrils, and throat. The examination also includes close attention to how your teeth look, how your breath smells, and the condition of the skin and soft tissues in the head and neck. Your healthcare provider should ask questions about your eating habits and digestion, your dental health, and any pain or discomfort in the head and neck region. This examination should include a discussion of the risks of smoking and chewing tobacco.

If the physical examination and discussion uncover possible sinus infections, a sinus x-ray should be ordered and a referral made to an ear, nose, and throat specialist, if necessary. Survivors with headaches or migraines should be referred to a neurologist for a thorough evaluation.

If you have a history of indigestion, difficulty swallowing, or stomachaches, your healthcare provider at the follow-up clinic may order tests (i.e., an upper gastrointestinal or a barium swallow) to see how the stomach empties. Esophageal strictures or esophagitis should be evaluated and treated by a gastroenterologist.

You should get a complete dental examination and cleaning every 6 months if you are a survivor of childhood cancer. Your dentist should refer you to an orthodontist if you have problems with teeth crowding or improper bite.

> I was not told about late effects to the teeth before my treatment for Hodgkin's. As a matter of fact, my orthodontist left my braces in while I was on treatment. When they took them off, my gums were in such bad shape that they bled and bled. I was not given any fluoride during treatment. When they took off the braces, I had a lot of cavities along the front surfaces.

Two years off treatment, my radiation oncologist asked, "Still using your fluoride?" I had never heard that I was supposed to be using fluoride. When I started using fluoride gel, it made me kind of nauseated. So I switched to the over-the-counter liquid called ACT®. My dentist gave me a lot of good education, and I do really good mouth care now and plan to do it forever.

Medical management

Medical management of late effects in the head and neck depends on your symptoms.

Careful orthodonture is necessary if you have crooked teeth, crowded teeth, or an improper bite. Before beginning any orthodonture, the orthodontist will need to carefully examine a full x-ray of the entire mouth to evaluate root length and general health of teeth.

If your spleen was removed during treatment, discuss with your doctor and dentist the need to take antibiotics prior to invasive medical procedures (for example, a colonoscopy). If you have an endoprosthesis (device used to replace cancerous bone), you may also need to take antibiotics prior to dental work to prevent an infection. Be sure to mention the endoprosthesis and ask about antibiotics when you schedule any dental work or invasive procedures.

Sinus medication is usually the first treatment for chronic sinus problems. In some cases, the ear, nose, and throat specialist may recommend watchful waiting to see if you stop having infections as you grow. In other cases, surgery may be necessary to clear out your sinuses and allow for proper drainage of mucus through your nasal passages.

Frequent fluid intake, especially of water, and artificial saliva may be recommended if you have decreased salivary flow.

If you have esophageal reflux, you may be told to do the following:

- Eat several small meals instead of three big ones.
- Avoid eating for 3 hours before going to bed.
- Raise the head of your bed 4 to 6 inches (not with pillows, the head of the bed needs to be raised).
- Avoid exercising, bending over, or lying down right after eating.
- Lose any excess weight.

- Avoid foods that cause more reflux. Some of the most likely to cause problems are acidic foods such as tomatoes or citrus fruits, and spicy or fatty foods.

- Avoid coffee, tea, chocolate, and alcohol, as they can also worsen reflux.

- Avoid smoking, because smoke prevents the muscle at the bottom of the esophagus from closing properly. Tobacco also decreases saliva.

- Try esophageal dilation (i.e., widening of the esophagus). This procedure may be necessary if you suffer from esophageal strictures.

Problems with reflux require an examination by a gastroenterologist who has experience treating survivors of childhood cancer. Your gastroenterologist may recommend antacids (to neutralize stomach acid), motility medications (to help move food through the digestive system), acid suppressers (to reduce heartburn), or acid blockers (to prevent production of stomach acid).

Chapter 12

Heart and Blood Vessels

The human heart has hidden treasures,
in secret kept, in silence sealed.

—Charlotte Brontë
Evening Solace

CERTAIN TYPES OF RADIATION and chemotherapy can affect the cardio-vascular system (i.e., heart, blood vessels, heart valves, and pericardium). Problems can occur during treatment, or months to years after treatment ends. Because children, teens, and adult survivors can appear well and be active despite heart damage, it is important to know if you are at risk and to obtain careful follow-up treatment to identify and treat problems early. It is also reassuring to find out if your particular treatments did not increase your risk of any of these problems.

This chapter provides a brief description of how the heart, blood vessels, valves, and pericardium function and describes the types of damage that can occur from treatment for cancer. It then discusses signs and symptoms of cardiovascular late effects and how to detect any heart malfunctions. Although some of the symptoms and ways to identify these late effects over-lap, the four main types of damage are discussed separately. Each section ends with a brief description of medical management of cardiovascular late effects.

The heart

The heart is a four-chambered, muscular organ that pumps blood through-out the body. It is approximately the size of a clenched fist and is located beneath the breastbone (sternum) in the center of the chest cavity. It is a hollow organ with thick walls of cardiac muscle. A double-walled sac called the pericardium surrounds it and helps anchor it in place with connections to the diaphragm and sternum.

The heart has two sides, separated by a thick, muscular wall called the sep-tum. The two upper chambers of the heart are called the right atrium and left atrium. The lower chambers are the left and right ventricles. The atria receive blood coming in from the lungs and the body. They squeeze blood into the ventricles, which then pump it out to the lungs and body.

Valves in the heart prevent blood from flowing backward. The valve between the left atrium and the left ventricle is called the mitral valve, and the valve between the right atrium and right ventricle is called the tricuspid valve. Two other valves are located between the ventricles and the major blood vessels; one leads to the lungs (called the pulmonic valve) and the other to the rest of the body (called the aortic valve). Figure 12-1 shows the anatomy of the heart.

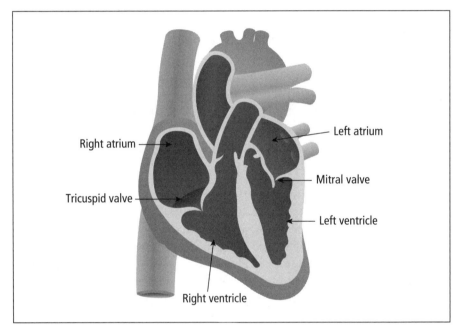

Figure 12-1. Anatomy of the heart

Heart muscle damage from treatment

The muscles in the heart are made up of cells called myocytes. By 6 months of age, an infant heart contains the adult number of myocytes. Further growth of the heart occurs from growth of these existing cells. Chemotherapy drugs called anthracyclines—daunorubicin (Cerubidine®), doxorubicin (Adriamycin®), epirubicin, and idarubicin—sometimes damage or destroy myocytes. The remaining cells enlarge and stretch to try to compensate for the damage. This can cause thin and stiff ventricular walls, which reduce the heart's ability to contract effectively.

My two sons both had Wilms tumor. Danny had 175 mg/m² (milligrams per square meter of body surface area) of Adriamycin® at 1 year old and Bobby had 300. They get echocardiograms every 3 years and will switch to a more frequent schedule when they start puberty. They are both doing great and neither has any late effects of any sort.

If the muscle of the heart is weakened, the heart may not pump as well as usual. This is called cardiomyopathy. Some survivors with early stage cardiomyopathy don't have any symptoms, while others have problems if the heart can no longer keep up with the demands brought on by growth, pregnancy, isometric exercise (e.g., weight lifting, pull-ups, push-ups), or activities of daily life.

Chemotherapy

The number of cells destroyed or damaged is related to the dose of anthracyclines, whether the heart was also irradiated, and other risk factors such as being female and age (children younger than age 2 are at highest risk and younger than age 5 are at high risk). In addition, there are other risk factors that are not yet known or understood.

Anthracyclines can also interfere with the rhythm of the heart and how signals are carried through the heart to make it beat regularly. Children treated with anthracyclines may be at risk for rhythm and conduction problems of the heart that can result in irregular heartbeats, called arrhythmia.

Some protocols incorporate drugs such as dexrazoxane (Zinecard®) to see if they will minimize damage from anthracyclines. During the last 3 decades, researchers have learned more about the long-term cardiac effects of anthracyclines, and lower cumulative doses are now being used whenever possible.[1]

My daughter was treated for rhabdomyosarcoma in the sinuses at age 9. She had radiation to the tumor (none to her chest) and relatively low doses of anthracyclines. Her echocardiogram at the end of treatment was normal. Since she was not at high risk for cardiac damage, the follow-up clinic did an echo 3 years later and found, to our horror, that her ventricles were very thin and her cardiac function was low (shortening fraction in the 20s). She is now enrolled in a clinical trial evaluating whether enalapril will prevent any further heart damage and improve heart function.

All survivors who were given anthracyclines should be periodically checked for cardiac damage for the rest of their lives. It is not clear what dose of anthracyclines is safe, but certainly higher doses at younger ages are more worrisome than lower doses at older ages. Also, many survivors with changes in the pumping ability of the heart have no symptoms and the changes may not at all interfere with life activities. Consequently, it is important for survivors to know about possible cardiac effects, be checked for them on a regular basis, and discuss any abnormal test results with their healthcare providers.

Anthracyclines are not the only drugs that can damage the heart. Very high doses of cyclophosphamide (Cytoxan®) given in preparation for a stem cell transplant may also cause heart damage. The walls of the left ventricle may thicken, leading to heart problems years or decades later. This rare complication may worsen if the child or teen also had radiation to the chest and/ or received anthracyclines.

The risk of developing heart problems may be greatest for survivors who had changes in their cardiac function noted on an electrocardiogram (EKG) or echocardiogram during or shortly after the end of therapy. Very long-term research studies are needed to determine who is most at risk.

Radiation

High-dose radiation can cause several late effects to the heart. Children or teens who received high-dose spinal radiation of more than 3000 centi-gray (cGy), chest radiation (for Hodgkin lymphoma or non-Hodgkin lymphoma), left flank radiation (for Wilms), or radiation directly to the heart are possibly at risk. Modern radiation techniques using lower total doses, hyperfractionation (smaller doses more often), and cardiac shielding (protecting the heart from radiation) are much less likely to cause damage. It is hoped that the use of proton therapy will reduce damage to healthy organs.

Whether the heart sustains injury after radiation treatment depends on several factors, including the following:

- Total radiation dose
- Dose of radiation fractions
- Amount and areas of the heart treated
- Presence of tumor in or next to the heart
- Chemotherapy drugs used

Age, weight, blood pressure, family history, smoking, and cholesterol levels do not change the likelihood of developing heart damage, but can magnify its effect later in life in those who have damage.

> I had 300 mg/m² of Adriamycin® and 2500 to 2800 cGy of mantle radiation to treat my Hodgkin's disease. I get echocardiograms periodically, and so far they have been fine. The echo technician always turns the screen around and explains what he's doing. I appreciate that.

Damage to the heart muscle from high-dose radiation can lead to restrictive cardiomyopathy and arrythmias. Restrictive cardiomyopathy is when the heart muscle becomes stiff and the heart cannot adequately fill with blood. This may lead to problems in the pumping action of the heart. Valves in the heart can also be damaged by radiation (see later section in this chapter about valve damage).

Signs and symptoms

Restrictive cardiomyopathy. Restrictive cardiomyopathy can develop months, years, or decades after treatment for childhood cancer ends. The early signs and symptoms of restrictive cardiomyopathy include the following:

- Increasing fatigue
- Decreased ability to exercise
- Shortness of breath, especially with exercise
- Feeling full after only a few bites of food
- Increased difficulties with regular activities of daily life

If you have any of the risk factors for heart damage, these signs and symptoms should prompt you to get a thorough evaluation of your heart. Fatigue alone can be caused by a multitude of things, but if it is getting worse or is accompanied by other symptoms, get it checked out.

Later signs and symptoms of restrictive cardiomyopathy include the following:

- Swollen lower legs and feet (called edema)
- Rapid or irregular heartbeat
- Rapid breathing
- Difficulty exercising
- Dizziness
- Chest pain

Arrhythmia. The electrical pathways that control the heart's rhythm can be damaged by treatment, which can result in arrhythmia (i.e., abnormally fast, slow, or irregular heartbeat). You may be asymptomatic or may have some of the following symptoms:

- Palpitations (a feeling that the heart is beating strongly)
- Rapid heartbeats
- Skipped beats
- Dizziness or lightheadedness
- Fainting

Some healthcare providers (doctors and nurse practitioners) are not aware of the risks for heart problems from your treatment for childhood cancer. If you find this to be the case, get a second opinion from a healthcare provider who is well versed in cardiac late effects associated with cancer treatment.

> My radiation-induced cardiac disease was misdiagnosed for years and I almost died. I counsel other survivors to seek out a cardiologist who has seen some irradiated hearts. It wasn't until I saw a very experienced doctor at a major medical center that my congestive heart failure was correctly diagnosed, although I had seen many cardiologists. It took someone who had seen many, many irradiated hearts to know what to look for.

> When I was in a medically oriented graduate program, they taught us this little saying, "When you hear hoofbeats, think horses, not zebras." That was to warn us to think about the most common things that go wrong with a person, not to think about the exotic or unusual. When someone my age (late 40s) ends up with an inflamed pericardium, viral pericarditis would be the horse. But with a history of mantle radiation, you have to think zebras.

The signs and symptoms for radiation-induced heart damage vary widely. Most damage is caused by higher doses (more than 4000 cGy) and older radiation techniques. Children and teens treated for Hodgkin lymphoma with mantle radiation using modern doses and heart shielding appear to be less likely to develop heart problems, but they still need to be followed over time to see if any long-term late effects develop. Some of the coronary arteries cannot be protected by shielding because of their location. Survivors who were treated in the 1960s and 1970s and those who received high doses of radiation to the chest need to be followed closely to monitor heart function.

Screening and detection

Survivors at risk for late cardiac damage are those who received anthracyclines and/or radiation to the heart (which can occur during radiation to the chest, whole lung, left kidney, and possibly the spine). Even if there are no symptoms, any survivor who received these therapies should have an annual examination to identify risk for cardiac deterioration, to help decide the best medical management, and to guide lifestyle choices. The minimum testing should include:

- Thorough medical history.

- Fasting blood levels of cholesterol, HDL, and LDL (only for adults).

- Physical examination.

- Chest x-ray.

- Echocardiogram.

- 12-lead EKG.

- Cardiac stress test, which may be used in survivors who have abnormalities noted on EKG and echocardiogram or in patients who received intensive treatment that may damage the heart.

> My daughter had Wilms tumor many years ago. Our clinic doesn't have a follow-up program per se, they just see us once a year and take blood and x-rays and ask if she's having any problems. Since her protocol back then was surgery and high doses of actinomycin D, vincristine, and Adriamycin®, I asked them last year to do an echocardiogram. They said they only do it if there's a problem, but I said it would make me feel better if they did it. We went around and around. I finally just put my foot down and said, "I want it." They did it, it was fine, and now I feel better.

The type of routine cardiac screening for survivors of childhood cancer depends on the treatment received. For cardiomyopathy, an echocardiogram is done (how often is based on a variety of factors). Cardiac magnetic resonance imaging (MRI) provides additional information for survivors diagnosed with cardiomyopathy. Routine screening for survivors who received treatment that could affect the heart must be performed for the rest of their lives.

Intervals between screenings may be longer for those at lesser risk. Ongoing research studies are helping to define the types of evaluations necessary and determine how often they need to be done. See Table 1 at the end of this chapter for more information.

In addition, any survivor at risk for cardiac problems should get a baseline evaluation and systematic follow-up testing when about to undergo increased stress to the heart. Following are examples of activities that stress the heart:

- Starting an exercise program
- Being pregnant
- Getting general anesthesia
- Taking growth hormone
- Doing isometric weight lifting (bench presses or squats)

Any changes in the EKG or other cardiac tests require a consultation with a cardiologist experienced in treating survivors of childhood cancer.

> I had Adriamycin® as part of my treatment for osteosarcoma. In my first year of college, I started having severe chest pains that would last from a few seconds to 5 or 6 minutes. Then my chest would ache for a long time afterwards. The pains would frequently wake me up at night. If I got upset it would hurt even more. I went back to my oncologist and he did an EKG and an echocardiogram. He said there was an irregularity, but it was nothing to worry about. I still get the pains once or twice a month.

In the example above, it would be a good idea to find out exactly what the "irregularity" was and to request a referral to an experienced cardiologist for further evaluation. Some survivors report that they have to insist on referrals because they are often young and healthy looking and may see healthcare providers who are not familiar with cardiac late effects from cancer treatment.

> My son's first Wilms tumor stretched from his diaphragm to his bladder. He had 2400 rads (cGy) of left flank radiation that included his spinal cord. When he relapsed, he had more radiation plus lots of cyclophosphamide. They could not shield his left ventricle that time because of the position of the tumor. He started getting pneumonia frequently, had a bad cough, and was really tired all of the time. We were worried so we got a second opinion from an expert in late effects (our hospital did not have a follow-up clinic at the time). She said that kids who had left side Wilms and received radiation do get some radiation to the heart. So taking that into account along with the Adriamycin®, whole lung radiation, and boost to the para-aortic area, she said he must have follow-up and we have to take seriously that heart damage is a possibility. So he had an echocardiogram and an EKG, and is scheduled for pulmonary function tests.

In the example above, the parents went to an expert and their son is getting appropriate follow-up. Many survivors with heart damage have no symptoms, so it is especially important to get thorough follow-up from a health-care provider with experience treating survivors of childhood cancer.

Medical management

Routine screening for damage to the heart is usually done by pediatric oncologists or internists. If abnormalities are identified (e.g., pericardial thickening, ventricular wall stiffness), a referral to a cardiologist with experience treating survivors of childhood cancer should be made.

> My son was diagnosed with high-risk T-cell ALL (acute lymphoblastic leukemia) in 1996. His white blood cell count was 465,000. He was supposed to get 360 mg of doxorubicin but only received 300. It did some damage to his heart and he was put on enalapril. After his last echo, the cardiologist said his heart was functioning in the normal range. He said he would have to be followed closely when he goes through puberty and the teen growth spurts, due to strain that the heart goes through at that time.

Treatment of cardiomyopathy from anthracyclines or radiation may include ACE inhibitors (such as enalapril) and beta blockers. Cardiac glycosides (such as digoxin) and diuretics, such as furosemide (Lasix®), are also used for survivors with congestive heart failure. In some rare cases of severely progressive disease, heart transplantation is considered.

> The wall of Clare's left ventricle has thinned due to Adriamycin® and her heart function is low normal. She had a dose well below the supposed threshold for heart changes, but they are now finding that some patients are having damage at the lower doses, though not many. No one knows the prognosis, but her doctors are optimistic that it is good. She is enrolled in a double-blind, placebo-controlled, randomized study using enalapril. After 10 months she is doing fine, and her heart function and wall thickness are stable, so we suspect she is really on the drug, but who knows.

Cardiac rehabilitation may also improve heart function and quality of life for survivors with heart damage.

> I started cardiac rehab back in the early spring after my last visit with the cardiologist, who had nothing to offer for either my pain or my increasing shortness of breath. I suggested a course of cardiac rehab, but he was very reluctant, saying that it was contraindicated in cases of restrictive cardiomyopathy. I pushed on with this plan with him and my insurance company.

The first sessions were ugly! It was hard to see just how little I could do and how easily I ran out of breath. But in the first two sessions I did learn that if I walked very slowly, I could walk for a very long time without becoming short of breath. Now we are talking a snail's pace here, but it was comforting to know and helped in my everyday life because I had a lot more energy and could last a lot longer if I just slowed myself down. I also made the first big discovery about my pain. Some of what I had been calling chest pain was really neck, shoulder, and back pain. And with that knowledge I could make some interventions to help with that. So I have started doing some of my old jazz dance relaxation exercises, and that pain has decreased noticeably. Progress is slow but steady.

Lifestyle counseling is necessary for survivors with heart damage. The discussion should emphasize eating a healthy diet, maintaining a normal weight, developing an exercise program, reducing stress, and not smoking cigarettes or using street drugs. Many healthcare providers caution survivors at significant risk for heart problems to limit isometric exercise as it can stress the heart, but they encourage aerobic exercise. Examples of isometric exercises are weight lifting, wrestling, football, and rock climbing.

Some over-the-counter medications include ingredients that can stress the heart; it's important to read labels and avoid taking medicines that have pseudoephedrine in them. Many illegal drugs (such as cocaine and various forms of amphetamines, including ecstasy and crystal methamphetamine) stress the heart and should not be taken. A rapid rise in blood alcohol levels can cause an irregular heartbeat, so excessive or binge drinking should be avoided. Some prescription drugs can be toxic to the heart. If you have cardiac problems, get a list from your cardiologist of medications to avoid. Pregnant survivors at risk for heart damage from anthracyclines should see an obstetrician who specializes in high-risk pregnancy, as well as a cardiologist.

Preventing heart problems

You cannot prevent the damage already done to the heart from chemotherapy or radiation. However, you can control some things that can lessen your risk of heart damage worsening as you age. To keep your heart as healthy as possible, you can:

• Not smoke (or quit if you smoke now).

• Not use drugs that stress the heart such as cocaine, ephedra, diet pills, or sport performance-enhancing drugs.

- Eat only healthy fats, and make sure they don't make up more than 30 percent of your calories.

- Maintain a healthy body weight.

- Exercise at least 30 minutes every day (but if you have heart problems now, check with your cardiologist before starting an exercise program and minimize isometric exercises).

- See a cardiologist if you are female, plan to get pregnant, and had anthracyclines and/or radiation to your heart.

Blood vessels

The human body has three types of blood vessels: arteries, veins, and capillaries. Arteries are large vessels that carry blood away from the heart. They branch into smaller arteries and then into arterioles. Arterioles eventually split into capillaries, which are vessels so small that blood cells have to flow through single file. The thin walls of the capillaries allow exchange of gases (i.e., oxygen and carbon dioxide), nutrients, and waste products. Capillaries merge into venules, which in turn merge into veins. Veins return blood to the heart.

The arteries that carry oxygen to the heart muscle itself are called coronary arteries.

Organ damage

The interiors of healthy blood vessels are usually smooth, but radiation can roughen them inside. These rough spots provide sites for fatty deposits (plaques) to develop in coronary arteries and other arteries and veins. Calcium deposits can harden the plaques, resulting in atherosclerosis (hardening of the arteries). When this happens in the coronary arteries in the heart, it is called coronary artery disease.

Survivors of Hodgkin lymphoma have been studied extensively due to the risk of vascular injury in the field of radiation (e.g., carotid arteries in the neck). An inflammatory process that damages the endothelial lining of the blood vessels is suspected. In these studies, survivors of Hodgkin lymphoma who did not have neck irradiation also had increased premature carotid artery disease and the reason is not yet understood.[2,3]

Atherosclerosis can cause three problems. First, the fatty deposits narrow the blood vessels, reducing flow of blood. Second, layers of plaque decrease the strength and elasticity of the arteries. Third, plaques roughen the lining of the vessel, allowing platelets to form clots at the rough spots. If a clot breaks free, it can block blood flow in narrow arteries, reducing or stopping the supply of oxygen to that area. When oxygen is slowed to areas of the heart, angina (chest pain) results. If the clot blocks a coronary artery completely, it causes a heart attack.

The tendency to develop atherosclerosis is related not only to treatment for childhood cancer, but also to family history, weight, and lifestyle choices such as diet, exercise, and smoking.

• Smoking vastly increases the risk of heart disease. The nicotine in cigarettes increases the heart rate and accelerates plaque formation that narrows arteries. It also damages the lungs, reducing their efficiency. Consequently, the heart must pump faster to deliver adequate oxygen to the cells of the body.

• A diet high in saturated fat (e.g., red meat, dairy foods, and eggs) can lead to high levels of cholesterol. This can increase the chance of developing fatty deposits in the arteries, making a heart attack or stroke more likely.

• Exercise helps maintain a healthy weight, increases lung capacity, and strengthens body muscles, including the heart. A note of caution is that if you received anthracyclines or radiation to the heart, you should consult your follow-up healthcare provider prior to starting an exercise program.

• High blood pressure (over 140/90 mm Hg) is a risk factor for heart disease and promotes atherosclerosis.

A healthcare provider who specializes in treating survivors of childhood cancer cautions:

> *A significant problem that we are just beginning to understand is the effect of cranial radiation and chemotherapy in promoting premature coronary artery disease. Leukemia (ALL) survivors, especially those treated with cranial radiation, have an increased incidence of obesity and are more likely to be physically inactive. Obesity and physical inactivity at a young age are significant risk factors for the development of high blood pressure, diabetes, and dyslipidemia (high LDL cholesterol, low HDL cholesterol, high triglycerides) and these aid in the development of premature coronary artery disease. Because of this, it is essential that survivors exercise, eat a prudent diet, and get regular follow-up.*

To slow the atherosclerotic process and help keep blood pressure low, you should:

• Eat a diet low in saturated fats, cholesterol, salt, and processed foods.

- Eat whole grains, fruits, and vegetables.
- Eat foods high in fiber.
- Exercise regularly (30 minutes every day).
- Keep body fat low.
- Limit alcohol intake (including beer).

Your physician may prescribe medications to lower your blood pressure.

Medical problems such as hypothyroidism, high blood pressure, high cholesterol, and diabetes can increase your risk of developing atherosclerosis.

Another problem that can occur after cancer treatment is development of thick and ropy blood vessels caused by chemotherapy damage. Currently, most children and adolescents get chemotherapy through implanted catheters. In earlier years, however, all medications were given through peripheral IVs (using a needle in an arm or hand vein). If the vein burst, the drugs leaked into the surrounding tissue, causing damage and scarring. Sometimes the scar tissue from such damage forms on the inner walls of the blood vessels, leaving them hard and inelastic.

> I was diagnosed with neuroblastoma when I was 5 months old in 1966. Back then they didn't have central lines so I had 3½ years of intravenous (IV) sticks. My veins got very hard so they placed IVs in my head, feet, and hands—pretty much everywhere they could find an open vein. My veins are still hard now, and I don't think anyone could ever get a needle into my left arm. The veins in that arm are like a solid rope. My right arm has softened up. Other than that, I have no side effects from all those years of treatment.

Raynaud's phenomenon can also develop in long-term survivors with vascular disease. This is when the fingers and toes become white or bluish due to spasms of the arteries leading to the hands. It is usually precipitated by cold or emotion, and affected individuals often have a genetic predisposition for developing Raynaud's. This may also occur in survivors treated with bleomycin. The condition is usually chronic, but it may improve slowly over several years in some survivors.

Signs and symptoms

Risk of coronary artery disease and heart attack is lower for patients who had lower doses of radiation (less than 4000 cGy) using modern techniques and higher for patients treated with high doses of radiation and no heart shielding. Signs and symptoms of coronary artery disease are as follows:

- Chest pain (or pressure-like sensation)
- Chest, neck, or jaw pain upon exertion
- Indigestion upon exertion
- Shortness of breath upon exertion

Symptoms of inadequate oxygen to the heart and heart attack are as follows:

- Crushing chest pain
- Pain or numbness down the left arm
- Shortness of breath
- Sweating
- Nausea
- Feelings of impending doom

Many of these signs and symptoms can be caused by other illnesses or conditions; however, it is prudent to get an evaluation if any of these symptoms are present.

Screening and detection

Screening and detection for coronary artery disease includes some of the tests described above for the heart. A stress test is also needed. Routine cholesterol screening for those at risk for coronary artery disease is also essential.

Medical management

Medical management should involve frequent surveillance for symptoms in at-risk survivors. A variety of medications and lifestyle modifications are used to treat coronary artery disease. Advanced coronary artery disease is sometimes treated with a coronary artery bypass graft (open heart surgery) or balloon dilation angioplasty.

Heart valves

The valves that control the flow of blood in the heart can become stiff or leaky after high-dose radiation to the chest (e.g., mantle radiation to treat Hodgkin lymphoma).

Signs and symptoms

Valvular disease may be asymptomatic or it may cause symptoms such as the following:

- Shortness of breath
- Fatigue
- Palpitations
- Rapid heartbeat
- Swelling of ankles
- Prominence of veins in the neck
- Cough
- Difficulty with exertion

Screening and detection

Regular and lifelong screening using an echocardiogram is done to check for possible valve problems caused by radiation to the heart. See Table 1 at the end of this chapter for recommended screening schedules.

> *I was treated for 10 years for leukemia and I had three relapses. In my 20s, I started having severe chest pains so I went to a cardiologist. He did a brief exam and said I had mitral valve prolapse and there was nothing that needed to be done. He gave me a pamphlet on my way out, and the pamphlet said mitral valve prolapse could only be confirmed with an echocardiogram, which I never had. So I asked my oncologist to recommend a cardiologist and I got another opinion. He ran a battery of tests and said my heart was fine. He thought it could be stress or esophageal reflux.*

Medical management

Medical management should involve frequent surveillance for symptoms in at-risk survivors. A variety of medications and lifestyle modifications may be used to treat heart valve damage. Severe damage to valves in the heart may require surgery to replace the valves. This care should be directed by a cardiologist.

> *I had 18 treatments of mantle radiation when I was 15 years old in 1971. I don't know how many rads. Heck, back then they didn't even tell you that it was cancer. I had a slight heart murmur for years that went from a whisper to a waterfall after a fever. When I lie on my side I can*

hear it: boom, squish, boom, squish. I had a transesophageal echocardiogram and it showed stenosis of the mitral and aortic valves. I take medicine to slow my heart rate, and the valve problem has not worsened. Eventually I'm going to need the valves replaced. Right now I can walk on flat surfaces for an hour, but I have a really hard time on inclines. I can't do heavy work like shoveling snow or raking leaves.

If you have valve damage or have had a valve replaced, you should take an antibiotic before dental work or any other invasive procedure (such as a colonoscopy). The antibiotic can help prevent endocarditis, a serious heart infection caused by bacteria entering the bloodstream during the procedure. The healthcare provider who will do the procedure (dentist or doctor) should write the prescription for you.

Pericardium

Pericarditis is an inflammation of the sac surrounding the heart. Acute pericarditis usually occurs during treatment or within the first year after treatment. Delayed acute pericarditis, a rare occurrence, usually resolves within a few months but may persist for years.

Constrictive pericarditis occurs when the sac surrounding the heart becomes tough and inelastic. This can result in an accumulation of fluid that can interfere with the heart's ability to pump efficiently. Constrictive pericarditis can occur years after treatment.

Signs and symptoms

The signs and symptoms of delayed acute pericarditis include the following:

• Fever

• Shortness of breath

• ST wave changes (elevation) on the EKG

The signs and symptoms of constrictive pericarditis include the following:

• Chest pain

• Wheezing

• Shortness of breath

• Decreased ability to exercise

> *I had nighttime coughing and I couldn't sleep at night unless the head of the bed was raised. The coughing and wheezing was much less during*

the daytime. In my case, the pericarditis was misdiagnosed over a period of 2 years as adult onset asthma and anxiety. Even when I was in severe cardiac failure, I was sent home from the emergency room twice because no one expected to see a healthy-looking 47-year-old with congestive heart failure. I had emergency cardiac surgery to relieve an impending tamponade of the heart and again was misdiagnosed as having viral pericarditis. It was only when I went to Stanford that they correctly diagnosed the radiation damage to both the pericardium and heart muscle. I had a thoracotomy (opened the chest) and they removed a piece of the pericardium to allow the fluid to drain. Mind you, this was all 26 years post-treatment: 5100 rads (cGy) to mantle, 3100 rads to para-aortic chain followed by four sets of MOPP (a combination of chemotherapy drugs).

Screening and detection

Screening for pericarditis is the same as for other cardiac problems. However, if you develop any of the symptoms listed above, you should see your health-care provider immediately to get an examination. Pericarditis can develop quickly and can be life threatening.

I had 4400 rads (cGy) of mantle radiation, 4400 to the mediastinum, and 4400 to the diaphragm and spleen area in 1968 to treat my Hodgkin's disease. My pericardium became so fibrous that I almost died. They kept me in the hospital for a month to stabilize me, and then I had the pericardium removed during open chest surgery. It gave me immediate relief from the pain and heart arrhythmia, but I had problems healing since my skin is so fragile from the radiation.

Medical management

Radiation-induced pericarditis is treated with medications and sometimes with surgery.

This medical information can be a two-edged sword. Key for me has been with each new health challenge to find out what things I can do to help myself. For example, when I was in the hospital waiting for my pericardial stripping, I made it my job to eat at least 2,000 calories a day. I had lost a lot of weight and had no reserves. It turned my whole attitude around to have something important to do that would make a difference in the outcome, even though all the meds and surgery were being done by professionals. With information there is always the potential empowerment of each of us to make a difference in whatever we are faced with.

Recommended test schedules

Although recommendations evolve as more research is done, the current recommendations for heart evaluations after taking anthracyclines and/or having radiation to the heart are contained in the following table, which is based on the Children's Oncology Group follow-up guidelines (*www.survivorshipguidelines.org*).[4]

Table 1: Recommended Cardiac Follow-Up

Age when treated with anthracyclines or radiation	Radiation to the chest	Total dose of doxorubicin, daunorubicin, epirubicin, and/or idarubin	Schedule for echocardiogram
Younger than 1 year old	Yes	None	Every year
		Any	Every year
	No	< 200 mg/m²	Every 2 years
		≥ 200 mg/m²	Every year
Ages 1 to 4	Yes	None	Every year
		Any	Every year
	No	< 100 mg/m²	Every 5 years
		≥100 to < 300 mg/m²	Every 2 years
		≥ 300 mg/m²	Every year
Ages 5 and older	Yes	None	Every year
		< 300 mg/m²	Every 2 years
		≥ 300 mg/m²	Every year
	No	< 200 mg/m²	Every 5 years
		≥ 200 to < 300 mg/m²	Every 2 years
		≥ 300 mg/m²	Every year

Chapter 13

Lungs

*The living body is a machine which
winds its own springs: the living image
of perpetual motion.*

—Julien Offroy de la Mettrie

TREATMENT FOR CHILDHOOD CANCER can affect how well the lungs function, which can involve your comfort, ability to exercise, and overall quality of life. This chapter begins with a description of the lungs and how they work. It outlines the types of damage that can occur from treatment and how healthcare providers identify and treat late effects involving the lungs. Several survivors describe how their lungs have been affected by treatment and how they cope with these late effects.

The respiratory system

The respiratory system consists of the lungs and various structures that allow air to enter the lungs. Most air enters the body through the nose. As it passes through the nose and nasal cavity, it is warmed, moistened, and filtered.

The pharynx (throat) is the area where the passages from the nose and mouth come together. This area leads to the esophagus (a tube to the stomach) and the larynx (which contains the vocal cords). When you swallow, a flap of tissue called the epiglottis covers the larynx to prevent food from getting into the lungs.

The larynx leads to the trachea—the main passageway to the lungs. The lungs are two organs that surround the heart and fill up most of the space in the ribcage. The lungs are divided into sections called lobes. The left lung is slightly smaller and has fewer lobes than the right lung.

The trachea branches into two tubes called bronchi, which divide into smaller and smaller tubes called bronchioles. These tiny tubes end in air sacs called alveoli. The air you breathe carries oxygen that moves across the air sac walls into blood in capillaries in exchange for carbon dioxide.

This carbon dioxide exits the body when you exhale. Figure 13-1 shows the respiratory system.

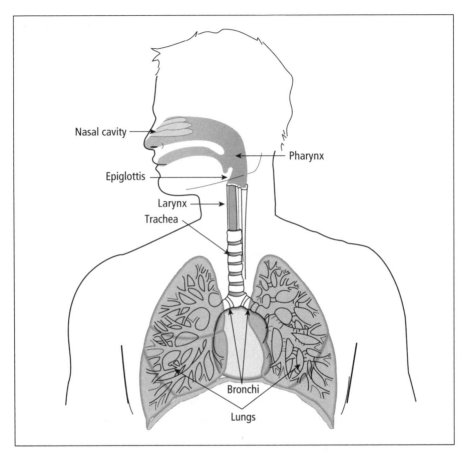

Figure 13-1. The respiratory system

Organ damage

A healthy adult's lungs can hold up to 6 liters of air. During quiet breathing, only about half a liter of air is exchanged. Lung damage from treatment can reduce your lungs' ability to expand and thus the amount of air they can hold (called restrictive lung disease). Lung growth and chest size can be affected in some survivors who were treated at a very young age. Treatment can also cause scarring in the lungs (called pulmonary fibrosis), which reduces the exchange of oxygen for carbon dioxide in the air sacs. Obstructive lung disease (narrowing of the airways) can also occur. A combination of these problems can develop after treatment for childhood cancer.

Lungs can be damaged by both radiation and chemotherapy. Certain types of chemotherapy drugs can intensify the damaging effects of radiation. Lung damage is common in survivors of transplants who develop chronic graft-versus-host disease. In addition, the parts of the body that house the lungs and help them expand and contract can be damaged by radiation. A study of more than 500 children and teens who were seen in a comprehensive follow-up clinic found that almost 13 percent of the survivors had some type of pulmonary late effect, although the vast majority of the problems were mild or moderate.[1]

Radiation

As shown in Figure 13-1, the lungs are in the chest. If the chest is irradiated during childhood or adolescence, the growth of bones in the area (spine, ribs, and sternum), as well as growth of muscles in the chest wall, can be slowed or stopped. Survivors who had mantle radiation, for example, often have smaller chests than do those treated only with chemotherapy. This reduces the area in which the lungs can expand and contract. Survivors who received radiation to one side of the body (e.g., those treated for Wilms tumor) can develop curvature of the spine (scoliosis) that can also affect the space occupied by the lungs. The incidence of scoliosis has been greatly reduced because recent protocols include the entire backbone (vertebral body) in the field of radiation, which results in a symmetrical reduction of growth.

A small number of children and adolescents who received high-dose radiation to the lung area develop radiation pneumonitis during treatment. They may recover from the pneumonitis on their own, or they may require treatment with corticosteroids for a period of time. If the pneumonitis worsens, it can result in pulmonary fibrosis. Pulmonary fibrosis occurs when lung tissue becomes scarred and loses its elasticity. The amount of air the lungs can hold (lung volume) is then reduced and the amount of gases exchanged (oxygen and carbon dioxide) is lowered.

Fibrosis can develop months to years after treatment, and it can either stabilize or continue to progress. Symptoms depend on the amount of lung involved. Fibrosis usually occurs in those who had tumors in the chest or lungs (e.g., Hodgkin lymphoma, Ewing sarcoma, primitive neuroectodermal tumors, or lung metastases from cancers in other locations) and were treated with radiation. It can also occur in survivors who received total body radiation (TBI) as part of their preparation for stem cell transplantation.

I had high-dose mantle radiation 27 years ago. I have become progressively more short of breath. My pulmonologist ordered a CT (computed tomography) scan that revealed little burn marks on my lungs. Conventional x-rays showed nothing. I also have areas of calcification where the Hodgkin's disease was in my lungs. I use three different inhalers: Ventolin®, steroids, and a long-term bronchodilator.

The risk of developing pulmonary fibrosis or other pulmonary late effects is highest in survivors who received:

- A total dose of 1500 centigray (cGy) or higher of radiation to the lungs.

- A single dose of 600 cGy or higher to the lungs.

- TBI of 1200 cGy.[2]

- TBI combined with any additional chest irradiation.

- Any radiation to the chest combined with bleomycin, busulfan, BCNU, CCNU, doxorubicin, or dactinomycin.[3]

Survivors who were treated in the 1960s and 1970s with very high doses of radiation to the lungs (for example, mantle radiation for Hodgkin lymphoma) can have very severe and sometimes life-threatening fibrosis. Children or teens who get relatively low doses of radiation—less than 1500 centigray (cGy) given in fractions—may develop mild or moderate restrictive pulmonary disease, but it usually does not affect daily life activities. Most of these survivors can participate in sports and lead active lives.

In early bone marrow transplants (BMTs), children were sometimes given 1000–1200 cGy of radiation in a single dose. These survivors have an increased risk of moderate to severe fibrosis. Currently, fractionated (getting smaller doses more frequently) radiation is sometimes used prior to stem cell transplants or for tumors requiring radiation to lung areas. Lower doses of radiation given daily do not usually cause lung problems that affect the ability to lead an active life.

I had a transplant 12 years ago when I was 7 years old to treat AML (acute myelogenous leukemia). I had total body radiation, but have had no lung problems since then.

• • • • •

Katie had TBI (total body irradiation) prior to her BMT at age 17 months. Her lung function tests at 5 years post-BMT were completely normal. She does not have restrictions on any activity. She loves athletics.

My 12-year-old daughter had a bone marrow transplant 5 years ago for AML. She got 1200 cGy of radiation in seven fractions. The transplant was in May, and by September she was crawling down the hallway croaking that she couldn't breathe. Her breathing was so loud you could hear it throughout the house. It was scary. She was diagnosed with scarred lungs. She had only 50 percent lung capacity.

When she finally went off the cyclosporine 2½ years ago, her lung capacity went up to 75 percent. Then she got mono, which did more lung damage, and she's now at 62 percent. Most of the time she's okay. If she gets a sinus infection, though, it goes down into her lungs, and we are back to the nebulizer and chest PT (physical therapy) every 2 to 4 hours around the clock for weeks. We all get pretty exhausted.

In one study it was noted that survivors of acute lymphoblastic leukemia (ALL), who were treated in the 70s and early 80s move a lower volume of air and have a decreased ability to exercise. Although not well understood, these late effects seem to be associated with lung infection during treatment, craniospinal radiation, and the chemotherapy drug cyclophosphamide.[4]

Chemotherapy

Pulmonary fibrosis can also be caused by some chemotherapy drugs, such as bleomycin, busulfan, carmustine (BCNU), and lomustine (CCNU). Survivors treated with these drugs can develop problems during treatment or many years after treatment ends.

Survivors most at risk for pulmonary fibrosis are those who had doses of:

- 600 mg/m^2 or higher of CCNU or BCNU.[5]
- 500 mg or more of busulfan.[6]
- 400 units/m^2 or more of bleomycin.[7]

Young age is also an additional risk factor for lung complications after receiving these chemotherapy drugs.

I had ABVD and 2800 cGy of mantle radiation 10 years ago when I was 15. They didn't do pulmonary function tests (PFTs) before treatment with the bleomycin. I had had asthma for years before I was diagnosed, so I don't know how useful the tests would have been anyway. I was diagnosed a few years ago with combined restrictive/obstructive defects.

Lung toxicity may increase if cyclophosphamide or radiation was given at the same time as bleomycin. An additional concern for those who received bleomycin is a life-long risk for respiratory problems during and after receiving general anesthesia.[8] Oxygen and fluids should be monitored closely by your anesthesiologist, and you should not be given high concentrations of supplemental oxygen. Too much oxygen to someone who was previously treated with bleomycin can cause edema (fluid buildup) in the lungs. This complication can be avoided with planning and communication ahead of time.

> When I needed oral surgery, I wrote my oral surgeon a letter in advance detailing my treatment history and included a copy of my summary letter from the hematologist who treated me. I said that if he had any questions, he should feel free to call me or the doctor. When I arrived for my appointment, he said he had indeed gotten the letter and there wouldn't be any problems. For confirmation, I said something like, "So basically, you do know that I was treated with ABVD (combination of four drugs including bleomycin) and mantle radiation for Hodgkin's in 1988–1989 and was splenectomized," and he said yes, that he wanted to take me off penicillin V for a few days and use a different antibiotic as prophylaxis since I would be at increased risk of infection compared to a "normal" 21-year-old. Everything went just fine! So far, I have yet to find a doctor this doesn't work well with.

> I find it really is crucial to talk and write about one's history in all of this. You just can't count on someone having reviewed your records thoroughly. I normally send a letter in advance with some relevant record copies, bring my records to the appointment, and discuss the situation with my doctor, ensuring that he did receive and read the letter and understands the situation. I'm a partner, not merely a patient.

Some parents report that their children developed asthma after treatment for childhood cancer. There is currently no research to support the theory that asthma is a late effect of treatment. There also has been an increasing incidence of asthma in the general population during the last 20 years. However, regardless of the cause, treatment is the same.

> We went for our checkup today and an echo of Alexander's heart. He has had an ear infection for the past week and a cold. Apparently that is not all that he has, because our oncologist has told us that he has asthma. Whenever he has a cold, it hits his lungs, and he has had pneumonia more than a few times while on treatment, and colds and pneumonia very often since. The doctor prescribed the Ventolin® and Beclovent®

puffers—two puffs four times per day. We were told that he would only need to use the inhalers whenever he has a cold. Hopefully it will remain in check by doing this and not become a daily regime.

Signs and symptoms

Signs and symptoms of pneumonitis are as follows:

- Cough
- Fever
- Shortness of breath
- Rapid heartbeat
- Painful breathing

Symptoms of lung fibrosis include the following:

- Chronic cough (with or without fever)
- Shortness of breath
- Painful breathing
- Tiring easily during exercise
- Increasing difficulty with activities of daily life

Screening and detection

Part of comprehensive follow-up care should be a discussion about any risks to your lungs from treatment. If you are at risk, you should tell your healthcare provider how you breathe at rest and while exercising.

If you took bleomycin, BCNU, CCNU, or busulfan; had chest, spine, or flank irradiation; or have any symptoms of fibrosis, you should have the following tests performed:

- Pulmonary function tests (PFTs)
- Chest x-ray
- Evaluation of chest wall growth
- Evaluation for scoliosis (curvature of the spine)
- Evaluation of trunk length and size of chest cavity

Current guidelines generally recommend monitoring during therapy, at the and at completion of therapy. If you have symptoms, or if the tests show abnormalities, you will be monitored periodically.

Most follow-up clinics do PFTs before and after administration of bronchodilators (medications given through an inhaler). If the chest x-ray or PFTs suggest fibrosis, a referral to a pulmonologist is usually made for further evaluation. Some treatment protocols include specific schedules for monitoring.

If you received bleomycin, you should have PFTs done before having general anesthesia. Make sure you tell the anesthesiologist about your cancer history, bleomycin treatment, and results of your PFTs.

Medical management

Some children and teens with pulmonary fibrosis respond well to bronchodilating medicines. If you have pulmonary fibrosis, you should maintain as active a lifestyle as possible to maximize your lung function. You should also be seen periodically by a pulmonologist.

All survivors who had pulmonary radiation or potentially lung-toxic chemotherapy should get a yearly influenza vaccine. They should also receive pneumococcal vaccine once they are off therapy and their immune system is functional—about 6 months to 1 year out from most conventional therapy, and later for those who had a stem cell transplant. This vaccine will not prevent all types of pneumonia, because many types are due to organisms not covered by these vaccines. An ounce of prevention—avoiding close contact with people who have a respiratory infection—is wise.

Careful management of upper respiratory infections is necessary if you have pulmonary fibrosis. If there are increasing signs of pulmonary distress, such as breathing difficulties, increased sputum production, or increased shortness of breath, call your healthcare provider.

> *Twenty-four years after my treatment for Hodgkin's, I had an enlarged liver. I had my first CT scan then and they found a pleural effusion. They tapped it (withdrew the fluid with a needle), but it was back within a week. They realized then that it had been a long-term problem. I had a pleuradesis, which means they went in and basically glued the pleural sac to the lung so fluid cannot get in between. It reduced the volume of my lungs, but improved my breathing.*

Survivors who had chemotherapy and/or radiation that can affect the lungs should have PFTs done and possibly see a pulmonary specialist prior to SCUBA diving.

You should not smoke cigarettes, marijuana, or anything else if you are a cancer survivor. This is especially important if you had any treatment that is potentially toxic to your lungs. Your medical management should include a frank discussion about the dangers of smoking. To protect your lungs, try to avoid fumes from chemicals, solvents, and paints and observe respiratory safety precautions in the workplace. For more information about keeping your lungs healthy after treatment for childhood cancer, visit *www.survivorshipguidelines.org/pdf/PulmonaryHealth.pdf*.

Chapter 14

Kidneys, Bladder, and Genitals

Prosperity is not without many fears and distastes; and adversity is not without comforts and hopes.

—Francis Bacon

THE KIDNEYS AND BLADDER are part of the body's system for clearing waste (the excretory system). In earlier years, damage to these organs from treatment for childhood cancer was far more common than it is today. Chemotherapy drugs that can be toxic to these organs are now given in lower doses or with protective agents and intravenous (IV) fluids that flush them through the excretory system quickly, minimizing damage. Organ shielding and use of lower doses of radiation have also decreased late effects. But some long-term survivors live with damage to the kidneys and bladder, and a small number of children on newer protocols still develop problems.

The genitals are organs in the body's reproductive system. Hormones that affect this system are covered in Chapter 9, *Hormone-Producing Glands*. Late effects to the vagina, uterus, prostate, and nerves that control sexual function are covered in this chapter.

Signs and symptoms, detection, and medical management of late effects to the kidneys, bladder, and genitals are discussed. Survivors share stories of their experiences and how they cope with damage to these parts of the body.

Kidneys

The kidneys, the main organs of the excretory system, are located at the bottom of the ribcage near the back of the body. These two bean-shaped organs are each about the size of a fist.

Blood enters the kidneys from branches off the aorta (the main blood vessel that carries oxygen-rich blood from the heart). The kidneys regulate blood pressure, filter waste products from the blood, and control the amount of water, minerals, and vitamins in the blood that returns to the body. Inside each kidney are millions of microscopic structures that filter out large particles, such as white and red blood cells and most proteins, allowing them to return to the bloodstream. What remains in the kidney after this process is the yellow liquid called urine. Urine flows from the kidneys through long tubes (ureters) into the bladder, where it is stored until it is eliminated from the body by urination. Figure 14-1 shows the location of kidneys and bladder within the body.

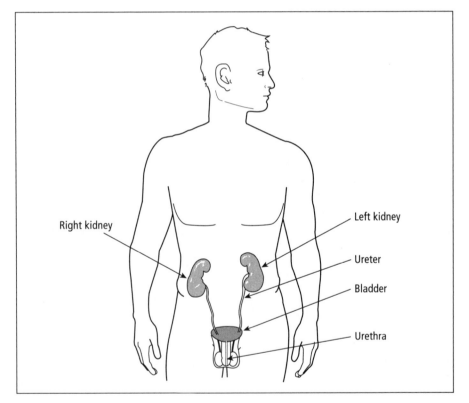

Figure 14-1. Kidneys and bladder

Organ damage

The kidneys can be impacted by surgery, chemotherapy, and radiation. The majority of children with Wilms tumor have one kidney removed. If they only receive a short cycle of chemotherapy and no radiation, the remaining kidney usually functions with no major problems. The remaining kidney enlarges and does the work of two kidneys. Protecting the remaining kidney is discussed later in this chapter, under "Medical management."

The vast majority of survivors of childhood cancer have good kidney function. The few long-term effects that do develop are rare. These include nephritis, high blood pressure, renal artery damage, and tubular necrosis.

Radiation

Radiation delivered directly to the kidneys can cause dysfunction. Survivors who are at highest risk include those who received:

- Radiation to the whole abdomen for soft tissue sarcomas of the pelvis or abdomen; tumors of the kidney, abdomen, or pelvis; or abdominal lymphomas.

- Total body radiation (TBI) before undergoing stem cell transplantation (e.g., bone marrow transplant, peripheral stem cell transplant, or cord blood transplant).

Chronic nephritis (inflammation of the kidneys) can develop after 2000 centigray (cGy) or more of radiation to an entire kidney. If chemotherapy is given as well, lower doses of radiation (1000 to 1500 cGy) can cause injury. Chronic nephritis is also seen in stem cell transplant survivors who had TBI as part of their conditioning regimen. The likelihood of nephritis developing appears to depend on which chemotherapy drugs the survivor had prior to the transplant.

Chronic nephritis can develop during treatment or years after treatment is completed. It can lead to kidney failure or heart damage and thus requires close medical surveillance. Improved radiation techniques and kidney shielding have decreased the number of cancer survivors who develop nephritis.

The kidneys also help regulate blood pressure. High blood pressure (hypertension) means the heart is working overtime to push blood through arteries. High blood pressure can lead to heart disease, hardening of the arteries (atherosclerosis), or stroke.

> Lisa had high-dose Cytoxan® and six doses of total body irradiation prior to getting her bone marrow transplant. A year later her hemoglobin and platelets started to drop. It took months to figure out that it was kidney damage. The kidney doctor said that if the radiation damages the kidneys, it usually shows up between 6 months and a

year post-transplant. Her kidney filtration rate was only 40 percent. She'd retain fluid in her feet and she developed high blood pressure. Her potassium also got high. Just when we thought things were fine, boom, we got hit with this.

She started out taking four bicarbonate pills a day, medication for her high blood pressure, and weekly injections. One of the jobs the kidneys do other than filter is to produce a chemical that tells the bone marrow to make red blood cells. Her marrow was full of precursor cells, but they weren't developing into red cells. When the kidney damage is great enough, not enough of this chemical is released, so a drop in hemoglobin occurs. So she began getting Epogen® (a drug used to treat anemia) injections on a weekly basis. It takes about 6 weeks to see the hemoglobin go back up, and it took weeks to figure out the exact dosage required to maintain her hemoglobin level. I assumed the damage was permanent and the injections would be a lifelong thing.

Suddenly, about a year later, we noticed her hemoglobin was too high and we started inching down her injections. Then we stopped the injections and waited to see what happened. Her hemoglobin levels continue to inch up at a really slow rate. She also had high creatinine and BUN (blood urea nitrogen) levels, and electrolyte imbalances, but all that seems okay for the moment.

Another rare late effect in long-term survivors who were treated with radiation to a field that included one or both kidneys (this includes Hodgkin lymphoma survivors who had their spleens irradiated) is renal artery damage or blockage. The main symptom is very high blood pressure that occurs years after treatment.

Chemotherapy

High doses of cisplatin can affect the kidneys. Some children or teens who received cumulative doses of more than 450 mg/m^2 of cisplatin can develop acute renal toxicity during treatment.[1] Over time, a kidney can sometimes repair itself. In other cases, survivors need to take replacement magnesium. Cisplatin damage usually becomes apparent during or within a year after treatment. Carboplatin is less toxic to the kidneys; however, in combination with other therapies, it can also impact renal function.

Jamie had acute renal failure on treatment, which resolved without dialysis, thank goodness. After the catheter was removed, Jamie suffered horribly for 2 weeks with kidney stones. His lab reports showed extremely high levels of uric acid and creatinine in his urine. This has since normalized. His first glomerular filtration rate (GFR) showed his kidneys functioning at 52 percent. Two months later, function was at 75 percent, and in the next 2 months it was at 95 percent. A huge improvement.

High doses of cyclophosphamide and/or ifosfamide can cause necrosis (death) of tubules in the kidneys. If these drugs are given with radiation to the pelvis or abdomen, or if combined with other drugs that can damage the kidneys, the risk of kidney problems increases. These changes usually occur only in survivors who have had multiple relapses and received extremely high doses of these drugs.

My daughter was treated for rhabdomyosarcoma. One of the chemotherapy agents she received was ifosfamide, which caused renal tubular acidosis. The oncologist told me the ifosfamide affected her kidneys' ability to process electrolytes. Her serum bicarbonate level was low, so her body's pH was low. With a low pH, you don't grow. She takes two supplements, Bicitra® and Neutraphos®, which keep her levels on the high side. This has met with some success. Though she still has a long way to go to catch up, she is now growing at a normal rate.

Some chemotherapy drugs, when combined with radiation, can increase the risk of late effects to the kidneys.[2] These drugs include the following:

• Ifosfamide

• Cytoxan

• Cisplatin

• Carboplatin

• Dactinomycin

Persistent problems usually only develop in survivors who had severe kidney problems during treatment.

My daughter was born with neuroblastoma. Her first two pea-sized tumors and her adrenal gland were removed when she was 1 month old, but she relapsed 3 months later. The new tumor was treated with Cytoxan® (cyclophosphamide), VP-16, cisplatin, Adriamycin®, ifosfamide, and vincristine in different combinations for over a year. Although the tumor stopped growing on chemo, it could not be surgically removed. It sat right on top of her left kidney and flattened it out. The tumor partially blocked the ureter and she started getting bladder infections. We monitored her kidney closely, and it failed after 5 months. She had a nephrostomy tube placed in 1993 and surgery a few months later to reroute her ureter around the tumor. She has had no problem with her bladder or kidneys since. She's now 8 years old.

Signs and symptoms

Signs and symptoms of kidney damage include the following:

- Fatigue
- Anemia
- Excessive urination during the night (nocturia)
- Weakness
- Retaining fluid (edema)
- High blood pressure
- Poor growth (this can be a sign of very poor kidney function)

Screening and detection

Survivors who received chemotherapy that can cause kidney problems need an evaluation of kidney function after the end of treatment. Survivors who were treated with chemotherapy and radiation to the abdomen or a kidney need an evaluation of kidney function either annually or every other year. Your evaluation should include the following:

- Physical exam
- Health history, including questions about frequency of urination, painful urination, and bedwetting
- Blood pressure
- Urinalysis
- Blood tests for BUN and creatinine levels

For a complete list of the tests you should have based on your treatment, you and your healthcare provider can refer to the Children's Oncology Group's survivorship guidelines at *www.survivorshipguidelines.org*.

Medical management

If you have long-term kidney toxicities from treatment, you should be seen by a pediatric or adult nephrologist (kidney specialist). Because damage to the kidneys can resolve over time, expert medical care is needed while waiting to see if recovery occurs. In the very rare cases in which progressive kidney failure occurs, dialysis and/or kidney transplant may be necessary.

If you had radiation to one or both kidneys, regular checks of your blood pressure should be part of your medical care. You should visit your healthcare provider's office or your school clinic several times a year to have your blood pressure checked. Steps you can take to help keep your blood pressure in the healthy range are maintaining a normal weight, exercising daily, and eating less salt.

The primary concern of survivors with only one kidney (after treatment for Wilms and occasionally neuroblastoma) is protection of the remaining kidney. The kidney is naturally very well protected within the body. However, you should talk with your healthcare provider about the sports you play. Your healthcare provider may recommend that you avoid contact sports or use a kidney guard if you do participate. Each family needs to balance quality of life issues with protection when making decisions about sports activities.

> My son Danny had Wilms when he was an infant and they took out half his kidney. He's now 10 and is a sports fanatic. He plays football, and I got him an abdominal protector that clips to the bottom of his shoulder pads. It is a hard shell with padding inside. It goes all the way around his abdominal area and hooks in the front. When Danny started wearing it the other boys all wanted one too. Instead of being the oddball, he began a new fad. I call him "the kid in armor."

Survivors with one kidney should also know the signs of urinary tract and kidney infections and seek treatment quickly to protect their single kidney. If you have burning upon urination, blood in the urine, painful urination, an urgent need to urinate frequently, or flank pain on the side of the remaining kidney, go to your healthcare provider as soon as symptoms develop.

There are certain categories of drugs, including some types of antibiotics, that can affect renal function. If you only have one kidney, don't use over-the-counter, herbal, or other medications without first discussing them with your nephrologist. Many of these are toxic to the kidneys, including nonsteroidal anti-inflammatory drugs (e.g., aspirin, ibuprofen, and naproxen) for pain, fever, or inflammation. Remind your healthcare provider anytime she gives you a prescription that you have only one kidney.

Survivors with only one kidney need to make sure their healthcare providers know of their special circumstances. Putting a card in with your driver's license that says you have only one kidney and/or wearing a medical alert bracelet will assist you in the unlikely event that you need medical care and are unable to tell emergency responders that you have a single kidney.

Bladder

The bladder is a muscular bag located in the lower pelvis. The ureters from the kidneys carry urine to the bladder. Urine collects in the bladder until it is full. When the muscle of the bladder signals the brain that it is full, the brain orders muscle contractions that squeeze the urine out of the bladder. The urine flows through a tube called the urethra to the outside of the body.

Organ damage

The vast majority of survivors of childhood cancer have good bladder function. However, bladder damage, including hemorrhagic cystitis, fibrosis, or a bladder that doesn't grow to a normal size, can occur after treatment with cyclophosphamide or ifosfamide and/or radiation.

> Katie started the BMT (bone marrow transplant) conditioning during the final days of April. She had total body irradiation and Cytoxan®. Day 0 was May 6. We made arrangements to go home on June 6, and wham, she started peeing blood. It was hemorrhagic cystitis from the Cytoxan®. We stayed for another 2 weeks, Katie was pumped with fluids, and the problem resolved and has not returned.

Radiation

Survivors who had tumors in the bladder or pelvic area may have received high doses of radiation (4000 cGy or more) that can scar their bladders. A scarred (fibrotic) bladder does not stretch to hold urine or contract well to empty. A bladder that does not grow (or shrinks due to fibrosis) may meet the needs of a preschooler, but will be too small for an older child. Thus, intervention may be necessary years after treatment even though the injury to the organ has not progressed. Radiation can also cause narrowing (strictures) in the urethra, which causes difficult, painful urination.

Treatment for tumors in the bladder or pelvic area once included total removal of the bladder and placement of a urinary diversion (surgery that allows urine to flow out of the body through a tube in the abdominal wall). Newer treatments combine chemotherapy with removal of part of the bladder. In the majority of cases, survivors retain functional bladders.

Chemotherapy

Hemorrhagic cystitis occurs when the tiny blood vessels that line the inside of the bladder wall are irritated, causing the vessels to leak blood into the bladder. This condition is caused by cyclophosphamide (Cytoxan®) or ifosfamide. Children who were given MESNA (a bladder protector) or who received cyclophosphamide by IV with lots of fluids to flush it through the bladder rarely get cystitis. Survivors most at risk for hemorrhagic cystitis are those who:

- Received cyclophosphamide and/or ifosfamide for long periods of time with minimal flushing through the system.

- Had hemorrhagic cystitis during treatment and the problem persists. It does not tend to spontaneously occur years later.

Signs and symptoms

Signs and symptoms of hemorrhagic cystitis are blood in the urine, lower abdominal pain, frequent and painful urination, an urgent need to urinate, and difficulties with urination.

Radiation damage to the bladder can cause bleeding ulcers and scarring in the bladder. Survivors with this condition may have little or no bladder control (wetting or leakage) or may have to urinate very frequently.

Screening and detection

All survivors who had therapies that can harm the bladder should have a baseline and then yearly urinalysis. An assessment of the function of the urinary system also includes asking questions about the following:

- Incontinence

- Urine dripping

- Difficulty starting urination

- Painful urination

- Inability to completely empty the bladder

Survivors with hemorrhagic cystitis are at risk for bladder cancers and thus need education about signs and symptoms, as well as yearly evaluations.

> I'm 34 and had neuroblastoma when I was an infant. Last March, I started passing blood in my urine, and it was misdiagnosed as prostatitis. It took a while before I went to a urologist, who did a cystoscopic exam and discovered a 1-inch malignant tumor in my bladder. He said he thought it might be caused by the abdominal radiation and cyclophosphamide I had so long ago.

Medical management

If you had treatment that could damage your bladder, and your urine test shows blood, it should be repeated in a week. If it is still positive, you should request a referral to a urologist with experience treating survivors of childhood cancer.

Survivors with chronic bladder infections need to drink lots of fluids. This can be challenging for parents of younger children. The following are suggested ways to encourage young children to drink more.

- Fill water bottles halfway, add a drop of food coloring, then freeze. Then add cold water to fill and add a different color.
- Use different kinds of cups with crazy-shaped straws.
- Flavor crushed ice with juice.
- Freeze juice in ice trays and add to drinks.
- Make juice popsicles.

Some survivors are at risk for cavities and obesity, so drink juice and energy drinks in moderation. It is important to brush your teeth often.

> We let her design her water bottle the way she liked it. She painted it and considered it her personal water bottle. It was insulated and helped to keep the water really cold.

Bladder-stretching surgery for survivors with scarred bladders has not been very successful. At some large, university-affiliated children's hospitals, new surgical techniques are being developed to increase bladder size (called bladder augmentation) by stitching in pieces of tissue from other parts of the body. If you have a fibrotic bladder, occasional visits to specialists in the field at large pediatric hospitals can alert you to the newest developments in treatment.

Children who had surgery to provide a urinary diversion need physical and psychological support as they grow. These services can be found at a comprehensive follow-up center.

Genitals

Genitals are human reproductive organs. The female organs are the ovaries, uterus, and vagina. Ovaries, the organs that release eggs and produce sex hormones, are discussed in Chapter 9, *Hormone-Producing Glands*. The uterus is an organ with strong, muscular walls. The structure at the bottom of the uterus that connects it to the vagina is the cervix. The vagina is a muscular, tube-shaped organ. It is sometimes called the birth canal because it is the opening through which a baby is born. Figure 14-2 shows the location of female genitals.

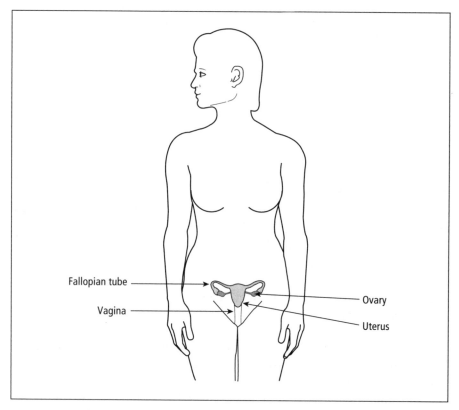

Figure 14-2. Female genitals

The testes are the male organs that produce sperm cells and the hormone testosterone. The testes are in a sac called the scrotum, located behind the penis. Each testis is made of coiled tubules called seminiferous tubules. Cells in the tubules produce sperm, which is stored in a structure called the epididymis. The prostate is a walnut-sized gland located just below the bladder. It makes fluid that is mixed with sperm cells to produce semen. The penis is the male organ through which sperm cells leave the body during sexual intercourse. Figure 14-3 shows the location of male genitals.

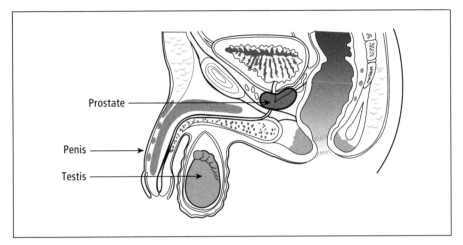

Figure 14-3. Male genitals

Organ damage in females

Very few girls get tumors in the vagina or uterus. However, some female children or teens with tumors in the pelvic area (i.e., rhabdomyosarcoma, Ewing sarcoma, osteosarcoma) get high-dose radiation that can affect the growth and development of the vagina and/or uterus. Lower doses of radiation, when used with some types of chemotherapy that enhance radiation (e.g., dactinomycin and doxorubicin), can cause the same long-term effects as high-dose radiation alone.

Some female survivors who had abdominal tumors treated with radiation have permanent changes in the size and function of the uterus. These late effects are more likely in girls treated before puberty with more than 2000 cGy of radiation. The uterus of a girl treated after puberty usually is not damaged unless more than 4000 cGy of radiation is used. Radiation can stunt the growth of the uterus and can also cause it to become scarred (fibrotic) and less elastic. This type of damage to the uterus can cause miscarriages of pregnancies or low birthweight children. It occurs most often in survivors of Wilms tumor who had more than 2000 cGy of abdominal radiation and in Hodgkin lymphoma survivors who had radiation to the abdomen and chemotherapy (but not either alone).

> *I had radiation to my right flank for Wilms when I was 2 years old in 1962. I've had three healthy baby boys, all over 7 pounds. The doctors were shocked when they found one of my fallopian tubes was badly damaged from the radiation. It didn't ever cause me any problems.*

Girls or teens who had more than 4000 cGy of radiation to a field that included the vagina can develop fibrosis (when the tissue gets scarred and tough and doesn't stretch well) and diminished vaginal development. This problem can also occur after lower doses of radiation if radiation-enhancing chemotherapy drugs (e.g., dactinomycin) are also given. Fibrosis can affect the size and flexibility of the vagina, which can alter sexual function and the ability to deliver babies vaginally.

Signs and symptoms in females

Signs and symptoms of uterine damage include the following:

- Small uterus (your gynecologist will tell you this)
- Inability to get pregnant
- Difficulties with menstruation such as irregular periods or heavier than normal flow
- Miscarriage
- Low birthweight babies

Signs and symptoms of vaginal damage include the following:

- Abnormal vaginal bleeding
- Vaginal dryness
- Inability to have intercourse due to a small vaginal opening
- Painful intercourse

Organ damage in males

Males children or teens who had high-dose radiation to the abdomen for rhabdomyosarcoma, Ewing sarcoma, or osteosarcoma are at risk for damage to the prostate gland and the nerves that control sexual functioning. Boys or teens with testicular cancer or relapsed leukemia (in the testes) usually have a testicle removed and the area irradiated.

> I had testicular cancer when I was 17, back in 1976. They removed the testicle, then did a retroperitoneal lymph node dissection to check for spread. They did find cancer in two lymph nodes. I had radiation for 6 weeks, then chemotherapy for a year.

Low doses of radiation to the prostate can slow or stop the development of this organ. High doses (more than 5000 cGy) can cause the organ to atrophy (shrink). Because the prostate produces part of the fluid that makes semen, damage to it can reduce or eliminate ejaculation. Nerve damage from surgery or radiation can affect the ability to have an erection and can also affect ejaculation.

Survivors who had radical lymph node dissections (removal of many lymph nodes in the groin) sometimes accumulate excessive fluid in the testicles (called hydrocele).[3] This late effect has been seen in long-term survivors of Hodgkin lymphoma, Wilms tumor, and paratesticular rhabdomyosarcoma.

Signs and symptoms in males

Signs and symptoms of prostate damage include the following:

- Decreased volume of seminal fluid (ejaculate)
- Small or atrophied prostate (your healthcare provider will tell you this)

Signs and symptoms of damage to nerves that control sexual function include the following:

- Inability to have an erection
- Inability to maintain an erection
- Inability to have an orgasm
- Having orgasms without ejaculation

Screening and detection for males and females

Frank discussions with your healthcare provider about changes in your sexual organs or sexual function are essential to identify and treat these late effects. Many people (including some healthcare providers) feel uncomfortable talking about sex and sexuality. However, sexuality is a vital part of your life that influences your sense of self and quality of life. Find a healthcare provider you trust who is comfortable discussing these issues so you can explore all of your options to address late effects involving your genitals.

> The radical lymph node dissection I had to see if my testicular cancer had spread damaged the sympathetic nerve that controls ejaculation. I'm normal sexually in every way except I can't ejaculate. This side effect was not explained well by the surgeon at the time. There I was, 17 and sitting in the room with my parents, when he said, "You might have problems with ejaculation." That's all. I didn't have a clue what he was talking about. It really worried me at the time. I thought I might never have an erection again. Twenty-two years later, I realize that the big loss is fertility. I still struggle with that.

Unfortunately, doctors are very uncomfortable talking about this type of late effect. No one asks me about erections, ejaculation, or the problems they cause. These things have changed my life in a big way and I have no one to talk to about it.

Healthcare providers for males should take an age-appropriate history that focuses on any problems with libido (sex drive), sexual function, or fertility. For males, the prostate gland is felt manually, and sometimes an ultrasound of the organ is done to evaluate size. Late effects involving the testicles are covered in Chapter 9, *Hormone-Producing Glands*.

Healthcare providers for female survivors should take an age-appropriate history that focuses on any problems with libido, sexual function, or fertility. Female children and teens need regular evaluation of their sexual development to ensure that puberty is proceeding normally. Women and sexually active teens should have a yearly pelvic examination. This exam may need to be done under anesthesia or sedation for women or teens who have small vaginas or vaginal fibrosis. The uterus can be evaluated using ultrasound, computed tomography (CT) scan, or magnetic resonance imaging (MRI). Abdominal radiation that included the ovaries requires extensive evaluation, outlined in Chapter 9, *Hormone-Producing Glands*.

A nurse practitioner who cares for survivors of childhood cancer said:

I have talked to many survivors with problems with sexual performance. Teenagers come in after becoming sexually active with both physical and psychological problems about sex. Many adults have lived for years with late effects that impact their ability to have satisfying sex. I talk to them openly and honestly about the issues. I ask them candid questions about sexual functioning, which include their satisfaction with their sex life, performance issues, and libido.

Sometimes we find a physical cause for sexual difficulties such as low testosterone or estrogen. Other times it involves their feelings about their appearance or it reflects problems in the relationship. Whatever the cause, it is our job as healthcare providers to initiate the conversation and help make them feel comfortable sharing these intimate details of their lives. That enables us to get them the help that they need and deserve.

Medical management for females and males

Female teens and women with late effects that alter sexual functioning or fertility need to be referred to a gynecologist and/or endocrinologist for further evaluation, testing, and treatment. Women or female teens with vaginal late effects may need vaginal dilations or reconstructive surgery. Survivors should consult a gynecologist with extensive experience doing these procedures. A woman with a small uterus or who has uterine fibrosis needs counseling about pregnancy. Pregnant women who had pelvic radiation should get their prenatal care from an obstetrician who specializes in high-risk pregnancies.

> At the age of 7, I was diagnosed with AML. After countless rounds of chemotherapy followed by total body radiation, I received a life-saving bone marrow transplant from my older brother, Nathan. As a result of the intensive cancer treatment, I experience chronic health issues such as a cardiomyopathy, endocrine dysfunction, and cataracts in both eyes. When I was 24, I was diagnosed with a secondary cancer—papillary thyroid cancer—a result of the total body radiation I received.

> Due to the total body radiation and the cyclophosphamide that I received as a child, I was told that I would be sterile. Coming from a large family, I had always dreamed of having a child of my own. On April Fool's Day, when I was 28 years old, I was taking a routine pregnancy test prior to a medical procedure to scan for thyroid cancer and discovered I was pregnant! Twelve weeks pregnant!

> I was fortunate to have both a fabulous oncologist and OB/GYN who managed my high-risk pregnancy. My cardiomyopathy was exacerbated by the pregnancy, leading to increased hypertension, which was controlled by beta blockers. The total body radiation I received led to impaired uterine growth and a shortened cervix. Despite a cervical cerclage being placed in addition to being on bed rest, at 25 weeks gestation my daughter—Hope Isabella—arrived weighing 1 pound 7 ounces.

> After 111 days in the NICU (neonatal intensive care unit) fighting for her life, she came home and continues to grow strong. To me, Hope is the epitome of a medical miracle. She is a wonderful example of how far we have come scientifically. She was born from an early BMT survivor who wasn't supposed to live to see her 8th birthday, and who was certainly not expected to be able to bear children. But, she also represents how far we have left to go to maintain cure rates while reducing late effects of treatments.

Male teens or men with late effects that alter sexual functioning or fertility need to be referred to a urologist and/or endocrinologist for further evaluation, testing, and treatment. Males who had a testicle removed may want to discuss having a prosthesis implanted. Those who develop a hydrocele usually have the fluid surgically drained.

I had my urine tested to see if I had retrograde ejaculation (ejaculate backing up into the bladder), but there were no sperm there. The only way to see if I'm fertile is to biopsy the remaining testicle. Since there is a small chance of damaging the testicle, I haven't had that done. The technology has improved so much that they say they only need a few sperm to fertilize an egg. But each time would cost $10,000 and would only have a 30 percent chance of success. I wish I was just back to the way I was before.

• • • • •

When the doctors told me that I probably was infertile, it was the most devastating part of the whole experience. By the time they told me about sperm banking it was too late. My urologist looked at the results and said, "No way, buddy." When I was dating, I told my future wife that I was told I'd be infertile. But in the back of my mind, I always had hope. My wife stayed on the pill until we thought we were ready to be parents. The first month she went off, she got pregnant. We have an 18-month-old boy, and my wife is pregnant again. It's wonderful. He's a miracle.

Any survivor with sexual problems that result from treatment for childhood cancer needs both medical and psychological follow-up. A team approach that provides psychological help to address concerns about body image, fertility, or sexuality is crucial.

I've never told any of my girlfriends what type of cancer I had. I have huge abdominal scars so I have to say something. I usually tell them I had intestinal cancer. I still struggle about the infertility. I'd love to have a family, but just can't discuss it with girlfriends. As soon as we start getting serious, girlfriends usually bring up kids, and I just don't want to go there. I can't seem to find a way to have that conversation.

Centers with comprehensive long-term follow-up programs have multi-disciplinary teams that include psychologists and social workers who are familiar with survivors' sexual issues and concerns. They can provide information, support, and one-on-one assistance with how to address these issues in relationships.

Chapter 15

Liver, Stomach, and Intestines

Food is an important part of
a balanced diet.

—Fran Lebowitz

THE LIVER, STOMACH, AND INTESTINES are part of the body's gastrointestinal (GI) system. This system extracts useful nutrients from food to help the body grow and function well. Different parts of this system perform different jobs. Some areas mix and store food, some help in chemical breakdown, and others absorb nutrients and store waste materials.

This chapter starts with a discussion of the functions of the liver. It outlines signs and symptoms of damage to the organ, how to screen for and detect late effects, and recommended medical management if problems arise. Next, the functions of the stomach and intestines are explained. Finally, a brief discussion of an uncommon late effect—gallstones—is included. Several survivors share stories of the late effects they developed and how they coped with them.

Liver

The liver is the body's largest internal organ and one of the most complex. This wedge-shaped organ is located beneath the rib cage in the upper-right part of the abdomen.

The liver performs thousands of functions that are essential to life. It converts food into energy, removes toxins (e.g., alcohol and drugs) from the body, keeps blood clotting normally, and manufactures proteins. It regulates the supply of essential minerals and vitamins and also produces bile, a fluid needed for proper digestion. In addition, the liver helps filter many chemical substances and waste products from the blood.

Figure 15-1 shows the location of the liver, stomach, and intestines.

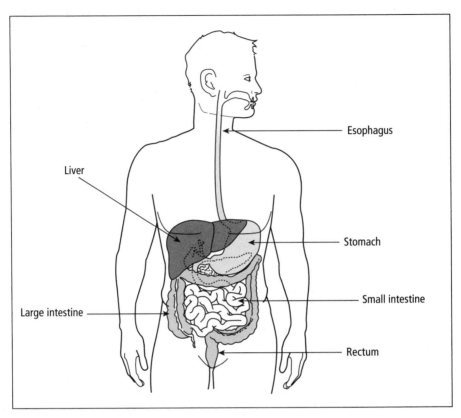

Figure 15-1. Liver, stomach, and intestines

Organ damage

Inflammation of the liver is called hepatitis from the Latin word for liver, *hepar*, and the Greek word *itis*, meaning inflammation. There are many possible causes of liver inflammation in childhood cancer survivors, including infection by viruses and damage from radiation and/or chemotherapy drugs. However, inflammation of the liver is relatively rare in survivors, especially in those treated in the last decade.

Hepatitis A

Hepatitis A is an infection caused by the hepatitis A virus, which is usually spread by contamination of food by human waste. Approximately 150,000 cases are diagnosed in the United States each year. It is most common in international travelers, sexually active homosexual men, intravenous drug users, and daycare workers. Most healthy people who get hepatitis A have no long-term consequences from the infection. There is an effective vaccine that prevents hepatitis A infections. This type of hepatitis is not a late effect of childhood cancer.

Hepatitis B

Hepatitis B is an inflammation of the liver caused by the hepatitis B virus (HBV). Approximately 1 million Americans have chronic hepatitis B infections, including survivors who received blood transfusions prior to 1972 (blood products were not screened for this virus before 1972). There is now an effective vaccine that prevents hepatitis B infections. The blood supply for transfusions is now well screened, and healthcare workers are routinely vaccinated.

Hepatitis C

Hepatitis C is an inflammation of the liver caused by the hepatitis C virus (HCV). HCV was spread by blood transfusions that were received prior to effective testing of blood products, and is currently spread by sharing needles for illicit intravenous drug use, and, less commonly, through sexual intercourse. Approximately 3.2 million people in the United States are infected with the HCV, making it the most common chronic blood-borne infection in the United States. There is no vaccine for HCV.

Before July 1992, there were no available laboratory tests to identify blood carrying HCV, and some children and teens with cancer received infected blood. Because more effective tests for the virus have been used by blood banks since July 1992, the current risk of getting HCV from a single blood transfusion is very small—only 1 per 2 million units transfused.

If you are infected with HCV, there are five possible outcomes:

- Your body's immune system may eliminate the virus and you will have no further problems (this happens in 15 to 25 percent of persons infected).[1]

- You may have a lifelong infection, but your liver will sustain no damage.

- You may develop liver inflammation, with or without symptoms.

- You may develop progressive inflammation and scarring of the liver. When this scarring (fibrosis) is spread throughout the liver and causes lumps, it is called cirrhosis. This process occurs over many years and usually results in symptoms. It can eventually lead to liver failure.

- In rare cases, liver cancer develops, but only after years of inflammation from chronic hepatitis C and cirrhosis.

Liver Fibrosis

Liver fibrosis (excessive formation of scar tissue) develops from liver inflammation, which has a variety of causes. Risks for development of liver fibrosis due to radiation are as follows:

• The amount of the liver that was irradiated

• The radiation dose

• Younger age at treatment

• Certain chemotherapy drugs (i.e., dactinomycin and doxorubicin) given in addition to radiation[2]

Survivors at highest risk are those who had 2,000 cGy or more to the entire liver.[3]

Chemotherapy can also cause liver fibrosis. Early protocols for acute lymphoblastic leukemia that gave daily oral methotrexate for 2 to 5 years caused liver fibrosis in up to 80 percent of children.[4] Very few children who received lower doses of methotrexate develop fibrosis. However, survivors of leukemia who have HCV and were treated with methotrexate are at increased risk for liver fibrosis.[5] Much less frequently, mercaptopurine (6-MP), thioguanine (6-TG), and dactinomycin can affect the function of the liver.

Survivors of stem cell transplantation (e.g., bone marrow, peripheral stem cell, or cord blood transplants) may have several risk factors for chronic liver disease, including HCV infection, iron overload, and chronic graft-versus-host disease (GVHD). One large study of more than 3,000 patients from the Fred Hutchinson Research Center estimated that 20 years after transplant, 3.8 percent of survivors had developed chronic liver disease.[6] Liver damage can develop rapidly in transplant survivors.

The risks for liver fibrosis are:

• Liver toxicity during treatment (high results on liver function tests many different times).

• Chronic viral hepatitis.

• Liver irradiation (abdominal radiation on the right side).

• High doses of drugs that can cause liver toxicity (e.g., methotrexate, 6-MP, 6-TG, dactinomycin).

• Stem cell transplantation.

Signs and symptoms

Because HCV can silently damage the liver, you may not be aware of the infection until the late complications of liver disease cause symptoms many years later. Though most people with HCV have no symptoms at the onset of the infection, some may experience the following:

- Jaundice (yellowish eyes and skin)

- Fatigue

- Loss of appetite

- Fever

- Nausea and vomiting

- Pale or clay-colored stools

- Dark urine

- Generalized itching

- Diarrhea

Signs and symptoms of liver fibrosis are as follows:

- Nausea and vomiting

- Fluid buildup in the abdomen

- Enlarged liver or spleen

Screening and detection

Your regular yearly examination should include a discussion about your liver and history of blood transfusions. You should get your blood tested for HCV if any of the following apply to you:

- You have been notified that you received blood from a donor who later tested positive for HCV.

- You received any blood products before 1993.

- You had a solid organ transplant before 1993.

- You have a history of illicit intravenous drug use.

- You have signs or symptoms of liver disease (for example, abnormal liver enzyme tests or an enlarged liver).

> *I had multiple blood transfusions in 1974, 1980, 1981, 1982, and 1984.*
> *In January 1998, I was at my internist's office getting blood work done.*
> *I told the doctor that my husband and I were going on our vacation to*

Cancun, Mexico, in the summer. He suggested I get a hepatitis test to see if I needed to get a hepatitis vaccination.

Lo and behold, the blood work came back positive for hepatitis C, antibodies for hepatitis B, but negative for hepatitis A. He then ran another blood test to determine the viral load (how much of the hepatitis C was in my system).

After that I was referred to a hepatologist at Baylor-Dallas. He did a liver biopsy in April 1998 to determine how much damage had been done to my liver and ran blood work to determine what genotype (or subtype) of hepatitis C I had. I had the genotype 2B, which is one of the easier ones to treat. This type often goes into remission with treatment.

In February 1999, I started on the combo treatment called Rebetron®, which is made up of interferon injections and capsules called ribavirin. The FDA had just approved it. So from February to August I endured these treatments, and the disease is now in remission. The viral load for hepatitis C is now undetectable.

Most institutions recommend three blood tests (ALT, AST, and bilirubin) on entry to a long-term follow up program. Stem cell transplant survivors should also have a serum ferritin test. All survivors treated prior to 1972 should be tested for hepatitis B and survivors treated before 1993 should be tested for hepatitis C.[7] During your annual physical examination, your healthcare provider should palpate (feel) your abdomen to check for an enlarged liver. Any abnormal findings should result in a referral to a gastroenterologist for further evaluation and treatment.

A small number of survivors who have had chronic HCV and develop cirrhosis may develop a type of liver cancer called hepatocellular carcinoma. The chance of developing this cancer is greatly increased in those who drink alcohol. To screen for this type of cancer, survivors with cirrhosis periodically need a blood test (called alpha-fetoprotein) done.

Medical management

There is no specific treatment for acute HCV. Rest may be recommended during the acute phase if symptoms are severe. The acute infection usually disappears 3 to 4 months after symptoms begin.

Chronic HCV can be treated with a number of medications. Interferon alpha, which stimulates the immune system to fight the infection, and ribavirin, an antiviral antibiotic, are usually given together. This combination treatment is effective in up to half of patients. Treatments for HCV are evolving and improving, so keep in touch with a specialist if you have HCV to learn of the newest options.

Some people who have had HCV infections for many years need a liver transplant, because the liver becomes so damaged that it can no longer perform its crucial functions.

If you have HCV or chronic liver fibrosis, you can do the following to protect your liver:

- Don't drink alcohol—it greatly increases damage to the liver. This includes even occasional beer or wine.

- Don't take over-the-counter medications, such as Tylenol® (acetaminophen) or Advil® (ibuprofen), herbal or dietary aids, or prescription medications, without first discussing them with your healthcare provider. Many of these can cause more damage to the liver. Read labels of other over-the-counter drugs to make sure they don't contain acetaminophen or ibuprofen.

- Get vaccinated against hepatitis A and B.

- See your healthcare provider regularly.

HCV can be spread to a partner by sexual intercourse, so it is important to use barrier protection, such as condoms. Because there is no vaccine against HCV, a spouse (or sexual partner) of a survivor with HCV can also get the infection. Therefore, your spouse (or sexual partner) should be periodically screened for HCV. Rarely, HCV can be transmitted to an infant during pregnancy. It is important that female survivors with HCV tell their obstetrician and family physician about the infection.

Counseling should be provided if you test positive for HBV or HCV to help you learn about and cope with these chronic diseases. Many people with HCV infections find comfort participating in support groups, which are available in many communities because HCV is so widespread.

For more information about HCV, read the frequently asked questions on the U.S. Centers for Disease Control and Prevention hepatitis C website at *www.cdc.gov/hepatitis/index.htm* or call (800) CDC-INFO (800-232-4636). The American Liver Foundation has an informative website at *www.liverfoundation.org*. Other helpful organizations are listed in Appendix B, *Resources*.

Stomach and intestines

When you eat, food travels from the mouth, through the esophagus, and into the stomach. The stomach is a muscular sac that contracts to mix food with digestive secretions. Glands in the stomach secrete acids and enzymes to help break down food and mucus to lubricate the digestive tract and coat the stomach wall.

Approximately 3 hours after arriving in the stomach, partially digested food passes in small amounts into the 20-foot-long small intestine. As it moves through the small intestine, digestion of proteins and carbohydrates is completed, fats are digested, and nutrients are absorbed into the bloodstream. Undigested material passes into the large intestine, also called the colon. In this 5-foot-long organ, water and vitamins are reabsorbed, leaving behind undigested material called feces. The feces move into the rectum, then out of the body through the anus.

Organ damage

Survivors of childhood cancer sometimes develop fibrosis (excessive formation of scar tissue) or chronic enterocolitis (inflammation of the intestines). Fibrosis can occur anywhere from the esophagus to the rectum, causing thickening of the inner walls that can cause strictures or obstructions (see Chapter 10, *Head and Neck*, for a discussion of esophageal strictures). Fibrosis can also occur outside of the GI tract in the form of adhesions (when different structures in the abdomen stick together). Fibrosis and chronic enterocolitis can be caused by the following:

- Radiation (3,000 cGy or higher)
- Abdominal surgery
- Chemotherapy (when given with radiation)
- Chronic GVHD
- Infection

Fibrosis and chronic enterocolitis can cause adhesions, obstructions, ulcers, diarrhea, constipation, lactose intolerance, and malabsorption problems.

Intestinal damage can appear months to decades after treatment ends. The colon and rectum are more often damaged by radiation than are the stomach and small intestine.

Survivors who received low doses of radiation have a very low incidence of GI damage, while those who had multiple abdominal surgeries and higher radiation doses (e.g., abdominal rhabdomyosarcoma, Ewing sarcoma, Hodgkin lymphoma, Wilms tumor treated in the 1960s and 1970s, or neuroblastoma treated in the 60s or 70s) are at higher risk.

I had 7 weeks of radiation to the abdomen 12 years ago to treat Hodgkin's disease. I was 13 years old at the time and went from 108 pounds to 76. The radiation tightened up and atrophied parts of my colon. I get bouts of partial obstructions. I have constipation, excruciating pain, and vomiting. When I feel it starting, I take mineral oil, and use suppositories and enemas. I listen to my bowels with a stethoscope and when the bowel sounds are absent, I know I'm in trouble. Sometimes I need to go to the hospital for fluids and big enemas, and once I needed surgery. They took out the most damaged part of my intestine at that time. I try to prevent these problems with diet, because I already have adhesions from my surgeries, and more surgeries will just make that worse. My doctors and surgeon are top-notch and that really helps.

· · · · ·

My 5-year-old son was treated for rhabdomyosarcoma of the prostate. He had a radical prostatectomy, radiation to the tumor bed, and chemotherapy. Since radiation, he has not regained bowel control. He has 10 to 15 bowel movements a day. He often can't make it to the toilet and it is a lot of mess for all of us. What amazes me is how little help we have had in finding solutions to what seem to be medical problems. We were very pleased with how his cancer treatment went. Now it seems that it was a breeze compared to the chronic health problems he experiences.

Chronic enterocolitis can cause acute abdominal pain and vomiting years after abdominal radiation. If you develop these symptoms, seek medical help and make sure you tell the healthcare provider about your prior radiation.

A common concern among families of Wilms tumor survivors is stomach pain. My son, Lucas, who is 11 years off treatment, has stomach pain and also has some bowel issues that come and go. Lucas avoids certain foods and activities out of concern that it might trigger the stomach pain. He's had so many tests done to try and figure out what is causing it and everything comes back normal. On paper, he is the model of health. And, yet, here's a 13-year-old who has a bucket that he keeps by his bed and carries around the house with him just in case the stomach pain might come along and cause him to throw up (it does not happen all the time with the pain, but it happens frequently enough). He's had a colonoscopy, blood work, ultrasounds—everything looks great. Oncologist says it's probably scar tissue (strictures) in or near the bowel. Surgeon blames the chemotherapy (vincristine in particular) because it causes neuropathy in the GI system. Both the oncologist and surgeon say the abdominal radiation is a contributing factor to poor bowel motility. What is frustrating in all of this is that, currently, we have no test (diagnosis) that confirms anything. Does it affect his quality of life? Yes. Is it serious, life threatening, and the end of the world? Probably not.

Another problem that can develop is slow emptying of the stomach and reflux of food back into the esophagus. These effects can occur after radiation or in survivors who had long-term problems with severe vomiting while on treatment. Reflux is a chronic problem. Barrett's esophagus (changes in the cells of the esophagus) can occur in association with reflux in those whose GI tracts were irradiated. For more information about late effects to the esophagus, see Chapter 11, *Head and Neck*.

Ever since my 4500 cGy of mantle radiation in 1968, I've had a lot of heartburn. All they had then to treat it was Tagamet®—not all the choices that are now available. I was sleeping on lots of pillows to keep my head elevated, but I still had heartburn. When the problem was identified, I started esophageal dilation and better medications. I now have precancerous cells in the stomach. I have endoscopies every 6 months to biopsy it.

A rare late effect that results from nerve damage is a change in the GI tract's ability to move food through at a normal rate (called dysmotility).

Melissa has gastric atony (lack of muscle tone in the stomach and failure to contract normally, slowing movement out of the stomach) due to nerve damage from vincristine. It might also have been affected by her severe pancreatitis or craniospinal radiation. She had really bad problems with reflux, also. She's had a jejunostomy tube in her small bowel for 3 years. Her tastes are really altered, too. Sweet and sour are mixed up—she says cake tastes too sour. And she used to love ice cream, but now it just doesn't taste right to her.

Lactose intolerance means the body can't absorb the sugar (lactose) contained in milk and other dairy products. Fibrosis from radiation, certain antibiotics, and some chemotherapy drugs can cause lactose intolerance in some individuals. The parts of children's or teens' intestines that break down lactose stop functioning properly, resulting in gas, abdominal pain, bloating, cramping, and diarrhea. Some people have a genetic predisposition for developing lactose intolerance. If you have this problem, discuss it with your healthcare provider. A nutritionist can provide you with information about low-lactose diets and alternate sources of protein and calcium.

The role of chemotherapy drugs and the development of GI late effects is not well understood. Certain drugs (i.e., dactinomycin, Adriamycin®, daunorubicin) are known to increase the effects of radiation and thus may increase the likelihood of GI problems.

A very small number of survivors have permanent colostomies or gastrostomies. Survivors with alterations of their GI tracts should have a gastroenterologist as part of their primary treatment team.

> My daughter was born in 1991 with neuroblastoma and Hirschsprung's disease. When she was 1 month old, the surgeon had to remove part of her bowel and put in a colostomy. He removed three small tumors at the same time. We still go back every few months for follow-up and see a variety of specialists, including the gastroenterologist.

• • • • •

> My daughter has a jejunostomy button and still gets tube feedings at night, many years after her treatment for relapsed leukemia. We use Pediasure® and it gives her about 800 calories a night. It's the only way she keeps any weight on her. She eats during the day, but only a very few types of food. She can't tolerate dairy products.

Signs and symptoms

Signs and symptoms of damage to the stomach and intestines are as follows:

- Chronic diarrhea
- Chronic constipation
- Nausea and vomiting
- Persistent or severe abdominal pain or cramping
- Blood in the stool
- Anemia
- Loss of appetite
- Problems gaining weight or loss of weight
- Malabsorption

The primary symptom of malabsorption is failure to grow and thrive. It often is accompanied by persistent diarrhea. This problem usually begins during treatment and persists. Malabsorbtion does not suddenly occur years after treatment.

My son was diagnosed with hepatoblastoma when he was 1, and he has major GI problems. Whenever the poor child eats all he can do is scream. He has only gained 2 pounds in the 14 months since treatment ended. He still looks so frail and weak. He has energy, but I have no idea where he gets it from. I do give him vitamins.

Small bowel obstructions generally begin abruptly. The signs and symptoms include abdominal pain, nausea, vomiting, and loss of appetite. The pain is sometimes described as crampy. It may be in one specific area but is more commonly generalized. If the obstruction is complete, you cannot pass gas or have a bowel movement. Vomiting is caused by the increased pressure from the obstruction. The abdomen will become distended and if tapped will sound like a drum. If this happens, you need to get medical attention right away because it can be life threatening.

Screening and detection

Your annual follow-up appointment should include a thorough physical examination and health history. If you haven't reached your full adult growth, your height and weight should be plotted on a growth chart. Your healthcare provider should ask about your diet, any stomach or abdominal pains, and whether you have chronic diarrhea or constipation. If you have persistent symptoms, you should be referred to a gastroenterologist for further evaluation.

The doctors used to call my son's stomach pains a mystery illness. They have performed every test on that child. They have gone down, up, and sideways. The barium enema was fine, the upper GI was fine, the scans were fine. They put him to sleep (thank goodness) for the colonoscopy and the endoscopy. They showed he had colitis.

These kids are so little and all they can say is, "It hurts." He will eat something and immediately double over in pain. We try to stay away from the things that we know will cause the most pain, but sometimes it's everything that goes into his mouth.

Certain abnormalities can be detected only with laboratory tests. A complete blood count will show if you have anemia. Some follow-up clinics check serum total protein and albumin levels every 3 to 5 years for survivors at risk for enteritis. You are at risk if you had one or more abdominal surgeries, abdominal radiation, or chronic GVHD after a stem cell transplant.

Medical management

Survivors with chronic GI problems need to consult with a gastroenterologist.

> *My son has frequent, uncontrollable bowel movements after radiation, chemotherapy, and surgery for rhabdomyosarcoma of the prostate. Our oncologist told us to use steroid suppositories. It was terribly invasive and didn't help. After months of just enduring and lots of advice about "being tough" with a 4-year-old who was pooping his pants, I self-referred him to rehab medicine. I was thinking that they could help with a bowel program for him, and I was very desperate. They had me take data for a while and then had me give him an anti-diarrheal. Again I didn't see improvement.*
>
> *All of these problems really affect his quality of life. He is in a mixed regular education/special education placement for kindergarten because of bowel and bladder concerns, even though he is in the 99ᵗʰ percentile in language and 95ᵗʰ percentile in cognitive skills. There are no options for first grade. We do have a very good pediatrician who has just referred us to the GI clinic. He wants to find out if my son has intact sphincter function.*

Some bowel obstructions resolve with time, bed rest, and fluids. If the obstruction is complete, the symptoms will continue and surgery may be necessary. Surgery to relieve obstructions or to remove damaged sections of the intestine is relatively high risk and should be done by a surgeon with extensive experience doing bowel surgeries and working on radiated tissues.

> *I work hard to prevent the partial bowel obstructions I am prone to getting. I don't eat pizza or cheese. Cheese, especially the processed kind, is the worst for blockages. I eat lots of fruits and veggies and take plenty of fluids. I also take mineral oil and try to prevent hard stools.*

Many GI problems require low-fat, gluten-free, lactose-free, or low-residue diets. These are best undertaken under the guidance of a gastroenterologist and nutritionist.

> *I had my stomach removed in 1982 and a new one formed out of part of my small intestine. I am lactose intolerant and can't have many dairy products. I also have to steer clear of really acidic items like orange juice, because it irritates the esophagus. Roughage like lettuce gives me problems too.*

It was a trial and error situation for many years learning what my "new stomach" could handle and what it couldn't handle. There are now post-gastrectomy diet plans available at most hospitals that have dietitians. I spoke to the dietitian when I had another surgery in 1997 and she showed me the suggested diet plan. It was pretty much what I had already learned on my own. Back in 1982, that type of surgery wasn't real common and definitely not in a young girl.

Gallstones

An uncommon late effect after treatment for childhood cancer is gallstones, which are solid lumps of cholesterol or bilirubin that form in the gall bladder. Survivors who are most likely to develop gallstones are those who:[8]

• Had abdominal radiation that included the gall bladder.

• Had a stem cell transplant.

• Have cirrhosis of the liver.

Some people with gallstones have no symptoms, and the gallstones are discovered in routine x-rays. Asymptomatic gallstones are usually not treated. However, if a gallstone blocks a bile duct, then pain develops in the mid right abdomen or upper right abdomen. Other symptoms include fever, nausea, vomiting, and clay-colored stools.

If you have these symptoms, you should see your healthcare provider immediately. Gallstones are usually diagnosed with an abdominal ultrasound or CT scan. In the past, open surgery was done to remove the gall bladder. Now, the gall bladder is removed using laparoscopic surgery, which uses smaller incisions and usually results in a much shorter hospital stay.

Chapter 16

Immune System

The courage of life is often a less dramatic
spectacle than the courage of the final moment;
but it is no less a magnificent
mixture of triumph and tragedy.

—John Fitzgerald Kennedy
Profiles in Courage

THE IMMUNE SYSTEM is the body's defense against harmful organisms and substances. It is made up of a variety of cells, organs, and systems, ranging from individual white cells to the entire lymphatic system. One of its primary functions is to fight infectious diseases such as influenza and the common cold. The immune system identifies foreign substances and neutralizes, eliminates, or breaks them down into harmless components.

Radiation, chemotherapy, stem cell transplantation, and removal of the spleen can result in decreased immune function (called immunosuppression) and decreased production of blood cells (called myelosuppression). This chapter discusses the lymphatic system (which includes the spleen and lymph nodes) and bone marrow. It describes the damage to these organs, the signs and symptoms of damage, how to screen for late effects, and medical management of these effects. Throughout the chapter, several survivors share their stories and advice about late effects of the immune system.

Spleen and lymphatic system

The spleen is part of the lymphatic system—a body-wide network of vessels and organs. The tonsils, thymus, and spleen are organs composed of lymphoid tissue. The tonsils, located in the back of the throat, filter and destroy bacteria. The thymus, a small organ beneath the breastbone, plays a role in helping white blood cells mature. The spleen is an organ in the upper abdomen that removes old red blood cells and platelets from the blood. It also stores red blood cells and performs other important functions of the immune system. Figure 16-1 shows the various parts of the lymphatic system.

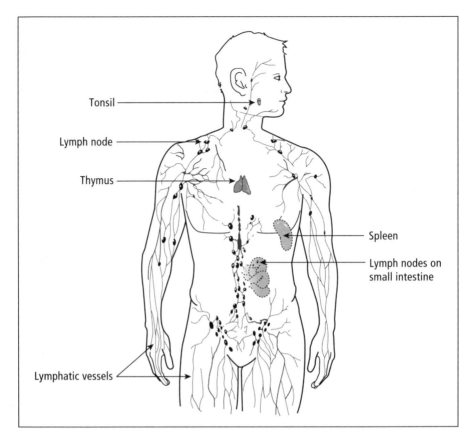

Figure 16-1. The lymphatic system

Organ damage

Much is still not known about immune status and risk of infections in childhood cancer survivors. By far, the best-documented threats to the body's immune system are removal of the spleen or high-dose (4000 centigray [cGy] or more) radiation to the spleen. Both of these treatments have been used to treat thousands of children and teens with Hodgkin lymphoma. Patients with non-Hodgkin lymphoma are also sometimes treated with high-dose radiation to the spleen. In this book, the term "asplenia" refers to either the absence of the spleen or a spleen that no longer functions after high-dose radiation.

> *I had 4400 rads (cGy) of mantle radiation, 4400 to the mediastinum, and 4400 to the diaphragm and spleen area in 1968 to treat my Hodgkin's stage IIA. CT (computed tomography) scans show no evidence of a*

spleen. My immune system still works okay, so maybe whatever's left of the spleen still supplies some service. I'm glad to still have it. The kidney on my left side is atrophied as well. I have lots of other problems, but my immune system has held up.

Susceptibility to infection is also a problem for survivors treated for chronic graft-versus-host disease (GVHD) after a stem cell transplant (e.g., bone marrow, cord blood, or peripheral blood).[1] The doses of total body radiation used to prepare children for transplantation do not destroy the spleen, although they do destroy bone marrow function. This is discussed later in the "Bone marrow" section of this chapter.

Signs and symptoms

Susceptibility to viral and bacterial infections is the hallmark of survivors with lowered immunity due to asplenia. These infections can progress rapidly and, in some cases, are life-threatening. Signs and symptoms of infection are as follows:

- Fever

- Sore throat

- Cough

- Shortness of breath

- Enlarged lymph glands

- Fatigue

- Chills

- Red vesicles that break open, then crust over (i.e., chicken pox)

- Red vesicles that travel in lines along the paths of nerves (i.e., shingles)

> *Ten years ago, I had a splenectomy, 2500 and 2800 cGy of mantle radiation, and ABVD (combination of four chemotherapy drugs) to treat my Hodgkin's. I get sick frequently. So far, I have not had overwhelming sepsis, but I have had many illnesses that required daily communication with the doctor to monitor them. During my illnesses, I spend from 1 to 3 weeks in bed, and it's about a month before I'm back to full energy level. I always know when something is starting because I get a weird feeling. I feel shaky, slightly short of breath, and my balance is off. Within a day or two, the sore throat, fevers, and severe illness start. I've learned to start the antibiotics when the feeling starts, and then the illness has a shorter course. It happens from two to four times a year.*

Screening and detection

Survivors without spleens or with nonfunctional, irradiated spleens need an annual exam that includes a detailed history of infections and illnesses. Methods to screen for and detect infections that require antibiotics and/or hospitalization should be part of a plan that you and your healthcare provider work out.

Medical management

Survivors with asplenia are at increased risk for bacterial infections that overwhelm the immune system very quickly. Infections with certain types of bacteria can become life-threatening in a matter of hours.[2] For this reason, children with asplenia are given daily preventive penicillin (or erythromycin if they are allergic to penicillin) and their parents are told to call the doctor immediately if the child develops a fever of 101°F (38.3°C) or higher. The Children's Oncology Group's (COG's) guidelines recommend that survivors with a temperature above 101°F (38.3°C) be given a long-acting, broad-spectrum antibiotic (e.g., ceftriaxone) and be closely monitored while awaiting the results of blood cultures.[3]

If you are an adult survivor with asplenia, your follow-up program will likely instruct you to call your healthcare provider immediately if you develop a fever higher than 101°F (38.3°C). Because bacterial infections are very dangerous for survivors who have asplenia, you will be prescribed long-acting, broad-spectrum antibiotics even before tests show what type of organism your body is fighting.

> *Post-splenectomy infection risks are not commonly understood by the general public, and sometimes not even in the medical profession. My oncologist is fantastic as far as response to possible post-splenectomy sepsis, but I find that even some experienced physicians don't get it. I've called in at my general practice doctor's office before with chills and a temp of 102°—on prophylactic penicillin V, I might add—only to be told that: (a) they might be able to work me in about a week later if someone canceled; (b) no, I couldn't speak with or leave a message for the doctor; (c) no, I couldn't speak with or leave a message for his nurse; and (d) they were booked and no, they couldn't possibly see me earlier than 1 week or more away. And that was my GP, whom I was supposed to call for that kind of thing.*
>
> *It's so much easier dealing with my late effects oncologist. I can call the office, tell the secretary who I am and what's wrong, and she says she'll page him to call me. I then actually get a quick callback, and he*

evaluates whether I need to come in or just do the antibiotics at home and come in if I get any worse. It really bothers me to have doctors who handle it otherwise because I'm very aware of how lethal this can be. I don't mind talking to the nurse; I don't mind some waiting, but I know that certain situations warrant major attention.

You should have a thorough discussion with your primary care provider when you are well about her approach to dealing with patients with asplenia. You should have a plan to follow in case of illness and fever. For additional information about testing and intervention for asplenia, you and your healthcare provider can refer to the COG's survivorship guidelines at *www.survivorshipguidelines.org.*

Because fevers can develop any time, such as when you are on vacation or traveling for business, make a plan for dealing with illness when away from home. One way to do this is to carry a wallet card with pertinent information about your history and risk and/or wear a medical alert emblem. An example of a wallet card for asplenic patients is shown in the information resource ("Health Link") called "Splenic Precautions" at *www. survivorshipguidelines.org.*

The following are additional suggestions for survivors with asplenia:

• Get the pneumococcal vaccine (prevents some types of pneumonia)

• Get the Hib vaccine (to prevent Hemophilus influenza B)

• Get the meningococcal vaccine (to prevent meningitis)

• Get the annual flu vaccine

• Make sure your healthcare providers know you don't have a functioning spleen before you have dental work or an invasive procedure such as a colonoscopy

Lymph nodes

The lymphatic system is composed of vessels, nodes, and organs. Lymph vessels are delicate tubes that branch, like blood vessels, into all parts of the body. They carry lymph—a thin, colorless fluid that contains white blood cells called lymphocytes. Throughout the network of vessels are groups of small, densely packed areas of tissue called lymph nodes. Clusters of lymph nodes are found in the neck, underarms, and abdomen. White blood cells are stored in lymph nodes, and from there they are sent out to attack substances or organisms they identify as foreign to the body.

To maintain blood volume, the fluid that routinely leaks from capillaries is collected by the lymphatic system, cleaned, and returned to the circulatory system. Two ducts under the collarbone connect the lymphatic system with large veins in the circulatory system (See Figure 16-1). Muscular contractions move lymph through the vessels, and one-way valves direct the flow.

Organ damage

Some children and teens with cancer have lymph nodes removed for biopsy. In some cases, this can result in permanent late effects, such as:

- **Hydrocele.** Occurs when fluid collects in the scrotum (most often in males who had abdominal surgery).

- **Lymphedema.** Occurs when lymph backs up into an extremity, causing swelling, pain, and loss of function (very rare with modern therapy).

- **Impotence.** Occurs in males when lymph node removal or radiation interferes with the nerves that control erections (very rare with modern therapy).

- **Ejaculation problems.** Occurs in males who had a radical pelvic lymph node dissection (very rare with modern therapy).

Lymphedema in survivors is generally caused by obstruction due to infection or scar tissue. The most common locations are in the pelvis and legs, or under the arms. Extensive information about lymphedema is available online at the National Cancer Institute's website at *www.cancer. gov/cancertopics/pdq/supportivecare/lymphedema/Patient* and the National Lymphedema Network's site at *www.lymphnet.org*.

Impotence, hydrocele, and problems with ejaculation are covered in Chapter 14, *Kidneys, Bladder, and Genitals*.

Signs and symptoms

Signs and symptoms of lymphedema are as follows:

- Limb feels full or heavy
- Skin feels tight
- Affected area feels painful and hot
- Limb has decreased flexibility
- Limb has swelling

- Indentations remain in skin when it is pressed (early in the process)

If untreated, the area can become very swollen and the tissues may harden.

Screening and detection

If you have lymphedema, your healthcare provider should take a history and do a careful evaluation of the involved areas. The history should include information about surgeries, radiation, infection, and when the lymphedema started. The circumference of the limb should be measured and circulation checked. Bring a list of your medications to show your healthcare provider, as other medical conditions such as diabetes, kidney problems, high blood pressure, congestive heart failure, or liver disease may contribute to the problem.

Medical management

Medical management of lymphedema includes treatments such as the following:

- Keeping the affected limb raised
- Wearing custom-fitted clothes that apply a uniform pressure
- Using manual lymphatic drainage

> Before I had to quit work I was a massage therapist trained in manual lymphedema drainage. It is a light massage technique that manually moves lymph out of your arms. The lymphedema may never go away but it can be improved and maintained better through these kinds of techniques. Look for a physical therapist or massage therapist in your area who specializes in this kind of massage.

Healthcare providers should educate you about additional ways to prevent or control lymphedema, such as the following:

- Proper skin care
- Diet
- Exercise
- Ways to avoid injury or infection (for example, no blood drawing from the affected limb)

Bone marrow

Bone marrow, the spongy material that fills the long bones in the body, is a blood-forming tissue. It produces white blood cells (which fight infection and disease), red cells (which carry oxygen and nutrients to body tissues), and platelets (which help form clots to stop bleeding). Decreases in cell production can cause lowered immune function, anemia, or bleeding problems.

Organ damage

Radiation to the bone marrow can affect blood cell production long after treatment ends. The amount of damage depends on the radiation dose and the amount of bone marrow in the radiation field.

Chemotherapy can also cause long-term effects in bone marrow function. Although the blood counts of most survivors return to normal within weeks after therapy ends, a few survivors treated with chemotherapy have problems with low blood counts for years after treatment.

My daughter was on a high-risk protocol for ALL (acute lymphoblastic leukemia). She went off treatment over 5 years ago. She had a CBC (complete blood count) 1 month after treatment ended, and all her counts were normal. They have stayed normal ever since. She rarely gets sick: I can't remember the last cold she had. In fact, we almost never see the pediatrician anymore because she just has her yearly follow-up visits with the late-effects oncologist.

· · · · ·

My daughter was diagnosed with average-risk ALL when she was 7 years old. She was treated with chemotherapy only. She has been off treatment over 2 years and her blood counts have never returned to normal. She had a CBC before she got sick, so we have a baseline. On that test, her platelets were 450,000. Since her treatment ended, they have never gone over 100,000. Her white blood cell count stays around 3.0 and her ANC (absolute neutrophil count) fluctuates between 600 and 1200. Her hematocrit is okay at around 38.

She catches every bug that goes around and has a hard time getting over them. For instance, last winter she got the flu and was sick for 4 weeks. She gets a lot of colds and they last 2 weeks. She has never regained her energy. She used to go out and ride her bike in the neighborhood for 2 or 3 hours. Now she can only manage a block or two before she comes back in and lies down. The doctors kept saying it takes some kids' immune

*systems longer to bounce back than others, but on our last visit the
oncologist said, "I don't think it's ever going to come back."*

Children who have undergone a stem cell transplant have lowered immune
system function for months after treatment. The bone marrow of these children has been destroyed by chemotherapy and/or radiation to allow the
healthy marrow or stem cells to grow. Re-establishing the immune function
takes time. All stem cell transplant recipients have profound impairment of
the immune system for up to a year. Transplant teams give families specific
instructions about ways to prevent infections during that time.

*Our daughter (age 9) had a peripheral blood stem cell transplant to
treat her Ewing's sarcoma. It's been several months and her white blood
cell count is still low, but we have come to the conclusion that we can't
make her live in a bubble anymore. We are careful to avoid potential
risks, though, such as being around large crowds of people.*

Graft-versus-host disease (GVHD) is a frequent complication of allogeneic
stem cell transplants (when stem cells come from a donor). It does not
occur with autologous (when stem cells come from the patient) or syngeneic transplants (when stem cells come from the patient's identical twin). In
GVHD, the bone marrow or stem cells provided by the donor (graft) attack
the tissues and organs of the child receiving the transplant (host). There are
two types of GVHD: acute GVHD and chronic GVHD. Acute GVHD occurs
within the first 100 days and chronic GVHD occurs or persists after day 100.
Patients can develop one type, both types, or neither one. Approximately
30 to 50 percent of survivors who have a related human leukocyte antigens
(HLA)-matched transplant develop some degree of GVHD. The incidence
and severity of GVHD are increased for children or teens who receive unrelated or mismatched marrow, but are decreased if cells that cause GVHD are
reduced prior to infusion. The majority of GVHD cases are mild, although
some can be life-threatening.

*JaNette's transplant was on May 5 and her ANC was up to 1000 on
May 30. That's when her graft-versus-host started. It doesn't look like a
regular rash, more like pinpoint red dots under the skin. It's very itchy,
and then it starts to peel. She looked like she had leprosy! She had very
little internal graft-versus-host disease. She's a year and a half post-
transplant, and she still broke out in a rash the last time they tried to
taper her off the cyclosporine.*

Chronic GVHD delays the return of normal immune function. Even when survivors with chronic GVHD have normal numbers of T and B cells, they may still be at risk for infection. Up to one-third of survivors with chronic GVHD develop serious, life-threatening infections.[4]

Signs and symptoms of GVHD

GVHD primarily affects the following parts of the body:

- Skin (itchy rash, discoloration or tightening of the skin, hair loss)
- Eyes (dryness, light sensitivity)
- Mouth and esophagus (dryness, tooth decay, difficulty swallowing)
- Intestines (diarrhea, cramping, weight loss)
- Liver (jaundice)
- Lungs (shortness of breath, wheezing, coughing)
- Joints (decreased mobility)
- Delayed immune response

Children or teens who underwent autologous stem cell transplants do not develop GVHD, but they can have a delayed immune response. The signs and symptoms of infection are fevers, sore throat, and shortness of breath, often accompanied by fatigue. However, fatigue by itself is not a symptom of infection. In addition, chicken pox and/or shingles can pose a threat to life if they are contracted when a child or teen is immunosuppressed.

> *Yossi had a small pimple near his eye on day 517 after his allogeneic BMT. The doctor thought it was a sty, and we put in antibiotic drops and started him on warm compresses. But by that afternoon, it had spread all around the bottom of his eye, near his nose and his lip. All on his left side. It was shingles. He went in the hospital for IV (intravenous) acyclovir for several days, then came home. After a few days the left side of his face looked pretty bad, but it stopped hurting and itching. He jokes that he is "Two Face."*

Screening and detection

Survivors of stem cell transplantations receive a multitude of tests that evaluate immune system function. Your institution will have its own list of tests and schedules, but it should include tests for both immune function and GVHD.

Medical management (after transplant)

Stem cell transplant survivors with GVHD may be treated with corticosteroids and other medications. All stem cell transplant survivors get prophylactic antibiotics for at least 6 to 12 months, and those with chronic GVHD continue to take antibiotics until all GVHD therapy has ended. If the survivor has low levels of IgG, she may get monthly IV IgG until her serum levels are normal for 2 months.

Prior immunizations are no longer effective after stem cell transplantation. Each treating institution has its own schedule for re-immunizing children and teens. Generally, survivors with no GVHD are given inactivated polio, influenza, and DPT (diphtheria-pertussis-tetanus) immunization after the first year. The MMR (measles-mumps-rubella) vaccine is usually given after the second year (survivors with GVHD do not receive the MMR). Find out when you (or your child) should get each immunization and talk with a healthcare provider about ways to avoid exposure to diseases until you are fully immunized. You also need to know how the treating institution manages chicken pox and shingles after a transplant.

Medical management (after treatment for any cancer)

Children who were treated when very young often miss immunizations and need to get them after treatment ends and their immune systems return to normal. Different institutions have different recommended schedules for re-immunizations. For example, your survivorship program may ask about immunization status and, if any are missing, advise that your child's pediatrician update them based on the Centers for Disease Control and Prevention (CDC) immunization schedules (see *www.cdc.gov/vaccines/recs/schedules/default.htm*). The U.S. guidelines recommend re-immunization no sooner than 3 months after standard chemotherapy and no sooner than 12 months after a stem cell transplant.[5] Both girls and boys are advised to receive the human papillomavirus (HPV) vaccine based on current recommendations.[6] Parents should check with their child's treating institution to find out the preferred immunization schedule for their child.

In addition, chemotherapy and radiation used to treat any childhood cancer can render prior immunizations ineffective. Recent studies in the United Kingdom have supported a strategy of re-immunizing all children after chemotherapy or stem cell transplantation, although a small number of patients do not achieve protective antibody levels after re-immunization.[5]

More research is needed to better understand whether patients should be screened for antibodies against vaccine antigens (meaning whether immunizations given prior to treatment are still effective).[7]

> My 13-year-old son Lucas was treated with surgery, chemotherapy, and radiation for Wilms tumor when he was 1 year old. I read a study about how chemotherapy can wipe out previous immunizations, so last year I had the oncologist check Lucas' titers. They were drawing blood anyway, so they just added that to the form. The results came back and, sure enough, Lucas needed to be re-immunized for about half of his vaccinations (even though everything was done on schedule and even though we waited over a year for him to be off treatment to get other vaccines and followed the schedule after that for years). So he's 12 years old and I'm thinking that he's "protected" because I've done everything we were supposed to do for vaccines, and it turns out that he wasn't as protected as I thought he was. A few other parents I know have done it now, as well. Some of their kids were fine, but a few had also had low or nonexistent immunity to illnesses for which they had been vaccinated.

> I am not saying one way or another that any parent has to or should get their child vaccinated. All I am saying is that for those parents who have had their child vaccinated and the child has undergone chemotherapy, it might be a good idea a couple of years off treatment to get their titers checked (during routine blood work) to make sure the child is still protected or needs to be re-immunized.

Chapter 17

Muscles and Bones

There are only two ways to live your life. One is
as though nothing is a miracle. The other is as
though everything is a miracle.

—Albert Einstein

LONG-TERM SURVIVORS of cancer may experience a number of complications to their muscles and bones. Radiation and surgery can alter both appearance and function of any part of the body. This chapter discusses the major late effects to the muscles and bones from amputation, limb-salvage procedures, radiation, and chemotherapy. It covers osteonecrosis, osteoporosis, osteoarthritis, and changes in body shape and size. Signs and symptoms, screening and detection, and medical management of these late effects also are presented. Included are many survivors' stories about how they cope with late effects to their muscles and bones.

Muscles

The human body comes equipped with more than 650 muscles. These muscles, together with other connective tissues (tendons and cartilage), form the support system for the skeleton. The muscular system enables body movement through a process of contraction and relaxation.

There are three types of muscle: skeletal, smooth, and cardiac.

- **Skeletal muscle.** Also called striated muscle, it manipulates the skeleton to cause movement. Skeletal muscles are voluntary muscles because their actions can be controlled.

- **Smooth muscle.** Involuntary muscle is found in many internal organs, such as the bladder, arteries, veins, and digestive tract.

- **Cardiac muscle.** A type of involuntary muscle found only in the heart.

All of these types of muscles can be affected by radiation and/or surgery.

Damage to the muscles

The most common late effect after radiation is muscle and soft tissue under-development, called hypoplasia. Over time, the non-irradiated muscles became larger and stronger than treated muscles. For some survivors, hypo-plasia is a problem more of appearance than function. For others, particu-larly those who had high-dose radiation many years ago, the weakening of bone and muscle increases with age and can severely impact quality of life.

> I had 4320 cGy of mantle radiation and 3600 cGy para-aortic and peri-splenic when I was 13. When I finished treatment I was so thin there was no fat on me anywhere. When I regained weight, the irradiated parts did not change. The muscles in my chest and neck look like leather with veins. There is no fat and the irradiated areas did not grow. I lift weights and have built up the surrounding muscles, but no amount of exercise changes the areas in the radiation field.

• • • • •

> I had high-dose mantle radiation 27 years ago. I'm 45, but feel like I have the body of a million-year-old woman. My whole upper torso is weakened. This occurred gradually over time. In my 20s I could chop wood and stack it. Now I have trouble just walking around the grocery store. I have very little strength, and hunch over. All of the muscles of my back, chest, and neck are atrophied.

Survivors who didn't have radiation or muscle-removing surgery in most cases quickly regain muscle strength and endurance.

> I was diagnosed with leukemia at age 12. I was heavily into sports so it was pretty traumatic when I was diagnosed. I had played soccer since I was 6 and was on the basketball team. I was on the sports fast track, doing really well, but that was nipped in the bud immediately.

> After the intensive part of treatment, I started playing tennis and volley-ball. Then, after I finished treatment, I went back to playing soccer and basketball. In college I was on the national championship crew team. During treatment I thought my sports dreams were dashed, but I had no late effects in terms of my muscles or strength.

If you had radiation to one side of the body while you were growing (for example, to treat Wilms tumor), you may have less muscle and fat tissue in the areas that were irradiated. This difference between the two sides of your body is called asymmetry. The more weight you gain, the more noticeable this disparity may become.

I only weigh 105. I had right flank radiation in 1962 for Wilms tumor. Because I'm so thin you can hardly see any difference in my hips. My doctor told me if I was heavier, it would be more obvious.

I do have a slight scoliosis and that caused a problem when they tried to start an epidural during the birth of my second child. They went too far and entered the spinal canal. When I was in labor with the third, I told them the history and told them to be careful and everything was fine.

Some survivors who had radiation to muscle groups have persistent problems with muscle tone. Occasionally, lack of exercise during years of treatment can also cause loss of muscle tone.

I had neuroblastoma at age 9 months and was treated with radiation on my left side. The muscle tone is really different on that side. I look a bit lopsided, and I'm just not as strong on that side.

• • • • •

I really should exercise more because I've never had as healthy a body as I'd like to have. It's hard to discipline myself to exercise. I also don't have a strong back or good posture. A physical therapist told me that I had lain in bed for so many years as a kid that the muscles just aren't in as good as shape as they should be.

My back hurts much of the time. Especially lately, because my son weighs 27 pounds and likes to be picked up and carried.

The muscles across my chest have atrophied a bit, causing me to sort of lean forward. I'm really not comfortable sitting up straight. I have sort of a rounded back and a hunched appearance.

Signs and symptoms

Signs and symptoms of hypoplasia are as follows:

- Decreased muscle mass
- Asymmetry of muscle mass of treated and untreated areas
- Decreased range of motion
- Decreased strength of affected muscles
- Stiffness and pain

Screening and detection

An evaluation of late effects to the muscles includes a visual inspection of all muscle groups, looking for asymmetry, swelling, atrophy, fibrosis, and strength. Your healthcare provider should also assess your gait and posture.

Careful measurements and comparisons of irradiated and untreated areas are important. An evaluation of tone, size, and strength is done for all muscle groups. You should have range of motion evaluated for affected muscle groups in arms or legs.

You should discuss your ability to participate in daily activities such as going to work, school, and taking care of your home. Talk about any limitations such as problems walking up stairs. Tell your healthcare provider about what types of exercise you do and how often. If you have late effects to the muscles that alter your appearance, discuss whether this affects your life in any way. Comprehensive care includes helping you adapt to changes in your body's appearance.

Medical management

Reversal of late effects to the muscles isn't possible, but trying to prevent further deterioration is. The primary way to do this is through a reasonable exercise program that works on range of motion and muscle strengthening. A physical therapist can help you design an individualized program to suit your needs.

> I was very athletic when I was diagnosed with Hodgkin's in 1982. It was hard for me to accept the changes in my body—I stopped growing, the muscles in my chest, back, and neck were atrophied. I needed to feel healthy after going through all that so I started exercising. I wanted to be strong and I achieved that. Except for the irradiated muscle groups, I am in great shape.

· · · · ·

> I went to a physical therapist and she helped me plan an exercise program. I have scoliosis and am slightly overweight. My back was hurting and the program has made a big difference. I do 6 days a week of aerobic exercise—usually swimming or walking. I also work out with weights three times a week.

Body size and weight

Heights of survivors can be affected by radiation to the spine or alterations in hormone production (see Chapter 9, *Hormone-Producing Glands*). Changes in body weight also can occur in small numbers of survivors. Long-term weight loss can be caused by malabsorption and other gastrointestinal problems (see Chapter 15, *Liver, Stomach, and Intestines*). At the other extreme, some studies show that a percentage of survivors become obese.

Not much is known about who is at risk for large weight gain or why it occurs. Survivors who tend to remain fairly inactive and become obese are usually those who had central nervous system radiation (for brain tumors and leukemia). Some of the questions for which the answers are not known are:

• Are these survivors gaining weight because they are inactive?

• Are they inactive because coordination is poor so they choose not to participate in physical activity?

• Do they have more fatigue?

• Is something altered physiologically in the brain that affects the drive to get up and move?

• Is there a physiological change in the brain that postpones feelings of being full while eating?

• Has their metabolism slowed?

• Did they not get into a lifelong habit of exercise due to long periods of being sick and/or on treatment for cancer?

• Does the use of steroids during treatment contribute to the risk of obesity?

Although much is not known, studies show that survivors who were treated with 2400 centigray (cGy) or more of cranial radiation have an increased likelihood of being obese. Females (especially those treated at early age) are at higher risk, although males can develop this late effect, too. The weight gain tends to begin in the first year off treatment.

Screening and detection

Monitoring growth includes plotting your height and weight on a chart at regular intervals. Measurements should be taken every 2 to 3 months during therapy and for the first year off therapy, and then once or twice a year until growth is complete. Abnormalities in weight or height require a consultation with an endocrinologist experienced in treating survivors of childhood cancer. For more information about growth, see Chapter 9, *Hormone-Producing Glands*.

Medical management

If you are underweight or overweight, you need a consultation with a medical specialist (gastroenterologist or endocrinologist). A discussion with a dietitian can be very helpful in planning a healthy diet. Weight loss usually includes an increase in exercise and changes in diet. Family participation in physical activities also helps survivors maintain a normal body weight. Participating in organized weight loss programs, such as Weight Watchers®, is sometimes helpful.

> My daughter is a leukemia survivor who had cranial radiation. Treatment seems to have permanently altered her perception of taste. All that tastes good is sugar or salt.
>
> After treatment, I purchased a big poster of the food pyramid. Every week when I am making my shopping list, I tell her to pick two vegetables and fruits for the week. I buy whatever she picks, and she has to eat them. I tell her that even if it doesn't taste good, her body needs it.
>
> Her weight is fine and she looks great. She hates to exercise, though. She refuses to hike, bike, or play sports. So I do the same with exercise as I do with food. I tell her she needs to do at least one organized physical activity each season. She's taking ice skating this fall. I try to find teachers who are lots of fun so she will enjoy it.

Bones

The human skeleton contains 206 bones, all held in place by connective tissues such as ligaments and tendons. The skeleton gives structure to the body and protects the internal organs. Bones determine our size and shape. The skeleton also works as a factory, making various blood cells in the marrow of the bones. Bones also store minerals such as calcium and phosphorus for use by the body.

The structure of bones changes as children grow. The skeleton of the fetus in the womb is made up mostly of cartilage. As pregnancy continues, bone develops, but even when the child is born, there are still areas that are a combination of bone and cartilage. At the end of long bones, such as those in the arms and legs, there are growth plates. Growth plates have a high level of activity until the child stops growing.

Damage to the bones

Survivors of childhood cancer can develop a number of complications that involve the skeleton. These can be caused by surgery, radiation, and/or chemotherapy.

Amputation

If a malignant tumor extends to vital structures such as major nerves and blood vessels, then amputation of a limb may be necessary. Survivors who had only the lower parts of extremities (below the knee) amputated usually function well after some rehabilitation. Generally, amputees can ski, run, hike, and perform other physical skills very well. These survivors may experience phantom pain in the missing limb and develop problems with calluses or pain in the stump. Those who had entire limbs removed or other portions of the skeleton (such as the pelvis) removed sometimes have ongoing problems with function and pain.

> I had osteosarcoma when I was 8 years old. I had a hip disarticulation (amputation of the entire leg), then chemotherapy. Because it's sometimes uncomfortable to stand with the proper posture, I tend to slouch. This pulls my hip down and curves my spine into an S shape. It also pulls on my ribs and they draw closer together, causing pain and shortness of breath. It's hard to sleep sometimes. This is a chronic problem for me. Some weeks are good and some weeks are really hard.

· · · · ·

> When I had to have my leg removed when I was 16 because of osteosarcoma, I thought my life was over. I knew that I would never be able to do the things I wanted to do—especially ski. Boy, was I wrong. While I was still on chemo, one of the doctors and a couple of nurses took a group of us skiing. I went along, but figured I would never be able to do it. Well, I was wrong again. They taught us how to ski on one ski with special poles to help us balance. That trip was so important to me. I went to college, met the man of my dreams, and got married. We have two little girls, and I am very happy.

The Amputee Coalition of America (ACA) at *www.amputee-coalition.org* provides extensive information about organizations and resources for amputees.

Limb salvage procedures

Growing numbers of survivors have bone and/or joint reconstructions or rotations instead of amputation. In these procedures, bones are removed or realigned. In many cases these surgeries are very successful, and the survivor's limb works very well. Other survivors require multiple surgeries and cope with pain, infection, and functional limitations.

> I was on a national championship cheerleading team when I was diagnosed with cancer. I had an allograft and a knee replacement done when I was 16, then had chemotherapy. I do have limitations on my activity now—the knee doesn't bend all the way and I can't kneel or sit crosslegged. I fall occasionally. I baby that plastic knee. I want to take care of it so it won't need to be replaced anytime soon.

· · · · ·

*My daughter was diagnosed with osteosarcoma at age 12. They replaced
8 inches of her femur with a titanium rod and gave her an artificial
knee. She ignored advice to limit her physical activity. She went right
back to cheerleading and jazz dancing. She is 19 now, has full range of
motion and great strength. She is on her college diving team and practices 3 hours every day. Her goal is to get into the NCAA finals so she
can invite her surgeon to come and watch.*

Limb radiation

Radiation to a limb will impact growth if a child has not completed puberty.
If the growth plate is involved in the field of radiation, the untreated limb
will continue to grow, creating a length discrepancy in the child's limbs.
This can be particularly problematic if the affected limb is a leg. The growth
plate of the untreated leg may need to be surgically altered to stop growth
to help keep the legs similar lengths. In some cases, leg-lengthening procedures are performed on the treated leg. However, this is a more involved
process.

Survivors who had radiation to a limb may be at risk for fractures without
trauma, and fracture may occur after minor trauma that would otherwise
not cause a fracture in an untreated bone. Fractures occur most often in
children who received more than 4000 cGy to the bone.[1]

*My son was diagnosed with Ewing's in his left distal femur at age 11. He
had chemotherapy from February to April of 1994. They removed the
tumor and 6 inches of his femur in May.*

*They replaced the femur with donor bone, but neither end grafted. The
donor bone broke several times, and the surgeons tried several creative
methods to fix it. However, they ended up just putting a rod in. The
growth plate was damaged in the surgeries, so that leg stopped growing.
He was on crutches much longer than any doctor had hinted at, which
got very depressing and upsetting for him.*

*Since then, he has had to have surgery once to shorten his "unaffected"
leg. He still has a lot of bone pain, and a limp that gets more pronounced
each day. He dislikes walking because it causes him discomfort, and
seldom attempts to run. All in all, though, I think he is thankful that he
got to keep his leg.*

Spine radiation

Some children and teens with cancer get their entire spines irradiated. Others have a portion of the spine treated. Scoliosis, a sideways curvature of the spine, is caused by radiation to only one side of the spine (down the midline of the body). When the untreated part continues to grow, the spine curves like a bow. This was a common side effect of children treated in the 1970s for Wilms tumor, neuroblastoma, or rhabdomyosarcoma. However, spinal radiation delivered since the 1980s has included the entire spine in the field of radiation, as well as the side of the body affected by the tumor, thereby decreasing the risk or degree of scoliosis. These children have a shorter trunk, but better spinal alignment. The damage is more pronounced for children treated when younger than age 6 or during the growth spurt of puberty. A survivor whose whole spine was radiated also may develop scoliosis; this is thought to occur because damage to the muscles and soft tissue on the irradiated side of the body pulls the spine out of alignment.

> My 9-year-old daughter Terri had a laminectomy to allow space for the tumor, which takes up more than the width of a normal spinal cord. I think the removal of the vertebrae contributes somewhat to the scoliosis. The other causative factors could be radiotherapy to the cervical/ thoracic area and paralysis in her left arm.
>
> Terri cannot bend her left arm at the elbow or raise it up from the shoulder, although she does still have movement in her wrist and fingers; so the arm does get some exercise but never anything too weighty. Her spine seems to be gradually curving more and more as time goes on, probably due to the heavy usage of the right arm. Her muscles in her right arm are almost as big as mine.

Other factors that may increase the risk of developing scoliosis are changes to the spine from tumor, osteoporosis, and fusion of parts of the spine.

A rare side effect of radiation to portions of the spine is kyphosis, where the upper spine curves outward, giving a hunchback appearance. This can occur with scoliosis after radiation to portions of the spine. Severe kyphosis and/or scoliosis can affect the functioning of other organs, such as lung volume.

> I had high-dose mantle radiation in 1972. I developed kyphosis, which has become much more noticeable in the last 10 years. It feels like I have thrown out my back. I also have fibromyalgia all along my spine. The muscles and tissue in my upper back and neck are atrophied, making it hard for me to stand up straight. When I was at the doctor's recently, he

called in a medical student and said, "Look at this woman's back. This is the reason we don't give high doses of radiation to kids anymore."

If radiation to the whole spine is needed, current protocols attempt to spare adjacent tissues to decrease the risk of scoliosis and kyphosis. Better staging of solid tumors has also decreased the number of children and teens who require radiation.

Radiation to the whole spine can stop or slow the growth of the spine. A short trunk (measured from the top of the head to the rump) occurs most often in brain tumor survivors whose entire spines were radiated with more than 3500 cGy. Total body radiation given prior to stem cell transplantation (i.e., bone marrow, stem cell, or cord blood) can also affect the growth of the spine, as well as growth of other bones exposed to radiation.

> *My daughter was born with neuroblastoma in 1991 and relapsed 3 months later. The second tumor was very large and sat on top of her kidney. After the big chemotherapy blitz, the tumor stopped growing. But in the several years it was in there, it eroded two of her vertebrae. She had to have part of her spine rebuilt. The section of the spine the surgeon worked on was fused and is supported by metal rods. It's inflexible and doesn't grow. From her mid-back to her waist is rigid, but she can still bend over at the hips.*

> • • • • •

> *Terri had spinal surgery and spinal radiation in her thoracic and cervical regions. She is still growing taller and at a reasonable rate, although she is well and truly below the lowest percentile for her age group. We've been very lucky that this hasn't really affected her too much.*

Radiation to any bones can cause slowed or stopped growth, depending on the age of the child and the dose of radiation. For instance, radiation to the orbits of the eyes in survivors who had retinoblastoma or rhabdomyosarcoma usually stops bone growth of the treated orbit. Hodgkin lymphoma survivors who had high-dose radiation often have underdeveloped ribs, collarbones, shoulders, and pelvises.

> *I was 13 years old when I was diagnosed with Hodgkin's disease stage IIIA. I was treated with 9 weeks of radiation, no chemotherapy. I was a pretty big kid then—5'5" tall and 108 pounds. I only grew another inch after treatment, so I'm much shorter than I would have been (my dad's 6 feet tall). All of the bones that received radiation stopped growing— my ribs, spine, collarbones. My chest and shoulders are the same size as they were when I was 13.*

Exostoses (also called osteochondromas) are outgrowths of the bone that are sometimes seen in children who were treated with radiation. Young children who receive total body irradiation (TBI) can develop osteochondromas as they begin puberty.[2] An x-ray is needed to confirm the diagnosis. These growths often do not require intervention. However, in a small number of cases, removal is necessary due to location and discomfort.

Slipped capital femoral epiphysis (SCFES) is displacement of the capital femoral epiphysis and is associated with radiation to the femoral head. It is often seen at the beginning of the pubertal growth spurt. New evidence is beginning to emerge that children who receive TBI and growth hormone replacement may be at even higher risk of SCFES. If a survivor whose hip was irradiated has hip pain, immediate attention is required.[3]

Osteoporosis

Some childhood cancer survivors experience a thinning of their bones (low bone density). This makes it more likely that they will break bones or develop osteoporosis, a disease of the skeleton that results from too little new bone formation or too much loss of bone tissue. This late effect is not well understood. It is known that survivors who took high doses of steroids (e.g., prednisone, dexamethasone), received high-dose methotrexate, had cranial radiation, had high-dose radiation to bones, or have low growth hormone seem to be most at risk. Young women who have an early menopause and men with low testosterone production also have a higher risk of developing osteoporosis.

> My daughter Melissa developed severe osteoporosis during her treatment. The process might have accelerated because she was in bed for almost a year, doing no weight-bearing exercise, and taking steroids. When she came home from the hospital, she seemed to be getting a bit better so we let her ride her bike. She fell and started screaming. It turns out she had seven fractured vertebrae. She was given pain medications and was on an IV (intravenous) drug in the hospital 3 days a month to treat the osteoporosis. Now she's on Fosamax® and her bone density has improved. She's playing soccer this year.

· · · · ·

> Coley was treated from ages 2¹/₂ to 3 with carboplatin, vincristine, and 5-fluorouracil, and daily injections of GCSF [granulocyte colony-stimulating factor]. When she broke her leg two times, they said the chemotherapy more than likely made her bones brittle.

• • • • •

Taylor hurt his ankle from a jump off a fence. We thought it was a sprain, but they x-rayed it and they found he had bad osteoporosis. His nurse said, "He has bones like Swiss cheese." His case nurse and I asked the doctors to start regular bone density scans to see if it improves. If it doesn't, maybe they can help with some drugs. So now he will get yearly bone density scans.

Osteonecrosis

Osteonecrosis (ON) is a condition caused by the death of the small blood vessels that nourish the bones. Other names for this condition are avascular necrosis (AVN) and ischemic necrosis. It is usually caused by radiation to bones and/or use of high-dose steroids (e.g., prednisone or dexamethasone).

I was an athlete who played three sports prior to my AML (acute myelogenous leukemia) diagnosis and bone marrow transplant. The steroids saved my life but destroyed my bones. I have had surgery on my shoulders, hips, and knee joints. My shoulders and hips are much better, but my knees are still painful, and I have trouble getting around. The surgeon is hoping that soon he will be able to use live bone in experimental surgery to help me.

Osteonecrosis is generally seen early rather than late—often within the first year off therapy. Adolescent girls are especially susceptible. Magnetic resonance imaging (MRI) is the best tool for diagnosis. As bone deterioration progresses, the bone may become weak and may eventually collapse. The course of the disease is variable. Some survivors have osteonecrosis for years with only minor problems with pain or movement, while others require surgery soon after diagnosis. Osteonecrosis can be very painful and sometimes leads to osteoarthritis. The website for the ON/AVN Support Group International is at *www.avnsupport.org*.

My daughter had leukemia and then relapsed. She has seven collapsed vertebrae in her back and a hip joint that has avascular necrosis. They think these problems were caused by steroids and having her nutrition compromised for so long when she was hospitalized. She's in a lot of pain, so she takes pain medication daily. We give her extra calcium and encourage exercise. She played soccer last year. We've taught her to ride a bike, and we hike. She also takes Fosamax®. She went to physical therapy for a long time and has a good range of motion and can even bend over. But when she gets tired, she limps.

• • • • •

My 13-year-old daughter Lisa had a BMT to cure her AML. She required huge doses of steroids for over 8 months to treat graft-versus-host disease. She started having knee pain when the steroids first began, but we had no choice but to continue with them. The avascular necrosis was confirmed soon after she was weaned off the steroids. Both femurs and tibias at the knee joint are affected, and her femurs also have what appear to be hairline fractures in them, although they don't cause her any pain now. Her knees swell periodically, and we ice them and wrap them in Ace® bandages. It's painful for her to walk, but she still tried out for and made the basketball team, although she could only play for a few minutes per game because of the pain. Things got worse and she needed to use a wheelchair for a few months until the pain settled down. Now she's walking again, but with the elastic bandages. It's a hard thing because she was a great athlete before. She lettered in track and was the second highest scorer in basketball. Now she can't run, jump, do PE. They did an MRI recently, and it hasn't worsened and hasn't improved.

Osteoarthritis

Osteoarthritis is a type of degenerative joint disease. It is characterized by pain with activity that subsides when resting. Survivors who had radiation to joints are at risk. People who have late effects that increase stress on the joints may also develop osteoarthritis. Helpful information about arthritis can be found at the Arthritis Foundation's website—*www.arthritis.org*.

I've walked on crutches for 20 years because my leg was amputated. I have arthritis in the knee from all those years of pounding on it. I ski with a group of amputees, and one time I sprained my knee. When I went to see the orthopedist, it turned out to be the fellow who had amputated my leg many years earlier. He was thrilled to see me. He gave me knee exercises to do to keep the knee strong. But he also told me he'd need to scope it in a couple of years to see how bad the arthritis is. He warned that I would eventually need a knee replacement. I'm trying to delay that as long as possible, hoping the technology continues to improve. I'd like the first replacement joint to last the rest of my life.

Signs and symptoms

Signs and symptoms of leg length discrepancy include the following:

• Difference in length and muscle mass between two limbs

• Limping

- Lower back pain
- Hip pain
- Scoliosis

Signs and symptoms of fractures include the following:
- Pain
- Deformity
- Swelling
- Bruising
- Loss of function

Signs and symptoms of spinal late effects include the following:
- Curved spine
- Uneven shoulder height
- Back or hip pain
- Limping
- Spinal shortening

Signs and symptoms of osteonecrosis, osteoarthritis, and SCFES include the following:
- Pain in affected joint
- Limping
- Impaired function

> I was diagnosed with acute lymphoblastic leukemia when I was 11 years old. I relapsed twice, then had a bone marrow transplant in 1988. Then I relapsed after the transplant. I was then put on a very experimental protocol at the National Institutes of Health, which cured me. I was on treatment for most of 14 years, and the majority of that time I was taking steroids.
>
> I have a big problem with osteonecrosis. Both hips went first, but only one hurt enough to treat. I had a surgery done on it called a core decompression. It relieved the pressure and the core grew into the bone. I was only 22 years old and wanted to buy time before I had the joint replaced.
>
> A couple of years later I started having problems with my shoulders, and they rapidly got worse than my hips. I have a high tolerance for pain,

so by the time I went in, both shoulders had collapsed. I had the left one replaced and that relieved the pain. The right one stopped hurting so I put off the surgery. I can use it but don't have full range of motion, and I can't do any heavy lifting.

Signs and symptoms of osteochondromas include the following:

- Hard lump on any boney surface
- Possible pain (depending on location)

Osteoporosis usually has no signs or symptoms, and bone density changes might not show up on regular x-rays unless the affected bone gets broken or infected. Advanced osteoporosis can cause the bones in your spine to compress, causing shorter height. It can also cause a hump on the upper part of the back.

Screening and detection

Amputation/Limb salvage

Survivors with amputations need an annual examination of the stump that includes a discussion about whether a prosthesis could be useful. Range of motion and function are evaluated. Survivors who had a limb salvage procedure should have both treated and untreated limbs measured every year (without clothes on to get accurate measurements), usually by an orthopedic surgeon. A baseline and then annual x-rays are needed until growth is complete to assess the growth plate. Survivors should also have a discussion with their healthcare provider if they have any back pain, limb pain, limping, or changes in muscle mass.

Scoliosis/Kyphosis

A scoliosis check needs to be done every year if you are at risk. Your back will be examined while you bend over with your fingers touching your toes and your knees straight.

If your child had radiation to his or her spine, several tests should be done to check for spinal abnormalities. Your child should have height checked while both standing and sitting, and the results should be plotted on a chart. Your child's healthcare provider should examine your child's spine every 3 months during puberty until growth is complete, and every year thereafter. A spine x-ray should be obtained for a baseline before puberty, then as needed.

Osteopenia/Osteoporosis/Fractures

If you had more than 4000 cGy radiation to any bones, they are at risk for fractures. Go to your healthcare provider if you have pain, swelling, or bruising in the areas that were irradiated. You may be at risk if:

- You went into an early menopause (periods stop).
- You are a stem cell transplant survivor who took high doses of steroids.
- You have any ovarian or testicular dysfunction.
- You are growth hormone deficient.
- You have a family history of osteoporosis.

Discuss your risk with your healthcare provider to see whether you need bone density studies. X-rays or computed tomography (CT) scans may be done to assess the amount of damage.

A painful joint should be evaluated by your healthcare provider. You may need an x-ray or CT scan to check for osteoarthritis and osteonecrosis.

Medical management

Amputation/Limb salvage

Medical management of amputations includes a visual inspection and checks for range of motion and muscle contractures. You should have your prosthesis checked (if you use one) and have a discussion with your healthcare provider about any advancements in technology.

> I wore a prosthesis for years because I was told by my parents, doctors, and physical therapists that I had to wear it. I think they wanted me to fit in with the other kids. But because I had such a high amputation, it was uncomfortable and painful.
>
> Finally, when I was 15, I just refused to wear it and I started using crutches. But I felt like I let them down and felt guilty about it for years.
>
> A doctor I met 10 years later told me if he had a high amputation he wouldn't wear a prosthesis. No one had ever told me that and it was so wonderful to hear. No one had ever said it was okay to use crutches or whatever was most comfortable for me. It was a relief just to hear one person give me permission to feel comfortable.

If you had limb salvage surgery or radiation and one limb is now longer than the other, discuss the treatment plan with your healthcare provider. Small differences in length of less than 2 centimeters (cm) usually don't require any treatment. Differences of 2 to 6 cm are treated with a shoe lift or surgery to stop the growth of the other limb. If the discrepancy is greater than 6 cm, other surgical steps may be necessary. These include shortening the untreated limb or lengthening the treated leg to restore a comfortable gait.

If you have an endoprosthesis, you need to take antibiotics prior to dental work to prevent possible infection that could spread to the prosthesis.

Scoliosis/Kyphosis

If you have any scoliosis or kyphosis, you should be referred to an orthopedic specialist with experience treating survivors of childhood cancer. If the curvature is noted during a period of rapid growth, such as puberty, do not delay seeing the specialist, because the curvature can increase rapidly during a growth spurt. Long-term survivors who have scoliosis or kyphosis often have back pain. The following may help make the pain more manageable:

- Physical therapy
- Using a brace
- Moderate exercise
- Pain medication

> I have severe pain from my kyphosis, fibromyalgia, and weakened back. I have tried over 15 different pain medications, including anti-depressants. You name it, I've tried it. They don't help much. I went to physical therapy and that helped quite a bit. I also did something called Pilates, which helped make the muscles that I still have a bit stronger.

If the curve in the back progresses (worsens) beyond 30 degrees (or curves 20 degrees with rapid progression), wearing a brace may be necessary. Curves greater than 40 degrees may require surgery. There are no standards for treatment of scoliosis after tumor surgery or radiation; the decision to use a brace or operate is individualized to the survivor's specific circumstances.

> The scoliosis was small, only around 12 to 15 degrees, and not sufficient to treat; however, the kyphosis was considerably larger and ended up being nearly 60 degrees. For that, I wore a Milwaukee brace 23 hours a day and did physical therapy exercises at home for over a year, then continued exercises and wore the brace at night for almost another year. No surgery for it. When I saw our pediatric orthopedist here after more than 10 years as a follow-up dropout, the curve had progressed to 69 degrees, which is more than 10 degrees worse than pre-bracing; however,

as that was when I was entering the growth spurt, I feel it was worth it. At this point, it's not a problem cosmetically, and the pain is manageable with exercise.

Osteoporosis

If you have osteoporosis, your yearly examination should include information that stresses the importance of:

- Weight-bearing exercise such as walking or running.
- A diet rich in calcium. This includes dairy products, shellfish, leafy green vegetables, and tofu. Your healthcare provider might also recommend taking supplemental calcium with added vitamin D.
- Adequate vitamin D. Some dairy products are fortified with vitamin D and the body makes some on its own when exposed to sunlight, but many survivors require supplementation.

> *I was told by my gynecologist that I should stay on the calcium tablets, and I was put on a nasal spray to help with the bone loss from the osteoporosis. However, I have severe allergies and the nasal spray gave me too many problems, so I am back to only taking the calcium tablets again. It becomes more of a problem because I am lactose intolerant and can't have milk or ice cream. I can eat yogurt and frozen yogurt. I tolerate pizza, lasagna, and macaroni and cheese in small portions.*

Osteonecrosis

Treatment for osteonecrosis may include:

- Activity modifications.
- Range of motion exercises.
- Electrical stimulation.
- Surgery to remove the inner layer of bone (core decompression). Sometimes a piece of healthy bone is put in when the inner layer is removed.
- Surgery to remove a wedge of bone (osteotomy) to reduce the weight bearing of the bone with osteonecrosis.
- Pain and/or anti-inflammatory medication.

> *Tim began having problems with his ankles at the end of his year of intense relapse therapy. He would have intense, intermittent pain. When*

the first MRI was done, it showed necrosis in the ankles, but nowhere else. The next year, the MRI showed necrosis still in the ankles and some involvement in the shins and knees, but none in the hips.

This fall, the orthopedic doctor hoped things might be better after being off the steroids for so long, but in fact, it looks like it may be increasing. The edema has gotten quite a bit worse. So we are watching it. Tim has not had further pain. He is on extra vitamin D and calcium supplements.

The ankle is not a good candidate for joint replacement. If Tim's necrosis gets worse, they will switch him to braces that include bracing along the front of the leg and, I think, the knee. The idea is to distribute some of the weight to the knee from the ankle. I would have them do MRIs of the knee before we did that.

• • • • •

My son Ben was diagnosed with acute lymphoblastic leukemia when he was 17. He was given painkillers pretty early in treatment for leg pain and headaches. Then, he was hospitalized for almost a month due to sepsis, and he was encouraged (and needed) to take more. As a caregiver and parent, I was totally unprepared when he became addicted to painkillers. I missed some pretty obvious warning signs and had no idea how serious a problem this can be until Ben nearly died from an overdose. Now I know that many things combined to increase Ben's likelihood of addiction—a possible genetic predisposition, access provided by legitimate physical pain, the emotional trauma of such a serious diagnosis, and he was at an age when so many people experiment with drugs.

By the time the avascular necrosis (AVN) was diagnosed, we were aware of his addiction and closely monitored the use of the painkillers. He had four surgeries at the end of treatment on his shoulders and hips, so of course had to continue to take painkillers, but with careful monitoring. After his last surgery, he went to residential rehab for a month. This spring, Ben is doing a "grand rounds" on his painkiller addiction at the hospital where he was treated. He's doing great now, but it was a process.

Fractures

If you get a fracture in irradiated bone, it most likely will occur where the bone was biopsied or at the site of tumor in the bone. These types of fractures may need surgery to insert a device to keep the bone aligned. Because the surrounding tissues were also irradiated, this presents a surgical challenge. Make sure this surgery is done by an orthopedic surgeon with experience operating on irradiated bone and tissues.

Osteochondromas

Osteochondromas are generally noted first by the survivor or a family member. Once the diagnosis is confirmed by x-ray, management will be determined by the symptoms. If there is pain or if the osteochrodroma is affecting other bone growth or joint function, a referral to an orthopedist is recommended.

Chapter 18

Skin, Breasts, and Hair

*It's no use going back to yesterday, because
I was a different person then.*

—Alice
Alice in Wonderland, by Lewis Carroll

THE HUMAN BODY IS WRAPPED in a waterproof covering called skin. Skin, hair, and nails are part of this covering, which is called the integumentary system. This system has several important functions. It protects the body by keeping fluids in and foreign organisms out. It insulates the body and helps regulate body temperature. Pigments in the skin help protect the body from sunlight's harmful ultraviolet rays. Nerve endings in the skin allow it to sense heat, cold, pain, and pressure.

Surgery, radiation, and chemotherapy can all cause short- and long-term changes in the skin, breasts, and hair. This chapter describes these changes, how they are diagnosed, and the most common methods used to manage them.

Skin

Skin is composed of two main layers: the epidermis and the dermis. The epidermis is a thin outer layer that is only 10 to 30 cells thick. The top layer of the epidermis is made up of dead cells full of keratin, a protein that keeps bacteria from entering the skin.

The thick, inner layer of the skin is called the dermis. Cells in the dermis produce melanin, a pigment that gives skin its color. Exposure to the sun increases the amount of melanin, causing a darkening of the skin. The dermis also contains nerve endings, blood vessels, and hair follicles. Sebaceous glands are usually attached to hair follicles in the dermis. These glands secrete oil that helps keep skin and hair from drying out.

Sweat glands produce a fluid containing water, salt, and waste products when the body is hot. When sweat evaporates, it cools the body. Blood vessels in the skin store blood to help regulate body temperature. During exercise, your skin appears flushed because the body pushes warm blood to the surface to cool off.

Organ damage

Skin can become discolored from some types of chemotherapy, higher doses of radiation, and graft-versus-host disease (GVHD), which occurs after some types of stem cell transplants.

> *My daughter had a BMT (bone marrow transplant) in March of 1995. She had no radiation. Conditioning was Cytoxan® and thiotepa. The thiotepa caused Paige to get what looked and acted like a very severe sunburn over her entire skin. It turned very dark brown and then all peeled off—all of her skin! It did heal with the rest of her body, and you would never know except for the softness and the brown mottled areas in her skin creases.*

$$\cdots\cdots$$

> *Robby has funky discoloration on his skin from the total body irradiation he had prior to transplant. He is brown-skinned, and has big freckles where the skin has lightened. He also has scars on his cheek, ear, and chin from shingles. They could eventually be helped with visits to the plastic surgeon, but for right now they don't bother him. He has also gotten quite a few moles all over his body, which now need to be watched.*

$$\cdots\cdots$$

> *I had Hodgkin's stage IIB and was treated with mantle radiation and ABVD (combination of four chemotherapy drugs). It came back 2 years later, and I had MOPP (another combination of drugs) and radiation again. I have a dark patch of skin in the hollow at the front of my throat. It always looks dirty—like I never wash my neck.*

Some children and teens treated with bleomycin or etoposide develop darkened areas of the skin (called hyperpigmentation). Pressure from trauma (such as removing a bandage from the skin) can result in darkened streaks in the traumatized areas. Bleomycin and etoposide can also cause darkening of the nail cuticles and creases on the palms. Dark bands on the nails may form as well. Doxorubicin (Adriamycin®), daunorubicin, and idarubicin can also cause darkening in skin creases, nails, palms, soles of feet, and face. These changes usually disappear over time.

> *Eric had very dark skin on the joints of his fingers and toes. Also, his knees were very dark. I hated it because he always looked dirty. His*

doctor told me that it was a side effect from the chemotherapy. It took a few months for it to disappear after treatment stopped.

Moles

Children or teens who had radiation therapy sometimes develop large numbers of brown moles on their bodies, often in unusual places such as the scalp, hands, or toes.

Garrett has a bunch of moles, all over. I even found myself digging in his belly button one night trying to remove what I soon discovered was a mole. He has them on the bottom of his feet, on his scalp, between his fingers, and everywhere else you can imagine. We have even observed some of them form (they started out looking like bug bites). We had the staff look at them, but they didn't seem surprised. We were told they were a direct consequence of the radiotherapy and should be monitored closely for unusual changes. Other than that, they said, "Don't worry, we see this all the time."

Scars

Most survivors have scars on their skin that serve as a daily reminder of their bout with cancer. Children or teens who had solid tumors may have extensive scarring from the tumor removal surgery. Those who had leukemia or lymphomas have scars from central line insertion and removal.

Chris has lots of scars in addition to the four big ones on his head to remove the tumor and put in the shunt. He has a scar from where the catheter was implanted, a hole from the G-tube (gastrostomy or feeding tube), and a scar in his belly button where he was checked to see that the shunt was placed correctly.

• • • • •

I had Wilms tumor in 1962 when I was 2 years old. I have a big scar that goes right around my waist. It's no big deal. I just don't wear bikinis.

• • • • •

Logan's scar is a giant Mercedes® symbol. Upside-down V with a 2-inch cut in the center going up the breastbone. He had a port and has a 2-inch scar from that. He has a scar from his G-tube that is deep and quite large and looks just like another belly button. He also has two drainage tube scars. But they're all beautiful to me. I tell him they're just his battle scars and he has a special tummy. But I hope they'll fade out some.

· · · · ·

I had cancer twice. I finished treatment for the second bout 6 months ago. I have a 3-inch-long bright red scar from the ports on my upper-left chest. I wore the push-up bra for months after the port was removed trying to keep the scar from stretching, but it didn't work. It looks awful and really limits the kind of clothes I wear. I like to look pretty and it bothers me. I was recently at a store in one of those big dressing rooms with mirrors all around. I felt like all of the women were staring at me. I ran out in tears.

Some children and teens who get severe cases of shingles have scarring along the nerve tracts. Mild and moderate cases usually heal without scarring.

Robbie has some scarring across one side of his face from having shingles after his bone marrow transplant. The biggest is the size and shape of a half dollar. Being fairly dark-skinned, the scar is very visible, and is actually darker than his regular skin. I told him he could go to a plastic surgeon if he wanted to, but he doesn't really want to go to any more doctors, and who could blame him.

Many survivors who had radiotherapy (except those who had cranial radiation only or total body irradiation) have permanent tattoos (small black dots) on their skin to outline the treatment areas.

Maybe others aren't as bothered as I was by the tattoos, but in my case they were always so public and sometimes led to the disclosure of my treatment that I wasn't ready or prepared to share with people. At least my staging laparotomy/splenectomy scar was hidden from view, but those darn little black spots were scattered across my body and two of them were right at the edge of most necklines of blouses.

One in particular seemed to catch everybody's attention, and on more than one occasion someone would wet the end of their finger and lean over to rub off the ink spot on my chest. I eventually had that one removed although my oncologist thought this was neither sensible nor necessary. But it did put an end to that particular intrusion.

Stretch marks

Some children and teens gain weight when they are on steroids (i.e., prednisone, dexamethasone) for extended periods of time. This can cause stretch marks. This is a variable side effect—some children gain weight but have no stretch marks, while others get them all over the body. Stretch marks sometimes fade with time.

My daughter gained 50 pounds while on high-dose steroids to treat her GVHD after her bone marrow transplant. Luckily, my daughter's skin never split, but now, 2 years later, she has massive stretch marks. They run down the inside of her legs, all the way to her ankles. They are everywhere on her thighs, hips, stomach, breasts, and arms. She has learned how to tolerate the stares and answer the questions about all the stretch marks.

Radiation injuries to the skin

Survivors of childhood cancer who had high-dose radiation frequently have acute skin problems (e.g., redness, peeling) during treatment. Chronic radiation injury to the skin and underlying tissues can occur months or years after the radiation is given. The signs and symptoms of radiation injury to the skin include the following:

• Dry skin

• Dark and/or light areas on the skin

• Thinning of the skin

• A spidery pattern of capillaries visible in the skin (telangiectasia)

• Ulcers on the skin

The first late effect to the skin after radiation is usually a loss of elasticity. Areas of the skin can become tough (called fibrosis) and the tissues can contract. In some cases, telangiectasia appears.

Radiation can also cause the skin to age faster. Skin in the areas radiated may become drier and more wrinkled and may develop age spots. These late effects are much more likely in survivors who had high-dose radiation. Late effects to the skin depend on dose per fraction (the amount of radiation given at one time) as well as total dose. The most damage occurs to skin and underlying tissue when radiation is given in fractions larger than 200 centigray (cGy). Current technology uses megavoltage (skin-sparing) radiation to avoid severe damage to the skin. Those who were irradiated in the 1960s and at some institutions in the 1970s with orthovoltage radiation are at higher risk for late effects to their skin.

I had 4500 cGy of mantle radiation in the 1970s to treat my Hodgkin's disease. The skin over my sternum always looks slightly reddened with deep wrinkles and creases, unlike the skin on any other part of my torso. I've heard some survivors call the thickened, wrinkled areas "chicken skin."

Tissue damage under the skin can make the skin tighter and more vulnerable to breakdown. Factors that contribute to ulcers in the radiation field are trauma, pressure, ultraviolet light (from sunlight or tanning beds), and exposure to intense cold.

I had my thyroid removed recently (casualty of Hodgkin's treatment). When I told my surgeon that it still hurt, he reminded me that because there is radiation damage at the vascular level I could expect to heal slower than a normal person. He teased me because I have no body fat on my neck or upper chest to help keep the skin loose. Then he told me I can take him off my Christmas card list because we are through with each other. He was so sweet and such a fine surgeon. The scar is already pencil-line thin.

• • • • •

I had 2800 cGy of mantle radiation 10 years ago. I never even had any skin problems, even irritation, while getting the radiation and I have no skin problems now.

Damage to glands

Radiation can also damage or destroy sweat glands, sebaceous glands, and hair follicles. Damage to these glands may be permanent.

Since my daughter's transplant she doesn't sweat at all. As a consequence, she can't tolerate heat or humidity. I first thought it was the skin GVHD problem causing it, but now the GVHD is gone and she still doesn't sweat. When she is hot she gets beet red and finds it hard to breathe. So she stays in the air conditioning. It's a problem because she's in the marching band at school and she can't march on hot days. She carries a water bottle and drinks cool water if the room is hot.

• • • • •

I only sweat on one side of my head and face now. When I work out, the right half of my face gets bright red and dripping wet. The hair on that side gets sweaty and yucky. I sweat on just the right half of the skin above my lip. I look really weird. It looks like I fell asleep with my face turned to the side and got sunburned. The left side of my face is perfectly white, dry, and looks like I haven't even exerted myself. My hair stays dry too. My oncologist told me to be careful about not getting overheated since half of my head can't release heat.

• • • • •

An effect that causes us all great humor is not sweating in the armpit that was heavily radiated and not having underarm hair.

Go figure—survivorship humor is very sick. I only sweat on the right side and have hair only on the right side. You'd think all these years I could have gotten a break on dry cleaning.

Itchy skin can persist for years after treatment with radiation. It is most common in those who had high-dose radiation or GVHD after an allogeneic bone marrow transplant.

Katie had itching on her torso for many years after BMT. We were told this was very, very mild GVHD. It was so mild, usually a good back scratch cured the problem.

• • • • •

I suffer from itching and incredibly long-lasting hives. When I went through my worst bout a couple of years ago, I discovered that a combination of Atarax®, Temovate® cream, and some kind of antihistamine with my steroids really helped.

Skin cancer

A serious late effect to the skin after treatment for childhood cancer is skin cancer (although it can develop in people who never had childhood cancer). Radiation increases the risk and shortens the development time of skin cancers. Skin cancers can arise in irradiated or non-irradiated skin, and exposure to the sun may hasten their development. Having a family history of skin cancers and getting older also increase your risk of developing skin cancers. See Chapter 19, *Second Cancers*, for more information about skin cancers.

Medical management

Careful evaluation of skin changes should be part of your yearly follow-up examination. In some cases, referral is made to a dermatologist for more frequent examinations. Any changes in color, scarring, dryness, fibrosis, or tightness should be identified and recorded in your medical chart. Reversal of late effects to the skin is not possible, but education about ways to slow the process can help.

You should protect your skin from the sun. If you had radiation, you have a definite risk of cancers of the skin, especially in the irradiated areas. Try to limit your sun exposure, and use sunscreen of at least SPF (sun protection factor) 30 when you are out in the sun. If you had radiation to the chest or back, always wear a shirt when in the sun. If you had radiation to the arms or legs, keep them covered. Anyone who had cranial radiation or who has thin hair should wear a hat when outdoors.

I wasn't supposed to go out in the sun after my transplant, but I did anyway. The sun aggravated the mild GVHD that I had and I turned blotchy. I had itchy light and dark patches on my stomach and face. I had to go back on steroids.

Scars need extra protection from the sun. Normal skin sloughs off if sunburned, but scars cannot do that. They may remain darker. If you are going out in the sun for extended periods with your scars exposed, it's best to put zinc oxide on them.

If you have lots of moles on your skin, be sure to inspect them regularly. The moles probably won't become cancerous, but it is best to keep an eye on them. Always point them out to your healthcare provider at your follow-up visits, especially ones he wouldn't normally notice—between your toes or on your scalp. Ask your healthcare provider to check areas you can't see. If moles change shape, color, or size, make an appointment with a dermatologist. Some dermatologists take photographs of a survivor's moles so they can do a yearly comparison. Moles need continued surveillance, and you should always use sunscreen to protect your skin and moles from ultraviolet rays.

If sebaceous gland damage makes your skin especially dry, using a moisturizing cream may make you more comfortable. Dermatologists sometimes treat scars, stretch marks, and other skin problems with medicated creams. If your scars and/or stretch marks bother you, check with your dermatologist to see if there are any medications available that might help them fade. You could also consult a plastic surgeon to learn about any surgical options for removal of scars and/or stretch marks.

My daughter developed a large keloid scar on her back after a chicken pox lesion was biopsied. She wanted it removed because it was itchy. The plastic surgeon said he could fix all the other scars too, from two central lines, two ports, and a gastrostomy. She said, "No, those are mine." She doesn't mind. She puts on her bikini and goes out on the beach with all the rest of the kids.

Make sure to tell your surgeon about your cancer history if she needs to operate on previously irradiated skin. Special precautions must be taken as the tissue might be fragile and slow to heal.

Breasts

Breasts arise from the epidermis during development in the womb. At birth, male and female breasts appear identical. During puberty, the female nipples, areolas, and breasts enlarge. The major part of female breasts is composed of mammary glands, which secrete milk after a child is born.

Organ damage

Radiation to a female's developing breast can affect its growth because the breast bud is very sensitive to radiation. A total dose of 1000 cGy can cause decreased breast development in the radiated area (called hypoplasia), and doses higher than 2000 cGy can stop all breast growth.[1,2]

If you had radiation only on one side (e.g., flank radiation that included the breast tissue) before puberty, the irradiated breast may not grow as large as the non-irradiated breast.

Young women who had radiation to the center of the chest for Hodgkin lymphoma or non-Hodgkin lymphoma may notice underdevelopment of the breasts on the parts closest to the center of the chest. This can give the illusion of breasts that seem especially far apart.

> *I was 16 when I had high-dose mantle radiation. That was the end of my youthful body. I had large breasts and after the radiation they never really regained their shape. They just flopped and have stayed that way ever since.*

When the developing breast is irradiated, it increases the risk of breast cancer. All survivors whose breasts were irradiated need lifelong surveillance for breast cancer (see Chapter 19, *Second Cancers*, for more information).[3,4]

The scientific literature does not contain much information about breast-feeding after radiation for childhood cancer. More information will become known as more survivors grow up and have children. Survivors of breast cancer sometimes have problems breastfeeding from the irradiated breast. If only one breast was irradiated, women are usually able to breastfeed normally from the other breast.

> *I was unable to nurse my second child, who was born 4 years after my treatment. I was told the milk glands were not working because of the radiation, like the sweat glands and the salivary glands.*

· · · · ·

I had mantle radiation to treat my Hodgkin's disease: 4000 rads to AP-PA (anteroposterior-posteroanterior) upper mantle, 400 rad boost to superior mediastinum, 4000 rads to para-aortic nodes. In addition, when the staging surgery was performed, one of my ovaries was moved to protect it from radiation in case I needed radiation to the abdomen. Fortunately, I didn't, and I have experienced relatively few significant side effects from treatment. I became pregnant 7 years after I was treated and I had no problems breastfeeding our daughter. Tammy is a healthy, happy almost-15-year-old.

Medical management

Your healthcare provider should carefully examine your breasts at each follow-up appointment if you had radiation to the chest area (mantle radiation for Hodgkin lymphoma, chest radiation for non-Hodgkin lymphoma, or total body irradiation prior to transplantation). You may need more frequent appointments during puberty.

Performing a monthly breast self-exam is one way to take care of yourself. This is especially important if your breasts were in the radiation field. Your healthcare provider should show you how to do a breast self-exam, as watching a videotape is usually not enough. You should do self-exams starting when you are a teenager and then every month for the rest of your life.

I think all follow-up clinics should have those synthetic breasts with lumps that survivors can feel to practice self-examination and to learn what lumps feel like. I was at a health fair and felt one of those things. Later, when I found my breast cancer during a self-exam, the lump felt exactly like that display breast. I think if survivors know what it feels like, they will be more likely to examine themselves and feel more comfortable speaking up.

Survivors at increased risk for breast cancer need to have their first (baseline) mammogram done 8 years after treatment or by age 25, whichever comes last. So, if you had mantle radiation at age 15, your first mammogram should be done at age 25. If you had mantle radiation when you were 19, you should have your first mammogram at age 27. Follow-up mammograms are done on a schedule determined by your risk. Many healthcare providers suggest mammograms every other year until age 40, then yearly.

If you have breast hypoplasia or breasts that did not develop, you may choose to use prostheses like the ones worn by women who have had breast removal surgery. Some survivors choose to leave their breasts as they are, and others have their breasts surgically enlarged. This surgery should be done by surgeons who are experienced and familiar with operating on irradiated tissue.

My daughter had one of the first transplants for AML (acute myelogenous leukemia) many years ago. I don't know how much radiation she got, but it was enough to stop all breast development. She had breast augmentation surgery while in high school. She was pleased with the results except that she gets keloid scars easily and those are pretty unsightly.

Hair

Hair and nails are made of dead cells from the epidermis (outer layer of skin). Individual hairs grow from living roots in hair follicles. Except for the root, the entire hair is made of dead cells. Nails grow from living roots underneath the cuticle (fold of skin at the base of nails).

Damage

Chemotherapy usually causes hair to fall out. When hair grows back after treatment, it can be a different color or texture than it was before diagnosis. Most survivors treated only with chemotherapy get a lush growth of hair after treatment ends.

Trevor had beautiful light-blond straight hair when he was diagnosed. He lost it twice, but now has the thickest, light-brown, wavy hair. Every time I take him in for his haircut, all the gals say, "Oh, I would love to have his hair!" So it came back totally different, but totally gorgeous. The only weird thing about it is the texture. The chemo made it coarse and dry. Trev's skin is also still very dry.

• • • • •

As a young boy, Joel's hair was blond and wild. It was thick and stuck up and out and every which way. As a baby, it used to look like he had a halo with all that blond fuzz around his head. The hair stylist who cut his hair struggled for years trying to figure out a way to cut it so it looked good, but no matter how much gel was used, as soon as it was dry it popped up. It became a part of him, his mischievous grin and wild hair.

After losing his hair during his treatment (ages 14 to 17), we joked that maybe he'd get good hair when it grew back. And it worked. His hair grew in a little darker, but also more fine and much more manageable. It would even lie down! The good hair has stayed, until losing it again this summer after relapse. It is just now coming back in and it looks even darker. Maybe it will be curly this time.

• • • • •

Jamie's hair was light brown and thick before diagnosis. When it grew back 9 months later, it was jet black and thin. It feels like velvet. I could spend hours rubbing his head, it's so soft!

Most children who have only chemotherapy prior to a stem cell transplant have full regrowth of hair. Very rarely, children who had busulfan and Cytoxan® to prepare them for a stem cell transplant have permanent baldness (called alopecia).[5] Children and teens who take cyclosporine for extended periods of time can have excessive hair growth.

My 6-year-old daughter had a bone marrow transplant when she was 4 years old. She stayed shiny bald for a long time. When it started to come in, it was very thin and it has never improved. It's very wispy and there is undergrowth, but the under part stays very short. She's starting to say she doesn't like the way she looks. So I got her a wig that looks pretty natural, but she was still so young that she tended to take it off out in public. We recently upgraded to the best synthetic wig you can get. She wears it to school and church and then immediately takes it off.

Radiation damages the hair follicles. The higher the dose, the more risk of permanent damage. Children or teens who had 1800 cGy or less radiation to the head usually have normal hair growth. Those who had more than 1800 cGy may have permanently thinned hair. Hair may not grow back in areas that had high-dose radiation (more than 3000 cGy). For instance, medulloblastoma survivors usually have bald areas on the back of the head where they got the most radiation. Survivors who had rhabdomyosarcoma of the parotid gland may have a hairless rim around the ears.

I can see exactly where they did the radiation to my son Chris' head. He looks like an older gentlemen who is losing his hair; he has a little there, but not much. There is a bald band from behind one ear in a strip to the other ear. We let his hair above grow longer to cover it. He has lots of scars to cover: where they did the ventriculoscopy in the front of his head, the shunt and brain surgery scars on the back side, and the VP (ventriculoperitoneal) shunt scar on the side.

• • • • •

Robby, being half-Indian, had black hair so dark it was blue. It was very soft and very thick. He never lost all of his hair during chemotherapy, but could pull it out in handfuls.

Prior to BMT, he had cranial-spinal radiation and all his hair fell out.
He was a little fuzzhead. When his hair finally came back in, it was still
very dark, but dark brown, and very stiff and coarse. He has many col-
ors of hair now—white, blond, red, and one big blond patch behind his
right ear. There is even some gray splattered throughout. Apparently the
radiation has damaged certain hair follicles. He now keeps it very short
and has some very strange cowlicks that never lie down.

• • • • •

My daughter Rachel's hair has stayed very thin and wispy in the years
since her bone marrow transplant. The hairdresser who cuts her wig
suggested we cut Rachel's hair short all over and try to mousse it and
it might look like a regular short haircut. Rachel doesn't like that idea,
as she likes long hair, even sparse long hair. And long to her is barely
touching her neck! She still is not happy with her hair.

• • • • •

My son had a BMT to treat his relapsed leukemia. He has no problems
with skin or hair, only that he seems every year to have more and more
moles. Other than that, he's got nice skin and is pretty hairy! Full head
of thick hair, facial hair, hair now growing on chest and legs.

Medical management

Permanent loss of hair cannot be reversed; however, in the last decade, plastic surgeons have worked on new techniques to transplant hair. These hair transplants use micrografts from parts of the head that still have thick hair growth. If you are interested in exploring this option, ask your doctor for a referral to a plastic surgeon with extensive experience using these new methods.

Survivors share the following tips about managing hair:

• If your hair is thin or wispy, ask your hair stylist to recommend hairstyles and hair products that can help the hair appear fuller.

• Don't dye your hair, as this can dry out and damage the hair shafts.

• Don't use perms. If you do, ask your hairdresser to use the most gentle type she has so you can minimize breakage.

• If you have very thin hair, it looks fuller if you keep it cut relatively short.

• If you have scars or bald spots on your head, you can grow your hair to cover the area.

Chapter 19

Second Cancers

Nothing is to be more highly prized
than the value of each day.

—Goethe

SURVIVORS OF CHILDHOOD CANCER may worry that treatment or genetic predisposition or the combination of the two will result in a second cancer. Second cancers are biologically different than a recurrence of the first cancer. The chance of developing a second cancer depends on a number of factors, including your original type of cancer, younger age at diagnosis, biological sex, types of therapy given, environmental exposures, genetic predisposition, and health decisions. Overall, for most survivors, the chance of getting a second cancer is very small.

This chapter begins with a discussion about what is currently known about the risks of getting a second cancer. Possible ways to prevent cancer and medical surveillance that may identify second cancers early are then discussed.

As you read this chapter, remember that for every story told here, the majority of survivors never develop a second cancer. The information in this chapter is meant to make you aware, not worried. You can use the information presented here to spark a discussion with your healthcare provider about your individual risk (if any). That knowledge can help you make healthy choices and get appropriate follow-up care to give you the best chance for a long and healthy life.

Risk of getting a second cancer

You may wonder whether you are at increased risk of developing a second cancer. For most survivors, the answer is no. But the risk is not the same for everyone. Factors that determine risk include your genetic predisposition and whether or not you received radiation and/or certain chemotherapy drugs. Your lifestyle and health behaviors can minimize or increase your risk, just as they can for people who never had cancer. For instance, if you had radiation to your chest, you have a small risk for developing throat and/or lung cancers. If you smoke, your chances of developing those cancers dramatically increase. If you don't smoke, don't drink alcohol, and eat a healthy diet, your risk decreases.

Although more is being discovered about the genetics of cancer, the relationship between genetic predisposition and the effects from chemotherapy drugs and/or radiation on developing second cancers is only partially understood. The lifetime risk of developing another cancer hasn't been determined, as most of the survivors studied are just reaching their second or third decade after cure.

> I had stage IV non-Hodgkin's lymphoma when I was 16. The tumor had metastasized to the bone by the time I was diagnosed. I had lots of radiation and chemotherapy. Nine years later I was diagnosed with breast cancer. Luckily, it had not spread to my lymph nodes. I had surgery, but no chemo or radiation and am doing fine now.

Much research is being done to maintain cure rates while lowering the toxicity of treatments to lessen the risk of second cancers. Research is also being done to identify those survivors most at risk so they can be followed appropriately. To find out your individual risk, talk to your healthcare provider during a follow-up visit. She will consider your original disease, the treatments you had, your age when treated, and your family history before discussing your unique situation.

> My daughter has a 30 percent chance of developing a secondary tumor because of her radiation for familial retinoblastoma. That's a pretty high number and it's very scary. The most likely to develop are osteosarcoma, soft tissue sarcomas, and melanoma. She's about to enter puberty, and we've been warned that they can show up as she gets older. She has checkups every 6 months.

· · · · ·

> My son was treated on an average-risk protocol for leukemia. The doctor said he is not at increased risk for another cancer, but we religiously go to our follow-up appointments. I consider it to be a type of insurance.

· · · · ·

> I was treated for osteosarcoma with chemotherapy when I was 8 years old. For many, many years, I was scared that I would develop a second cancer. I went to a survivor's conference and asked the doctors about it.

I was relieved to learn that for patients who had had my treatment, if it didn't happen within the first 5 years, chances were it never would. I think accurate information is really important to prevent unnecessary worry.

Genetic predisposition

Cancers with known genetic causes sometimes carry a greater risk of second cancers. For instance, survivors of the genetic form of retinoblastoma should be evaluated regularly for the rest of their lives, because they have a much higher chance of developing second tumors than do other survivors.

I had bilateral retinoblastoma when I was a baby, rhabdomyosarcoma at 12, and breast cancer at 22. At first, they thought the rhabdo might be from the radiation scatter from the retinoblastoma treatment, but the gene for retinoblastoma predisposes to other kinds of cancer. So it's possible I could develop cancer in any cell. My friends joke with me by saying, "If you don't cut this out, you'll have a Ph.D. in oncology." But I really don't want to get it that way. It's scary and tough and pretty hard not to get anxious.

· · · · ·

I was diagnosed with neuroblastoma when I was 9 months old, 33 years ago. It started on my left kidney. They removed my kidney and the tumor, gave me radiation and chemotherapy. Three years later I developed leukemia and was treated until I was 9 years old. I'm now 34 years old and was just diagnosed with bladder cancer. The doctors think it may be a late effect from the cyclophosphamide and radiation. In the follow-up clinic, I was never told that second cancers were a possibility. So this has really hit me—it has hit me hard.

Some types of cancer (colon, breast, and ovarian) run in families, so it is important to discuss your family history with your healthcare provider. Knowing your risk factors tells you a bit about the chance that you might develop that cancer. It does not determine whether or not you will get cancer again, because not all individuals with the predisposing gene get cancer. Survivors with many risk factors may live long and healthy lives and never get cancer again, while some people at low risk will get cancer. The facts your healthcare provider discusses with you are probabilities for large groups of people; no one can predict what will happen to you.

Survivors at highest risk for second cancers are those who:

• Were treated with radiation.

- Received high doses of alkylating agents: mechlorethamine (nitrogen mustard), cyclophosphamide (Cytoxan®), procarbazine, ifosfamide, melphalan, nitrosoureas (carmustine, lomustine), and/or epipodophylloxins (VP-16, VM-26).

- Have genetic diseases that carry an increased risk of cancer, such as, xeroderma pigmentosum, Klinefelter syndrome, Bloom's syndrome, Li-Fraumeni, von Recklinghausen's neurofibromatosis, or the genetic form of retinoblastoma.

If you are in one of the above groups, your follow-up care should be especially vigilant. This allows for earlier detection and treatment should you develop another cancer, increasing your chance for cure. It also gives you the opportunity to discuss ways of lowering your risks by making healthy lifestyle and behavior choices.

Wendy Harpham, a physician and cancer survivor, wrote in *After Cancer: A Guide to Your New Life*:

> *Knowledge of family risk can ruin one's quality of life if it causes a sense of hopelessness; knowledge of family risk empowers if it is used to maximize prevention and early detection.*

Treatment

Radiation and some types of chemotherapy can increase the risk of second cancers. Combined radiotherapy and chemotherapy may play an additive role in the development of second cancers. Some types of second cancers are very easy to cure; these include skin cancers and thyroid cancers. Second cancers that require more intensive therapies are bone and soft tissue sarcomas, non-Hodgkin lymphoma, brain tumors, and acute myelogenous leukemia (AML).

Radiation

In general, higher doses of radiation increase the risk of developing a second cancer. The radiation technology in the 1950s, 1960s, and 1970s delivered a lot of radiation to normal tissues around the tumor. More recent protocols have used lower radiation doses (in some cases), more precise techniques, and radiation given in smaller fractions, allowing the healthy tissue to repair itself. It is hoped that the use of the new proton therapy will significantly decrease the risk of damage to healthy tissue.

Radiation kills cancer cells and may also cause changes in normal cells that are exposed to the radiation. In some cases, second cancers develop in the irradiated areas. For instance, female survivors of Hodgkin lymphoma (formerly called Hodgkin's disease) treated in the 1970s and 1980s who had more than 3600 centigrays (cGy) of mantle (chest) radiation have a markedly increased risk of developing breast cancer, often at an early age.

> I'm still angry with my radiation oncologist who happily retired and never told me about my risk of breast cancer from the mantle radiation he gave me when I was 15. I discovered it by accident while doing research in the medical library while I was in graduate school. I came home and cried and threw the articles at the wall. I started doing self-exams, but I'd never been taught how to do them and found out later I was doing it wrong. When I finally found a doctor who specialized in treating survivors of childhood cancer, he carefully explained my risks in a very balanced way. He said he knew I was aware of my increased risk for breast cancer. Then he sounded apologetic and said, "We had to do the treatment to save your life and there is nothing we can do about that now. But we can do everything possible to detect it. It probably will never happen to you, but we need to do yearly mammograms, a yearly clinical breast exam, and you need to do monthly breast self-exams. If it does happen, we will catch it and treat it as soon as possible." It sounds crazy, but I really needed to hear someone acknowledge that the treatment is what put me at risk.

Some radiation (called "scatter") escapes into the areas surrounding the radiation field. Survivors who had radiation to the head or chest can develop late effects in the thyroid gland or salivary glands from scatter radiation. These areas, as well as the radiation field, should be routinely evaluated during follow-up appointments.

Thyroid tumors are a common second tumor following radiation delivered to the cranial/spinal region, head and neck, chest, or total body radiation given before a stem cell transplant. Younger children at time of treatment are at greater risk for thyroid tumors. Thyroid tumors can be either benign or malignant, and the malignant tumors are very treatable.

> My daughter had cranial radiation to treat high-risk leukemia. Her risk for thyroid damage is very low, but every year, the late effects doctor palpates her thyroid. She's never found a problem.

Radiation to the pelvis or abdomen (more than 3000 cGy) is associated with an increased risk of colon cancer. The current recommendation for follow up is to have a colonoscopy at age 35 or 10 years after the radiation, whichever occurs last.[1]

Chemotherapy

Several chemotherapy drugs are associated with second cancers in some survivors. Examples of these are:

- **Alkylating agents:** procarbazine, nitrogen mustard, cyclophosphamide (Cytoxan®), ifosfamide, melphalan, and nitrosoureas. High doses of these drugs can cause myelodysplastic syndromes (bone marrow abnormalities that are similar to leukemia) as well as AML. The peak incidence occurs 4 to 6 years after the drugs are given and gradually tapers off until 10 to 15 years have passed.[2]

- **Epipodophyllotoxins:** VP-16 (etoposide), VM-26 (teniposide). These drugs have been associated with AML that usually occurs within 3 years of treatment.[3]

- **Platinum analogs:** cisplatin, carboplatin. Research has not clarified the risk of second cancers after treatment with plantinum analogs such as cisplatin or carboplatin. Most AML or myelodysplastic syndromes occur when these drugs are given in conjunction with alkylating agents or epipodophyllotoxins.

Secondary leukemia in survivors treated with alkylating agents and/or epipodophyllotoxins usually occur in the first 10 years after treatment. Solid tumors tend to occur many years or decades after treatment ends.

> My son Jeremy was treated for Ewing's when he was 11 years old. The drugs he took included VP-16. Four years later he developed AML. He was put on chemo immediately and went into remission on day 7, and soon thereafter had a syngeneic bone marrow transplant from his identical twin brother. He's doing extremely well.

Children and teens who were treated with an immunosuppressant (e.g., cyclosporine or FK 506) have a small chance of developing disorders of the lymph system, including lymphoma. These disorders sometimes resolve without treatment when the immune system is no longer suppressed.

> My daughter Katy had taken cyclosporine for 6 weeks when we noticed swollen glands in her neck. She was put on two different antibiotics, but they kept growing. They finally swelled so much that they met in the midline and she was hospitalized for breathing difficulties. When they did blood work, we discovered that she had a positive EBV (Epstein-Barr virus) titer. Scans showed growths in her neck and her adenoids. The growths were removed surgically and examined by a pathologist. She was diagnosed with Epstein-Barr virus lymphoproliferative disorder. Within 6 weeks her scans were clean.

Risks following treatment for specific cancers

The information in this section describes risks for groups of survivors (not individuals). Some of the treatment-related second cancers discussed in the following list are attributed to treatments that are not considered the standard of care today. Many current clinical trials are focusing on maintaining cure rates while using less toxic treatments. Thus, in the future, it is hoped that cures will continue to increase while treatment-related second cancers decrease. All survivors, however, need lifelong surveillance for second cancers, either to provide reassurance that they are in the large majority of survivors who have no second cancers or to diagnose any problems early.

- **Hodgkin lymphoma.** Survivors of Hodgkin lymphoma have been studied extensively for many years. The treatments for Hodgkin lymphoma are very effective and have changed dramatically over the last 3 decades. The following information is about long-term survivors of Hodgkin lymphoma. Because treatments have improved, it is hoped that people treated on current protocols will have fewer second cancers. Researchers have found that breast cancer is the most common second cancer after treatment for Hodgkin lymphoma, and it accounts for 65 percent of second cancers in female Hodgkin lymphoma survivors.[4] Females treated between the ages of 10 and 16 and those who received more than 4000 cGy of mantle radiation have the highest risk of developing breast cancer.[5] Risk factors for developing leukemia are older age at diagnosis, treatment with alkylating agents, recurrence of Hodgkin lymphoma, and a late stage of disease at diagnosis.

- **Retinoblastoma.** Researchers at several institutions studied 1,604 survivors of retinoblastoma and found a substantial risk for second cancers in those who had the genetic form of retinoblastoma and had been treated with radiation.[6] All survivors who had tumors in both eyes (bilateral) have the genetic form. The second cancers that develop most often in retinoblastoma survivors are bone and soft tissue sarcomas. Bone sarcomas occur equally in and out of the radiation field, while soft tissue sarcomas mostly occur in the radiation field. Retinoblastoma survivors with the genetic form should be followed closely throughout their lives for second cancers.

- **Wilms tumor.** The National Wilms Tumor Study enrolled 5,278 survivors and found 43 who developed a second cancer. Fifteen years after diagnosis, the incidence of second cancers was 1.6 percent. Survivors who received more than 3500 cGy of abdominal radiation, were treated with doxorubicin, or were treated for a relapse had the highest risk.[7] These doses of radiation are no longer used to treat children newly diagnosed with Wilms tumor.

- **Brain and spinal cord tumors.** Children treated with radiation to the brain and/or spinal cord are at risk for development of both benign and malignant tumors. Meningiomas (tumors of the membranes that surround the brain) are the most common benign tumors and, depending on the location and symptoms, can either be followed with MRIs or be surgically removed. Malignant tumors usually require more intensive therapy. Children who received more than 3000 cGy and were younger than age 5 at time of diagnosis are at greatest risk.[8]

- **Ewing sarcoma.** Leukemia, sarcomas, and carcinomas can develop after treatment for Ewing sarcoma. Alkylating agents (e.g., cyclophosphamide, 5FU) and topoisomerase inhibitors (doxorubicin, VP-16) contribute to the risk of leukemia, and high-dose radiation increases the risk of solid tumors.

- **Rhabdomyosarcoma.** High-dose radiation and high doses of chemotherapy appear to increase the risk for developing a second cancer in survivors of rhabdomyosarcoma. Children who received radiation and dactinomycin have a higher rate of second tumors.

- **Acute lymphoblastic leukemia (ALL).** Several studies have found second cancers to be an uncommon late effect of treatment for childhood ALL. Second cancers very occasionally occur in the brains of survivors treated with cranial radiation when they were younger than age 5.[9,10]

- **Stem cell transplantation.** Child and teen survivors of stem cell transplants have usually received radiation and a variety of chemotherapy drugs. There are different risks for second cancers depending on previous treatment, cumulative doses of drugs, age at transplant, and other factors. Leukemia, thyroid cancer, skin cancer, and solid tumors sometimes develop after a stem cell transplant.[11,12]

One way to cope with the information your healthcare provider gives you about your risk for developing second cancers is to think in terms of the chance that you will not get a second cancer. For instance, if you have a 3 percent chance of getting a brain tumor because you had cranial radiation at a young age, turn that statistic around and focus on the 97 percent chance that you will not get another cancer. This change in perspective may help you file the information away in your mind and allow you to think of risk in a different way.

> *I figure I probably have a higher risk of bodily harm every time I drive my car than I do of developing cancer again. And I don't think of having an accident every time I step into my car. It is just a risk I accept in order to take my children to school, buy my groceries, and visit my friends.*

The small risk of another cancer is a price I paid for cure. A price I was very willing to pay.

Prevention

Once you know what your risk might be, what do you do then? Practical ways to deal with this potentially upsetting information are to do everything you can to prevent a second cancer, and then take steps to make sure that if anything develops, it is detected and treated early.

I had mantle radiation for Hodgkin's disease in the 1970s. Two small skin cancers grew under the edge of my left breast. Not any place that commonly saw the sun. But that's where they decided to grow! I try to be cautious about sun exposure, especially with the skin over my sternum, which is very strange-looking from the radiation.

· · · · ·

I had cranial radiation when I was 4 to treat high-risk leukemia. I know I have a tiny risk of a brain tumor, so when I had bad migraines at puberty, instead of just treating them with medication, I also had an MRI to check for tumors. No big deal, and no tumors. And after I went through puberty, no more migraines! I go to a really good follow-up clinic every year, and other than that, I don't think about it.

Although you cannot alter a genetic predisposition or undo the damage from radiation or chemotherapy, you can modify your risk factors by making healthy lifestyle choices to minimize your risk. There are numerous ways to prevent cancer that are outlined in Chapter 5, *Staying Healthy*. Some of these are:

- Don't smoke.
- Don't take illegal drugs or recreational inhalants.
- Drink alcohol only in moderation.
- Avoid exposure to the sun, wear a hat that covers the face, and use sunscreen, particularly on irradiated skin.
- Exercise regularly.
- Maintain a healthy body weight.
- Eat four to six fruits and vegetables a day.

Early detection

Taking control of your risk for second cancers includes periodic surveillance, as well as making healthy lifestyle choices. Your healthcare provider should do a thorough assessment every year and discuss with you any risks you have for second cancers. The specific tests done are determined by an assessment that considers the treatment you received for childhood cancer, any past or current behaviors that affect your risk, and personal or family history of disease.

Your follow-up examinations should include updating your family medical history, with special attention to cancers that have developed in first-degree relatives (your mother, father, brothers, sisters, and children). This valuable information can be missed if family medical history is not updated at regular intervals.

If you were treated with radiation, the area that was irradiated should be visually inspected. Areas where scattered radiation may have occurred also need to be examined. For instance, children who had cranial radiation sometimes develop thyroid problems from the scatter. Therefore, the necks of these survivors should be palpated (felt by hand) yearly. The results of a thorough physical evaluation and preliminary screening determine the need for any additional tests. It's very important that female survivors of Hodgkin lymphoma who had mantle radiation get frequent follow-up care that includes annual mammograms starting at age 25, or 8 years after radiation (whichever comes later). They also need to be taught breast self-examination because they can develop breast cancer at an early age.

> I had Hodgkin's disease when I was 15 and was treated with mantle radiation and ABVD (combination of four chemotherapy drugs). I find that knowing the possibilities helps me comply with appropriate measures—like breast self-exams, mammography (my first was at age 25), and lifestyle changes. Doing these things makes me feel more in control of my life—not that I can stop something from happening, but that perhaps I can notice a change early on and make a difference in terms of treatment or even survival. My thought is that a breast self-exam might mean I find a lump at 1.5 cm that could be 2.5 cm by the next physical exam. And that could mean a difference in my survival as well as my treatment. But I definitely don't sit around and worry.

Routine yearly examinations will not detect all second cancers. Healthcare providers rely on you to bring any concerns or abnormalities to their attention. Try to feel confident in your ability to notice if something does not feel right. If you have an ache or a pain that does not go away, it should probably be checked out. If you notice a lump in the area of your body that was irradiated, go have it evaluated. It probably will not be cancer, but having it evaluated will provide either reassurance or an early detection of a problem—both good outcomes.

There are steps you can take to identify and treat second cancers. For example, you can have your physician remove very small skin cancers, and you can stay out of the sun or use sunscreen routinely. If you had retinoblastoma and were treated with radiation to the orbit, it makes sense to examine the socket yourself regularly for any changes. By examining the orbit regularly, you are taking good care of yourself and making an investment in your future. Another way to think of this issue is to try to find a place in your life for your cancer history. Don't trivialize what's happened to you and your family—it was a significant part of your life and shaped your interests and character. And yet, your cancer history is only one part of who you are.

> *I try to put cancer in its place. I've learned everything I can and I know what my risks are. I have a little drawer in the back of my mind that I put that knowledge in, then I close the drawer. I stay aware for the signs and symptoms, and if any arise, I'll open that drawer and take action. But the rest of the time, I don't worry about it.*

Chapter 20

Homage

*The true meaning of life is to plant trees, under
whose shade you do not expect to sit.*

—Nelson Henderson

CELEBRATIONS OF LIFE. Perhaps you've attended one. Every year in early June, treatment centers across the country organize special events for National Cancer Survivors' Day with games, entertainment, and refreshments. At some events, college scholarships are awarded. Maybe there is a friendly softball competition between survivors and staff. Or the doctors agree to take a turn in a dunk tank, good-naturedly letting themselves be dunked by kids and teens. Always, there is a chance to renew the bonds forged by shared experience and to reconnect with staff members on a relaxing and fun day.

But survivorship isn't the only cause for celebration. We also celebrate the memory of all those who fought hard to survive but were ultimately overcome by cancer. Sometimes we remember in testimonials spoken from the heart, or messages written in memory books, or videotaped recollections, or in phrases and images sewn into patchwork quilts. All the children and families who came before gave priceless gifts that make survivorship, complicated as this book attests, possible today.

The truth is that there is no medicine in use today, no treatment regimen that now achieves remarkable survival rates, that wasn't at one time considered investigational. Most young people with cancer have participated in clinical trials over the past 40 years. Step by step, as each clinical trial answered questions about more effective and safer treatments, treatment improved, and cure became possible. This is the legacy of the children and teenagers for whom survival wasn't to be. And it's the legacy of the families who cared for them, hoped for them, and remember them always.

So in this book about life after cancer in childhood, we pay homage to the memory of these young people and their families. Whether or not we have photos on our walls, or a collection of artwork, videos, or cards that remind us of the unique spirit of each child, each of them left a lasting impression in our hearts, and they made a lasting contribution toward the end of cancer. They are not forgotten.

Appendix A
Survivor Sketches

THE SURVIVORS INTERVIEWED FOR THIS BOOK lead rich and fulfilling lives. To balance the challenges described in the text, we invited them to provide a glimpse of "the rest of the story." With warmth and humor, they did so. We feel privileged to know them.

Luc is an 18-year-old high school senior who excels in music. He surrendered a football and lacrosse career when he was diagnosed, and rather than focus on loss and limitation, Luc turned to music and studied guitar and piano. He plans to pursue a career as a music teacher. He cannot be described as an average teen. Rather than recapturing the 3-year chunk that was carved from his teenage years, he moved forward. His friends tend to be older and spiritually based. His music teacher described him as a remarkably mature young man with what she calls a gift to claim a room of unruly students and turn chaos into common sense.

Shannon is now 9 years old and in third grade. She hit her "5-year" remission in June 1999. She enjoys music and doing crafts. Shannon has made top cookie seller 2 years in a row for Brownies and enjoys sleepovers.

Elizabeth is an 8-year-old who was diagnosed with Wilms tumor at the age of 3. She loves school and church. Her favorite activities are swimming, bike riding, and playing with her mom.

Marilyn is a 50ish woman who survived unilateral retinoblastoma at age 2. Due to genetic concerns, she adopted a daughter (now age 25) and has one grandson. Marilyn is a residential mortgage lender and a national trainer/speaker for the mortgage industry. In her spare time, she quilts, gardens, and enjoys cross-country skiing. Depth perception is still an issue, so she is still not brave enough to try downhill skiing.

Taylor is now a 9-year-old boy who had T-cell acute lymphoblastic leukemia (ALL). He is currently enjoying the challenges of fourth grade. His interests include computers, chess and all other board and card games, playing with his friends, teasing his brother and sister, sports, and just being a kid like the rest of his friends again.

Brenna is a 5-year-old diagnosed with acute lymphocytic leukemia in early 1998. She lives with her mom and dad, Denise and Jerry, two brothers, one sister, and her bird. She enjoys dancing and art. When she grows up, she wants to be a ballerina or a doctor—so her oncologist can retire.

Bobby is a 12-year survivor of ALL, now doing well after 6 years of treatment including a bone marrow transplant. He and his family recently bicycled 3,900 miles across the United States to visit and encourage other children fighting cancer and their families. He is now 20 years old, in his second year of college, co-founder of a small non-profit organization dedicated to supporting children fighting cancer, and engaged to be married.

Casey, 19, is a 6+ year survivor of osteogenic sarcoma in her right distal femur. Her obsession with returning to cheerleading led to an extraordinary physical recovery and she is now a first-year student at Smith College. She relieves an intense academic environment with diving for the school team and riding horses.

Gina is now a survivor of ALL for over 12 years. She is 15 and completing the eighth grade. She enjoys voice lessons, piano lessons, singing in the school choir, and being part of the technical crew for the school's show choir. She is an excellent, hardworking student and is looking forward to driving a car soon.

Katy is a 6-year-old miracle child who continues to amaze her family daily in her recovery from her bone marrow transplant. She loves first grade, having friends sleep over, and playing "hospital." She wants to be a nurse when she grows up.

Garrett is a 4-year-old survivor of acute myelomonocytic leukemia (AMMOL) and an unrelated cord blood transplant. He loves looking for alligators and dinosaurs on family camping trips. He and his 6-year-old brother, Shawn, want to be race car drivers when they grow up.

Sharon, a 13-year survivor of an astrocytoma, has worked for the past 5½ years as a research assistant in a laboratory. She and her husband were married 4 years ago, and she has just started business school in search of a master of business administration degree at Temple University.

Zackary loved dolphins, music, Nintendo and life. Erin and Nick live in Utah where they work with Candlelighters to enhance the lives of kids with cancer.

Rachel is an active second grader, learning to play tennis and the piano. She is very independent and self assured. Her teachers are continually amazed at this because of all she has been through!

Rima, age 45, was treated for Hodgkin's disease in 1971. She is the child of a woman who died of Hodgkin's disease in 1958. She has been teaching elementary school for 21 years and has a supportive husband and one lovely miraculous daughter. She loves to read, walk, garden, and take hot baths, though not at the same time!

Paige was diagnosed with neuroblastoma at age 4 in 1994. She is a 5-year survivor and a spunky kid who likes to sing, be a clown on stage, eat candy, and watch TV. Paige plays soccer and basketball, does well in school, and loves her sister and brother.

Heather, a very bright, creative, and vivacious 8-year-old, was diagnosed with stage IV neuroblastoma when she was 14 months old. As part of her treatment, Heather underwent a bone marrow transplant. Today, she enjoys swimming, acting, singing, dancing, and playing with her friends, family, and two small dogs. To know Heather is to love Heather!

Kyle is a bright, happy and fun-loving 9-year-old who was diagnosed with a medulloblastoma (brain tumor) at the age of 4. He is in the third grade and although it is a struggle for him in some areas, he is doing well. He likes to play on the computer, draw, ride his adapted bike, and go to grandma's house, and he has always loved treehouses.

Elizabeth, a 32-year survivor of Hodgkin's disease, has been a legal secretary and successful massage therapist. She lives with her husband and two adoring labradors and enjoys the challenges of being a hospice volunteer.

Trevor is now almost 7 years old and has been battling leukemia for nearly 3 years. He is a bouncing, beautiful first grader who loves art, math, football, all of his friends, and Pokémon.

Nicholas is a 7-year-old conqueror of ALL. He's a serious first-grader and all-around family comedian. He enthusiastically collects and trades Pokémon cards, cheers for the Jacksonville Jaguars, and does gymnastics in his spare time. Nick's favorite toy remains Woody and the gang from "Toy Story," including Mr. Potato Head.

Lisa is a law student who hopes to pursue a career in child advocacy after graduation.

Alexander, 7 years old, was diagnosed with high risk acute ALL at the age of 2½ years. He is happy and doing very well in first grade. He is quite the social butterfly and is joyfully taking skating lessons and playing baseball and soccer. He loves making crafts with empty tissue boxes, paper towel and toilet paper rolls, string, and—much to his father's chagrin—any Scotch tape that is in his Dad's home office.

Susan is a 20-year survivor of Hodgkin's disease. Recently, late effects from her cancer treatment caused her to stop working. She now researches survivorship issues, lives a simple life, and takes care of her health. She is a writer, an advocate for animal rights, and mother to five cats and dogs.

Joel, 18, is a student and athlete who is looking forward to beginning college after a year off for treatment. He was diagnosed with ALL at age 14 in 1995. He relapsed in 1999 and was still in treatment as of December 1999.

Chris is a 9-year-old who had a medulloblastoma at age 5. He is a fourth grader who is making rapid improvements in his reading and writing abilities. He is active in Cub Scouts and enjoys bowling, playing with his friends, and playing in the snow.

Jamie is a 10-year-old boy with an ever-present smile and a wicked sense of humor. He has taught our family to explore and enjoy life to the fullest. He is a true cancer warrior.

Kevin is a 15-year survivor of Hodgkin's disease. Despite a recurrence in 1998, he and his wife live happily in Oklahoma with their three pet ferrets. Kevin has degrees in business and health care administration and is currently pursuing a degree in computer science. He enjoys reading, traveling, and keeping active in their church.

Jennifer, a 14-year non-Hodgkin's lymphoma survivor, is a world traveler for the moment until she figures out what she wants to be. She enjoys exploring the world, time with family and friends, and helping others as much as she can.

Katie is 9 years old and a survivor of juvenile chronic myelogenous leukemia. She enjoys amusement parks, horses, cartoons and her guinea pig. She lives in Virginia with her parents and three brothers.

Linda is a 28-year survivor of Hodgkin's disease. She is a child and adult psychoanalyst and works with survivors in her clinical practice. She also founded and runs the Long-Term Survivors internet discussion group. She lives, plays, and swims with her husband and standard poodle in sunny southern California.

Robby was diagnosed with high risk ALL at age 5½. He relapsed in his central nervous system at age 7½ and again 6 months later. He received an autologous bone marrow transplant at age 8½ and is now 4 years post-transplant and doing wonderfully. He attends a school for academically advanced students and is on honor roll. He enjoys video games, computer games, and talking on the phone to friends—a typical teen!

Jared is a very active and intelligent 10-year-old boy who has been past cancer for 8 years. His favorite sport is soccer. He is very sensitive to others' pain and knows that the Lord has healed him.

Jeremy was diagnosed with Ewing's sarcoma at age 11. He was diagnosed with secondary acute myelogenous leukemia (AML) at the age of 15. He is now a typical 17-year-old who works part-time in addition to being an "average" high school junior. He sleeps late on the weekends, has a messy room, and fights with his brothers. He has an infectious smile and is a wonderful reminder that our children are precious gifts from above.

Linda, a 23-year survivor of Hodgkin's disease, lives with her husband and teenage daughter in Missouri. She enjoys sewing and writing.

Kenny has now been off therapy since January 1998. He attends pre-kindergarten in Georgia and is currently pursuing every Pokémon card available. He is full of life!

Ardeth is a 36-year-old former assistant librarian and minister's wife who has been happily married for the past 12 years. She works for a local hospice agency and helps her husband as he pastors a local church. Ardeth's hobbies are researching genealogy and family history, collecting angels, playing the flute, oil painting, reading, and spending time with her pets—two dogs and a talking parrot.

Yossi Chaim is an 11-year-old boy who had a bone marrow transplant at age 9. He enjoys playing Game Boy, Pokémon, reading, and drawing. He hopes to be a cartoonist when he grows up.

Coley is now a healthy 7-year-old, who has survived the hepatoblastoma she was diagnosed with at age 2. She lives happily in Florida and enjoys the first grade, playing Barbie with her sister Chrissy, and trying to ride horses with her sister Anna. She even enjoys playing "wrestling matches" with her brother Sean and adores her brother Jason. She is very loved and very happy.

Mark is a 23-year survivor of testicular cancer who lives in Los Angeles. He's a mortgage professional and enjoys traveling, sporting events, and playing golf.

Brian is a 3½-year survivor of high-risk ALL. He is a happy 14-year-old high school freshman, who enjoys art, soccer and playing guitar. His brother Kevin was diagnosed with ALL at age 4. Now he is a busy 6-year-old, whose favorite subjects in first grade are art, PE, and lunch!

Terri is now 9 years old and 6 years out from diagnosis. Although her tumor has metastasized and she is diagnosed as terminal, she continues to battle on bravely and looks forward to being a vet when she grows up—by the grace of God.

Laurie, a 34-year-old neuroblastoma survivor, lives with her husband and children. She works in the medical communications field and is involved in a local bioethics committee and a national bioethics committee for pediatric oncology. In her spare time, she enjoys cooking, gardening, and activities with her family.

Steve, a 21-year survivor of osteosarcoma and an amputee, currently works as a health educator/counselor with cancer patients. Steve enjoys the many hobbies he has, such as exercising, fishing, and being outdoors. He volunteers as a counselor at a pediatric oncology camp. He feels blessed for all the wonderful friends and relationships he has had over the last 21 years.

Justin is an 11-year-old who was diagnosed at age 8 with a brain stem tumor. He has undergone radiation and is now doing well with very few symptoms of his disease. He is now in fifth grade. He enjoys playing his Nintendo 64. He lives in Washington.

Andrea is a 22-year-old two-time survivor. She finished her BA in 3½ years while receiving treatment. She plans on attending graduate school and hopes to one day get her Ph.D.

Shortly after the birth of her first son, **Teresa** began a career as a newscaster for both CBS and NBC affiliates. She now resides in her hometown of Indianapolis, where she is president and CEO of Teracom Media Group, a multimedia distributor of integrative health information. Teresa also is publisher of *Healthy Living* magazine, as well as the current host of the Healthy Living TV show and radio programs.

Clare is a 16-year-old survivor of rhabdomyosarcoma, which she was treated for at age 9. Now a junior in high school, she is doing well academically and plans to attend college. She enjoys playing the piano and clarinet, writing poetry, acting in high school musicals, listening to music, and spending time with her friends.

Carol, a 24-year survivor of Hodgkin's disease, was diagnosed after the birth of her first child. She is now retired due to ill health. She lives with her husband in Kent, England, and has two grown-up children.

Matthew is a 6-year-old who survived a malignant brain tumor (medulloblastoma) and its treatment at the age of 2. He loves classic Disney cartoons, Disney Beanie babies and videos, cookies, and going to the mall to walk for physical therapy; which includes a visit to the Disney store.

Melissa was diagnosed with ALL at the age of 3. She is now 10 years old and is in the fourth grade. Her favorite activities are making crafts, learning to play the fiddle, and telling jokes and stories. She is looking forward to starting horseback riding lessons.

Matthew was diagnosed with stage III favorable histology Wilm's tumor with some unknown malignant areas at age 1 and then relapsed at age 2½. He is now 5 years old and has been off treatment for 18 months and is doing exceptionally well. He loves Star Wars, Pokémon, playing with cars and Legos, and just in general running around and having fun.

Barb, a 9-year survivor of Hodgkin's disease stage IIIB NS, is a medical office assistant who lives with her husband in British Columbia, Canada. She enjoys outdoor activities and treasures the quiet times with her husband.

James, a 19-year-old survivor of ALL, is a sophomore engineering student at the University of Colorado, Boulder. He enjoys flying remote control helicopters and planes, riding his mountain bike, and computers of all sorts and colors.

Julie is a 3-year survivor of Hodgkin's disease, having been diagnosed just prior to her high school graduation. She is an art major in college specializing in graphic design. She particularly enjoys silk painting, weaving, quilting, and country music.

Nikhila was diagnosed with T-cell ALL when she was 9 years old. She is now 12 and enjoys art and writing stories and poems. Her passion is learning about and taking care of lizards!

Selah was 4½ when diagnosed with T-cell, high-risk, poor prognosis ALL. Treatment, including cranial irradiation, lasted 2 years, 2 months, and 2 days. Selah is now 13½, an honor student in junior high, and sees her doctors just once a year. No long term effects to date (unless excessive giggling is somehow related to leukemia!), and she is a joyful member of our family.

Eleven-year-old **Oliver** was first diagnosed with ALL at age 5 and underwent a bone marrow transplant age 8 after a relapse. He is a bright, funny child who loves his family, pets and friends, playing soccer and cricket, and even going to school!

Anne is a long-term (23-year) survivor of ALL. She is 28 years old, living with a college friend in a suburb of Philadelphia. She has a master's degree in social work from the Catholic University of America and has been practicing social work for 6 years. She enjoys her job working with neighborhood organizations in Philadelphia to help families connect with the services they need. She has close family and friend relationships and is happy with her life.

Gib is a survivor of ALL—in remission for 11 years. Proud father of 21-month-old Lucas (wasn't supposed to happen—so much for medical prescriptions). Gorgeous sweet wife. Attorney and advocate for childhood cancer survivors. Life is good!

Ann is a 5-year survivor of non-Hodgkin's lymphoma who lives in North Carolina with her husband. She is a computer programmer and enjoys cake decorating, gardening, and cycling in her spare time.

Preston is a 23-year-old who was diagnosed with leukemia (ALL) at age 10. He was successfully treated with chemotherapy, graduated from college, and now works for a large brokerage house in New Jersey. He enjoys sports and keeps fit by running each day, playing squash, and traveling around the country to ski with his friends.

JaNette is a 12-year-old who had a bone marrow transplant for AML when she was 6. A few chronic medical problems don't keep her from enjoying life—school, choir, friends, and youth activities!

Naomi, a 12-year survivor of AML (M5), is currently studying biology at the University of Ottawa in Canada. She is hoping to pursue a career in medicine to give back to the world of science that enabled her to survive her cancer. She spends her summers working as a counselor at Camp Trillium—a camp for children with cancer.

Carol, a 22-year survivor of Hodgkin's disease, lives with her husband Marv and a newly adopted kitten Roxy and their dog Stoney. She enjoys listening to music, reading, daily walks, and riding on the back of their Harley Sportster.

Dottie, a long-term Wilms tumor survivor, is a registered nurse and mother of three boys, two of whom are also Wilms survivors. She lives in Florida and enjoys the beach along with family days at the ball field.

Tim, who was diagnosed with ALL at age 8 and relapsed at age 12, is now a high school sophomore. He is taking classes such as pre-calculus and Latin. He enjoys computers—both games and networking. He also enjoys science fiction and fantasy reading, gulping down 700-page books with ease.

Lisa, now 16 and driving (!), was diagnosed with AML leukemia at 12 years, relapsed with bone marrow transplant at 13 years, and graduated eighth grade valedictorian. She continues to be a great pianist and excels in the band and choir programs at high school.

Kimbra, diagnosed with Hodgkin's disease at age 15, is now a 26-year-old librarian and writer. She loves reading, writing, and volunteering with children, and she recently married her pediatric oncology camp sweetheart, Darren, who was diagnosed with optic nerve germinoma at age 16. Her research interests include children's and young adult literature, clinical biomedical information for patients and clinicians, the Crusades, medieval and nineteenth-century medicine, and most important, long-term survivor issues.

Jennifer is 26 years old and works for Cancer Services of Allen County in Fort Wayne, IN. She likes to read, do crossword puzzles, jigsaw puzzles, and cross stitch.

Laura, a 34-year-old ALL survivor, lives in Washington with her husband and two children. She enjoys volunteering at a camp for children with cancer and a teen support group.

Tom, a 29-year-old survivor of ALL, is a dedicated volunteer who believes that his experience with cancer has made him a stronger and more caring person. Because he is sensitive to the needs of children and young adults with cancer, he devotes his time helping them navigate the path to emotional and social recovery. If given the opportunity, he would not trade his experience with cancer for a "normal" life.

Rachel is an active, happy 10-year-old survivor of ALL. She enjoys her friends and family. She once declared she was "giving up cancer for Lent."

Resources

A WEALTH OF INFORMATION and services is available from organizations, agencies, books, and the Internet. This appendix identifies and gives contact information for some of these resources.

Follow-up programs

Throughout this book we discuss the importance of comprehensive follow-up care for survivors of childhood cancer. One way to obtain state-of-the-art care is to see a specialist in late effects at a clinic for survivors. To find a survivors' clinic near you, visit *www.ped-onc.org/treatment/surclinics.html*.

The Children's Oncology Group's recommendations for screening and management of late effects of treatment for childhood, adolescent, and young adult cancers are available online at *www.survivorshipguidelines.org*.

Organizations

The following organizations and/or their websites provide services, information, and referrals for survivors of childhood cancer. The list begins with general organizations, and then specific-topic organizations are listed alphabetically.

American Childhood Cancer Organization (ACCO)
P.O. Box 498
Kensington, MD 20895-0498
(855) 858-2226 or (301) 962-3520
www.acco.org

ACCO (formerly Candlelighters Childhood Cancer Foundation) provides support, education, and advocacy for children and adolescents with cancer, survivors of childhood/adolescent cancer, their families, and the professionals who care for them.

The Association of Cancer Online Resources, Inc. (ACOR)

www.acor.org

ACOR offers a wide range of electronic discussion groups that provide information and support to patients, caregivers, and families. Some examples of the support groups are PED-ONC, PED-ONC Survivors, ALL-KIDS, GVHD support group for people post-transplant, LT-survivors (long-term survivors), and BMT-TALK. To find a list of the groups, go to *www.acor.org/mailing.html*.

ACOR's Site for Families of Survivors of Childhood Cancer

www.ped-onc.org/survivors

Hosted by ACOR, the Pediatric Oncology Resource Center offers articles about specific late effects of treatment for childhood cancer, an extensive section about education issues, links to informative websites and support groups, a list of clinics for survivors, and a bibliography of pertinent journal articles.

Beyond the Cure

www.beyondthecure.org

Beyond the Cure offers articles about school, medical issues, legal issues, relationships, health insurance, and more. The website also lists contacts by state for special education information. This organization holds Web conferences about different topics of interest to survivors and their parents; past webcasts are archived and available as audio files.

Cancer Care

275 Seventh Avenue
New York, NY 10001
(800) 813-HOPE or (800) 813-4673
www.cancercare.org

Cancer Care, a nonprofit organization, provides a variety of services, including counseling, education, referrals, publications, and financial assistance.

CancerNet

www.cancer.net

CancerNet is the patient information website of the American Society of Clinical Oncology (ASCO). The website provides information about late effects of childhood cancers, videos, and links to more information.

Chai Lifeline/Camp Simcha
151 West 30th Street
New York, NY 10001
(212) 465-1300 or (877) CHAI LIFE
www.chailifeline.org

National nonprofit organization dedicated to providing support service programs to Jewish families. Some of the many services provided are medical referrals, support groups, a respite program, negotiating insurance claims, financial aid, transportation, a kosher camp for children with cancer, and more.

Children's Oncology Group's (COG) Long-Term Follow-Up Guidelines
www.survivorshipguidelines.org

COG maintains and updates the comprehensive long-term follow-up guidelines that provide recommendations for screening and management of potential late effects of childhood cancer treatment. This document is available in a downloadable format (free) or in print format (for a charge). The website also has shorter "Health Links" about the different late effects; these are written for survivors.

CureSearch for Children's Cancer
www.curesearch.org

CureSearch is a national nonprofit foundation that supports children's cancer research and provides information and resources to all those affected by childhood cancer.

Ulman Cancer Fund for Young Adults (UCF)
6310 Stevens Forest Road, Ste. 210
Columbia, MD 21046
(800) 393-FUND (3863)
www.ulmanfund.org

A leading voice in the young adult cancer movement, the UCF supports, educates, connects, and empowers young adult cancer survivors. It raises awareness of young adult cancer issues and helps ensure all young survivors and their families have a voice and the resources necessary to thrive.

Family Voices
www.familyvoices.org

Family Voices helps families achieve family-centered care for all children and youth with special health care needs or disabilities. Especially helpful on its website is the state-by-state list of Family-to-Family Health Information Centers at *www.familyvoices.org/page?id=0034*. These centers provide help with health care, insurance, and access to community services.

Institute of Medicine Report on Survivorship After Childhood Cancer
www.iom.edu/Reports/2003/Childhood-Cancer-Survivorship-Improving-Care-and-Quality-of-Life.aspx

The Institute of Medicine (IOM) released the report titled *Childhood Cancer Survivorship: Improving Care and Quality of Life* in 2003. The report can be downloaded from the website for free or a printed copy is available for purchase. This lengthy report provides comprehensive coverage about all aspects of childhood cancer survivorship.

LIVESTRONG (formerly the Lance Armstrong Foundation)
2201 E. Sixth Street
Austin, TX 78702
(877) 236-8820
www.livestrong.org

LIVESTRONG funds research and provides support to individuals with cancer from diagnosis through survivorship, including a young adult alliance and a survivor empowerment initiative.

Leukemia & Lymphoma Society (LLS)
1311 Mamaroneck Avenue, Suite 310
White Plains, NY 10605
(914) 949-5213
www.lls.org/#/diseaseinformation/managingyourcancer/survivorship

LLS is the world's largest voluntary health agency dedicated to blood cancers. It funds lifesaving cancer research around the world and provides free information and support services.

National Cancer Institute (NCI)
(800) 4-CANCER
www.cancer.gov

The NCI website provides information about all aspects of cancer, including survivorship issues. NCI also provides a nationwide telephone helpline for people with cancer, their families, friends, and the professionals who treat them, and sends out informational booklets about a variety of cancer-related topics.

NCI articles about late effects of childhood cancer are available online at the Web addresses listed below. These articles provide comprehensive information about the late effects that treatments for childhood cancer have on the different body systems. They also provide links to more information.

www.cancer.gov/cancertopics/pdq/treatment/lateeffects/patient
www.cancer.gov/cancertopics/pdq/treatment/lateeffects/healthprofessional

NCI's Office of Cancer Survivorship (OCS) is on the Web at *http:// cancercontrol.cancer.gov/ocs*. Founded in 1996, OCS funds research on survivorship issues. OCS is dedicated to developing the infrastructure— such as databases and researcher networks—that supports the follow-up needed to study long-term survivors. OCS also supports programs to educate patients, physicians, and the public about cancer survivorship.

National Coalition for Cancer Survivorship
1010 Wayne Avenue, Suite 770
Silver Spring, MD 20910
(877) 622-7937 or (301) 650-9127
www.canceradvocacy.org

A nonprofit organization that addresses the needs of long-term cancer survivors and advocates for changes in healthcare to maximize survivors' access to optimal treatment and support. The coalition has an extensive publication list.

Patient Advocate Foundation
421 Butler Farm Road
Hampton, VA 23666
(800) 532-5274
www.patientadvocate.org

Provides help with insurance problems, publications, and referrals to attorneys.

Survivor Alert
www.survivoralert.org

Survivor Alert offers information about survivorship issues: who is at risk for late effects, how to get health insurance, how to get your medical records, and the importance of choosing a healthy lifestyle.

Amputation

Amputee Coalition of America (ACA)
900 East Hill Avenue, Suite 205
Knoxville, TN 37915-2566
(888) 267-5669 or TTY (865) 525-4512
www.amputee-coalition.org

The mission of the ACA is to reach out to people with limb loss; to educate and empower them to lead rich, productive lives; to advocate on their behalf; and to develop and disseminate the resources necessary to accomplish these goals.

Disabled Sports USA
451 Hungerford Drive, Suite 100
Rockville, MD 20850
(301) 217-0960
www.dsusa.org

Disabled Sports USA provides opportunities for individuals with physical disabilities to gain confidence and dignity through participation in sports, recreation, and related educational programs.

Education and Employment

Cancer and Careers
www.cancerandcareers.org

Cancer and Careers is a nonprofit organization that empowers and educates cancer survivors as they return to work or search for new jobs.

The Disability Rights Education and Defense Fund
3075 Adeline Street, Suite 210
Berkeley, CA 94703
(510) 644-2555 (voice) or (510) 841-8645 (FAX, TTY)
www.dredf.org

This organization answers questions about the Americans with Disabilities Act and explains how to file a complaint.

Cancer Legal Resource Center
www.disabilityrightslegalcenter.org/about/about.cfm

The Cancer Legal Resource Center provides free information and resources about cancer-related legal issues to cancer survivors, caregivers, healthcare professionals, employers, and others coping with cancer. It is a national, joint program of the Disability Rights Legal Center and Loyola Law School Los Angeles.

HEATH Resource Center at the National Youth Transitions Center
The George Washington University Graduate School of Education and Human Development
2134 G Street NW, Suite 220
Washington, DC 20052-0001
askHEATH@gwu.edu
www.heath.gwu.edu

HEATH is the national clearinghouse on post-secondary education for individuals with disabilities. It provides information about educational support services, policies, procedures, adaptations, and opportunities at American campuses and vocational-technical schools.

Job Accommodation Network (JAN)
www.askjan.org

This consulting service provides free information about how employers can accommodate people with disabilities. It also provides information about the Americans with Disabilities Act and how people with disabilities can start their own small businesses.

Learning Disabilities Association of America
4156 Library Road
Pittsburgh, PA 15234-1349
(412) 341-1515
www.ldanatl.org

A national, nonprofit organization that advances the education and general welfare of children and adults with learning disabilities.

National Dissemination Center for Children with Disabilities
1825 Connecticut Avenue NW, Suite 700
Washington, DC 20009
(800) 695-0285 or (202) 884-8441
www.nichcy.org

A clearinghouse that provides pamphlets and information about disabilities and the rights of disabled children and their parents.

Parent Technical Assistance Center Network
www.parentcenternetwork.org

Lists Parent Training and Information (PTI) centers by state. These PTIs provide training and assistance to families of children with disabilities, including help with IEP and 504 plans.

Facial differences

Let's Face It
University of Michigan
School of Dentistry/Dentistry Library
1011 North University
Ann Arbor, MI 48109-1078
www.dent.umich.edu/faceit

A national information and support group for people with facial differences.

Federal government agencies

Equal Employment Opportunity Commission (EEOC)
(800) 669-4000 or (800) 669-6820 (TTY)
www.eeoc.gov

The EEOC provides information about how to enforce rights under the Americans with Disabilities Act.

Department of Justice Civil Rights Division
Americans with Disabilities Act: ADA Home Page
(800) 514-0301 or (800) 514-0383 (TTY)
www.ada.gov

Specialists answer questions about Title I and Title II of the Americans with Disabilities Act.

National Women's Health Information Center, U.S. Department of Health and Human Services
(800) 994-9662 or (888) 220-5446 (TDD)
www.womenshealth.gov/illnesses-disabilities

Resource center for the nation's 10 million disabled women. Offers information about disabilities, laws, statistics, access to healthcare, financial assistance, abuse, parenting, sexuality, and links to advocacy groups.

Free (or low-cost) medications

NeedyMeds
P.O. Box 219
Gloucester, MA 01931
www.needymeds.org

NeedyMeds is a nonprofit organization that lists assistance programs to help uninsured or under-insured people obtain free or low-cost medications from patient assistance programs. Most medicines are provided by the pharmaceutical companies that manufacture them. This organization does not charge for its services.

Partnership for Prescription Assistance
(888) 477-2669
www.pparx.com

The Partnership for Prescription Assistance helps qualifying individuals without prescription drug coverage get the medications they need through the program that is right for them. Many people get their medications free or nearly free. This organization does not charge for its services.

RxAssist
www.rxassist.org

RxAssist is a Web-based medication assistance resource center that provides comprehensive, up-to-date information about patient assistance programs. It is part of the Center for Primary Care and Prevention at Memorial Hospital of Rhode Island.

Rx Outreach
P.O. Box 66536
St. Louis, MO 63166-6536
www.rxoutreach.org

Rx Outreach is a nonprofit charitable organization with the mission to provide affordable medications for people in need. It offers more than 400 different medications through its mail-order pharmacy to qualifying low-income individuals and families.

Genetics

Genetic Alliance
4301 Connecticut Avenue NW, Suite 404
Washington, DC 20008-2369
(202) 966-5557
www.geneticalliance.org

This nonprofit coalition of support groups, professionals, and consumers is dedicated to promoting the interests of children, adults, and families with or at risk for genetic disorders. It specializes in linking people interested in genetic conditions with organizations that provide support and information.

www.GINAhelp.org

This website provides an introduction, and answers, to common questions about the Genetic Information Nondiscrimination Act and its protections in health insurance and employment. This online resource was created by the Genetic Alliance, the Genetics and Public Policy Center at the Johns Hopkins University, and the National Coalition for Health Professional Education in Genetics through funding by The Pew Charitable Trusts.

The National Human Genome Research Institute
www.genome.gov/10002328

The National Human Genome Research Institute provides information on its website about the Genetic Information Nondiscrimination Act of 2008.

The National Society of Genetic Counselors (NSGC)
401 North Michigan Avenue
Chicago, IL 60611
(312) 321-6834
www.nsgc.org

NSGC assists consumers in locating genetic counseling services.

Hair loss

Locks of Love
234 Southern Blvd.
West Palm Beach, FL 33405-2701
(888) 896-1588 or (561) 833-7962
www.locksoflove.org

A nonprofit organization that provides hairpieces to financially disadvantaged children under the age of 21 suffering from long-term medical hair loss. (It does not provide hairpieces for temporary hair loss due to chemotherapy and radiation.)

Hearing impairment

The American Academy of Audiology
11730 Plaza America Drive, Suite 300
Reston, VA 20190
www.howsyourhearing.org

The American Academy of Audiology, representing nearly 11,000 audiologists, is dedicated to providing quality hearing care services through professional development, education, research, and increased public awareness of hearing and balance disorders. The website provides extensive resources for families.

American Society for Deaf Children
800 Florida Avenue NE, #2047
Washington, DC 20002-3695
(800) 942-2732 (voice, TTY)
www.deafchildren.org

A national organization of families and professionals advocating for high-quality programs and services to help parents make sound and informed choices to meet their children's needs.

Hearing Loss Association of America (HLAA)
7910 Woodmont Avenue, Suite 1200
Bethesda, MD 20814
(301) 657-2248 (voice, TTY)
www.shhh.org

HLAA helps people with hearing loss through information, education, advocacy, and support.

Hepatitis C/Liver

American Liver Foundation (ALF)
39 Broadway, Suite 2700
New York, NY 10006
(800) 465-4837 or (212) 668-1000
www.liverfoundation.org

ALF is a national, voluntary nonprofit health agency dedicated to preventing, treating, and curing hepatitis and all liver diseases through research, education, and support groups. Its helpline is available to answer questions about liver disease, including hepatitis.

Hepatitis Foundation International (HFI)
504 Blick Drive
Silver Spring, MD 20904-2901
(800) 891-0707 or (301) 622-4200
www.hepfi.org

HFI provides referrals to hepatologists (liver specialists) and gastroenterologists, as well as information about vaccinations, diagnosis, treatments, and caring for the liver. HFI also provides referrals to more than 400 support groups in North America.

Infertility

Fertile Hope
www.fertilehope.org

Fertile Hope provides support and information for cancer survivors at risk of infertility because of cancer treatments.

National Infertility Network Exchange
P.O. Box 204
East Meadow, NY 11554
(516) 794-5772
www.nine-infertility.org

A nonprofit organization that offers peer support for infertile couples, referrals to appropriate professionals, and educational materials.

The Organization of Parents Through Surrogacy
P.O. Box 611
Gurnee, IL 60031
(847) 782-0224
www.opts.com

Provides information about surrogate parenthood.

RESOLVE: The National Infertility Association
1760 Old Meadow Road, Suite 500
McLean, VA 22102
(703) 556-7172
www.resolve.org

RESOLVE's mission is to provide timely, compassionate support and information to individuals who are experiencing infertility issues.

Osteonecrosis (also called avascular necrosis)

The National Osteonecrosis Foundation
5601 Loch Raven Blvd., Suite 201
Baltimore, MD 21239
(443) 444-5985
www.nonf.org

A nonprofit organization that provides funding for medical research and education of patients, physicians, and other health professionals.

The ON/AVN Support Group International Association, Inc.
7408 Henry Ave.
Philadelphia, PA 19128
www.avnsupport.org

An online support group for people with osteonecrosis (also called avascular necrosis).

Sexuality

The American Association of Sexuality Educators, Counselors, and Therapists
1444 I Street NW
Washington, DC 20005
(202) 449-1099
www.aasect.org

The AASECT directs individuals to certified sexuality educators, counselors, or therapists in their area.

Sjögren's Syndrome

Sjögren's Syndrome Foundation
6707 Democracy Blvd., Suite 325
Bethesda, MD 20817
(800) 475-6473 or (301) 530-4420
www.sjogrens.org

This foundation provides practical information and coping strategies about how to minimize the effects of dry eyes and mouth. In addition, the foundation is the clearinghouse for medical information about Sjögren's syndrome.

Stem cell transplantation

Bone Marrow Transplant Information Network (BMT InfoNet)
www.bmtinfonet.org/after/top

BMT InfoNet provides support and information for patients and survivors of bone marrow, peripheral blood stem cell, and cord blood transplants. The section for survivors includes articles about medical, financial, emotional, educational, and practical issues. A resource directory of helpful organizations and agencies is included.

Center for International Blood and Marrow Transplant Research (CIBMTR)
www.cibmtr.org

CIBMTR leads research studies on transplants, collects data, and provides access to the data to researchers and patients. The website offers post-transplant guidelines, study summaries, and transplant and survival statistics. To access these resources, navigate to the Reference Center and then to Patient Resources.

Books

Books can be borrowed from your local library or ordered through interlibrary loan. Most libraries have a computerized database of all materials available in their various branches. A librarian can show you how to use this system, how to request a book from another branch, and how to place a book on hold if it is currently checked out. If a book is not in your library's collection, ask the librarian to try and obtain it from another library by requesting an interlibrary loan. This common practice allows you to borrow books, including medical textbooks, from university or medical school libraries. You can also purchase books from your local bookstore, your favorite online bookseller, or from the publisher.

General

Halvorson-Boyd, Glenna, and Hunter, Lisa. (1995). *Dancing in Limbo: Making Sense of Life After Cancer*. San Francisco, CA: Jossey-Bass.

Harpham, Wendy Schlessel. (1995). *After Cancer: A Guide to Your New Life*. New York, NY: W. W. Norton & Co.

Hoffman, Barbara, ed. (1996). *A Cancer Survivor's Almanac: Charting Your Journey*. Hoboken, NJ: John Wiley & Sons: Chronimed Publishing.

Genetics

Teichler-Zallen, Doris. (2009). *To Test or Not to Test: A Guide to Genetic Screening and Risk.* Waterville, ME: Thorndike Press.

Hearing impairments

Ogden, Paul W. (1996). *The Silent Garden: Raising Your Deaf Child.* Washington, DC: Gallaudet University Press.

Schwartz, Sue. (2007). *Choices in Deafness: A Parent's Guide to Communication Options, 3rd ed.* Bethesda, MD: Woodbine House.

Hepatitis C

Askari, Fred K. (2001). *Hepatitis C, The Silent Epidemic: The Authoritative Guide, rev. ed.* New York, NY: Plenum Publishing.

Everson, Gregory T., and Weinberg, Hedy (2006). *Living with Hepatitis C: A Survivor's Guide, 4th ed.* Hobart, NY: Hatherleigh Press.

Infertility

Aronson, Diane, ed. (2001). *Resolving Infertility: Understanding the Options and Choosing Solutions When You Want to Have a Baby, rev. ed.* New York, NY: Harper Resource.

Peoples, Debby, and Ferguson, Harriette Rovner. (2000). *Experiencing Infertility: An Essential Resource.* New York, NY: W. W. Norton & Co.

Learning disabilities

Hayden, Deidre, et al. (2008). *Negotiating the Special Education Maze: A Guide for Parents and Teachers, 4th ed.* Bethesda, MD: Woodbine House.

Kravets, Marybeth, and Imy F. Wax, eds. (2010). *The K & W Guide to Colleges for Students with Learning Disabilities or Attention Deficit Disorder, 10th ed.* New York, NY: Princeton Review.

Simpson, Cynthia, and Spencer, Vicki. (2009). *College Success for Students With Learning Disabilities: Strategies and Tips to Make the Most of Your College Experience.* Waco, TX: Prufrock Press.

Thompson, Sue. (1997). *The Source® for Nonverbal Learning Disorders.* East Moline, IL: LinguiSystems. (800) PRO-IDEA.

Limb loss

Winchell, Ellen. (1995). *Coping with Limb Loss.* Garden City Park, NY: Avery Publishing Group.

Riley, Richard Lee. (2005). *Living with a Below Knee Amputation: A Unique Insight from a Prosthetist/Amputee.* Thorofare, NJ: Slack Incorporated.

Seizures

Freeman, John M., et al. (2002). *Seizures and Epilepsy in Childhood: A Guide, 3rd ed.* Baltimore, MD: Johns Hopkins Press.

Sexuality

Schover, Leslie R. (1997). *Sexuality and Fertility after Cancer.* New York, NY: John Wiley Inc.

Statistics and epidemiology

Cancer Incidence and Survival among Children and Adolescents: United States SEER Program 1975–1995. Bethesda, MD: National Cancer Institute, 1999. Available online at *http://seer.cancer.gov/publications/childhood.*

Cancer Epidemiology in Older Adolescents and Young Adults 15 to 29 Years of Age, Including SEER Incidence and Survival: 1975–2000. National Cancer Institute. Available online at *http://seer.cancer.gov/publications/aya/index. html.*

Technical information about late effects

Baggott, Christina, et al., eds. (2011). *Nursing Care of Children and Adolescents with Cancer and Blood Disorders, 4th ed.* Glenview, IL: Association of Pediatric Hematology/Oncology Nurses, Chapter 20 covers late effects of childhood cancer and its treatment. Chapter authors are Wendy Hobbie, Claire Carlson, Jeanne Harvey, Kathleen Ruccione, and Ida Moore; pp. 694–763.

Ganz, Patricia A., ed. (2007). *Cancer Survivorship: Today and Tomorrow.* New York, NY: Springer. Chapter 7 discusses survivorship after treatment of childhood cancers.

Hoppe, Richard, et al., eds. (2007). *Hodgkin Lymphoma, 2nd ed.* Philadelphia, PA: Lippincott, Williams, and Wilkins. Chapters 23 to 27 cover late effects of treatment for Hodgkin lymphoma.

Pizzo, Philip, and David Poplack, eds. (2010). *Principles and Practice of Pediatric Oncology, 6th ed.* Philadelphia, PA: Lippincott, Williams, and Wilkins. Chapter 47 covers late effects of childhood cancer and its treatment, pp. 1368–1387.

Schwartz, Cindy, Wendy Hobbie, Louis Constine, and Kathleen Ruccione, eds. *Survivors of Childhood and Adolescent Cancer: A Multidisciplinary Approach, 2nd ed.* (2005). New York, NY: Springer.

The Internet

There is an astonishing amount of information available through the Internet. Libraries from all over the world can be accessed, and you can download information in minutes from huge databases such as PubMed and Cancerlit. Exchanges between individuals occur through bulletin boards and discussion listservs. However, the large numbers of people using the Internet has spawned thousands of chat rooms, websites, and FAQs (frequently asked questions), which may or may not contain accurate information. You might want to adopt the motto, "Let the buyer beware." It is wise to verify information prior to acting on it and to bring all questions or concerns you have to your healthcare provider.

Support

Internet support groups (also called listservs) are free, email discussions about specific topics of interest. Each subscriber receives a copy of an email sent by any member of the group. Some active groups generate dozens of messages a day. If you subscribe to the "digest" mode, you will receive one email containing all the messages posted that day. The Association of Cancer Online Resources, Inc. (ACOR), a nonprofit organization, manages the best cancer-related Internet support groups. Some examples are PED-ONC, PED-ONC Survivors, ALL-KIDS, GVHD support group for people post-transplant, LT-survivors (long-term survivors), and BMT-TALK. To find a list of the groups, go to *www.acor.org/mailing.html*.

References

Chapter 1: Survivorship

1. Mariotto, A. B., et al. (2009). Long-term survivors of childhood cancers in the United States. *Cancer Epidemiol Biomarkers Prev*, 18(4): 1033–40.

2. Mullan, F. (1985). Seasons of survival: Reflections of a physician with cancer. *N Engl J Med*, 313: 270–273.

3. Masera, G., et al. (1996). SIOP working committee on psychosocial issues on pediatric oncology: Guidelines for care of long-term survivors. *Medical and Pediatric Oncology*, 27: 1–2.

4. Corrigan, J. J., et al. (2004). American Academy of Pediatrics' guidelines for pediatric cancer centers. *Pediatrics*, 113(6): 1833–35.

5. Klausner, R. (Apr 1998). NCI Spotlights Survivorship. *The Bone & Marrow Transplant Newsletter*, 9(1), issue 41.

Chapter 2: Emotions

1. Bruce, M. (2006). A systematic and conceptual review of posttraumatic stress in childhood cancer survivors and their parents. *Clinical Psychology Review*, 26: 233–256.

2. Stuber, M. L., et al. (2010). Prevalence and predictors of posttraumatic stress disorder in adult survivors of childhood cancer. *Pediatrics*, 125(5): 1124–1134.

Chapter 3: Relationships

1. Sankila R., et al. (1998). Risk of cancer among offspring of childhood cancer survivors. *New England Journal of Medicine*, 338(19): 1339–44.

2. Signorello, L. B., et al. (2012). Congenital anomalies in the children of cancer survivors. *Journal of Clinical Oncology*, 30(3): 239–45.

Chapter 4: Navigating the System

1. Wolfson, J. K., et al. (2010). Health care reform 2010: expected favorable impact on childhood cancer patients and survivors. *Cancer J*, 16(6): 554–62.

2. Mariotto, B., et al. (2009). Long-term survivors of childhood cancers in the United States. *Cancer Epidemiol Biomarkers Prev*, 18(4): 1033–40.

3. Weiner, S. L., et al. (2010). Pediatric cancer: advocacy, insurance, education, and employment. In *Principles and Practice of Pediatric Oncology*, P. A. Pizzo & D. G. Poplack, (Eds.), pp. 1441–1450. Philadelphia, PA: Lippincott, Williams & Wilkins.

Chapter 5: Staying Healthy

1. Stolley, M. R., et al. (2010). Diet and physical activity in childhood cancer survivors: a review of the literature. *Ann Behav Med*, 39(3): 232–49.

2. Wasserman, A. L., et al. (1987). The psychological status of survivors of childhood/adolescent Hodgkin's disease. *American Journal of Diseases of Children*, 141: 626–31.

3. Hollen, P. J., Hobbie, W. L., et al. (2007). Substance use risk behaviors and decision-making skills among cancer-surviving adolescents. *J Pediatr Oncol Nurs*, 24(5): 264–73.

4. Tobacco Use: Targeting the Nation's Leading Killer At A Glance 2011. Retrieved April 21, 2012, from *www.cdc.gov/chronicdisease/resources/publications/AAG/osh.htm.*

5. Bradley, K. A., et al. (1998). Medical risks for women who drink alcohol. *Journal of General Internal Medicine*, 13(9): 627–39.

Chapter 6: Diseases

1. Smith, M. A., et al. (1999). Cancer incidence and survival among children and adolescents: *United States SEER Program 1975–1995.* Bethesda, MD: National Cancer Institute, SEER Program. NIH Pub. No. 99–4649.

2. Hunger, S. P., et al. (2012). Improved survival for children and adolescents with acute lymphoblastic leukemia between 1990 and 2005: a report from the Children's Oncology Group Journal of Clinical Oncology. *http://jco.ascopubs.org/content/early/2012/03/06/JCO.2011.37.8018.short.*

3. Bhatia, S., et al. (1996). Breast cancer and other second neoplasms after childhood Hodgkin's disease. *New England Journal of Medicine*, 334(12): 745–51.

4. Green, D. M. (2001). Congestive heart failure after treatment for Wilms' tumor: a report from the National Wilms' Tumor Study group. *J Clin Oncol*, 19(7): 1926–1934.

Chapter 7: Fatigue

5. National Comprehensive Cancer Network. (2012). *NCCN Clinical Practice Guidelines in Oncology: Cancer-Related Fatigue.* Retrieved April 21, 2012, from *www.nccn.org.*

6. Mulrooney, D. A., et al. (2008). Fatigue and sleep disturbance in adult survivors of childhood cancer: a report from the childhood cancer survivor study. *Sleep*, 31(2): 271–81.

Chapter 8: Brain and Nerves

1. Smibert, E., et al. (1996). Risk factors for intellectual and educational sequelae of cranial irradiation in childhood acute lymphoblastic leukaemia. *Br J Cancer*, 73(6): 825–830.

2. Brown, R. T., et al. (1996). A 3-year follow-up of the intellectual and academic functioning of children receiving central nervous system prophylactic chemotherapy for leukemia. *J Dev Behav Pediatr*, 17(6): 392–398.

3. Schatz, J., et al. (2000). Processing speed, working memory, and IQ: a developmental model of cognitive deficits following cranial radiation therapy. *Neuropsychology*, 14(2): 189–200.

4. Montour-Proulx, I., et al. (2005). Cognitive changes in children treated for acute lymphoblastic leukemia with chemotherapy only according to the Pediatric Oncology Group 9605 protocol. *J Child Neurol*, 20(2): 129–133.

Chapter 10: Eyes and Ears

1. Children's Oncology Group Long-Term Follow-Up Guidelines, Version 3.0, Health Link: Eye Health, page 4. *www.survivorshipguidelines.org.*

Chapter 11: Head and Neck

1. Gevorgyan, A., et al. (2007). Radiation-induced craniofacial bone growth disturbances. *J Craniofac Surg*, 18(5): 1001–1007.

2. Paulino, A. C., et al. (2000). Long-term effects in children treated with radiotherapy for head and neck rhabdomyosarcoma. *Int J Radiat Oncol Biol Phys*, 48(5): 1489–1495.

3. Liu, R., et al. (1990). Salivary flow rates in patients with head and neck cancer 0.5 to 25 years after radiotherapy. *Oral Surg Oral Med Oral Pathol*, 70(6): 742–749.

Chapter 12: Heart and Blood Vessels

1. Van Dalen, E. C., et al. (2007) Prevention of anthracycline induced cardiotoxity in children: The evidence. *Eur J Cancer*, 43(7): 1134–40.

2. Meeske, K. A., et al. (2007). Premature carotid artery disease in long-term survivors of childhood cancer treated with neck irradiation: a series of 5 cases. *J Pediatr Hematol Oncol*, 29(7): 480–484.

3. Cheng, S. W., et al. (1999). Irradiation-induced extracranial carotid stenosis in patients with head and neck malignancies. *Am J Surg*, 178(4): 323–328.

4. Shankar, S. M., et al. (2008). Monitoring for cardiovascular disease in survivors of childhood cancer: report from the Cardiovascular Disease Task Force of the Children's Oncology Group. *Pediatrics*, 121(2): e387–396.

Chapter 13: Lungs

1. Wasilewski-Masker, K., et al. (2010). Severity of health conditions identified in a pediatric cancer survivor program. *Pediatr Blood Cancer*, 54: 976–982.

2. Hobbie, W., et al. (2011). Care of the survivor of childhood cancer. In C. Baggott (Ed.), *Nursing Care of Children and Adolescents with Cancer and Blood Disorders, 4th ed.* Glenview, IL: Association of Pediatric Hematology/Oncology Nurses.

3. Huang, T., et al. (2011). Pulmonary outcomes in survivors of childhood cancer: A systematic review. *Chest*, 140(4): 881–901.

4. Jenney, M. E., et al. (1995). Lung function and exercise capacity in survivors of childhood leukaemia. *Med Pediatr Oncol*, 24(4): 222–30.

5. Children's Oncology Group Long-Term Follow-Up Guidelines, Version 3.0, page 12. *www.survivorshipguidelines.org.*

6. Children's Oncology Group Long-Term Follow-Up Guidelines, Version 3.0, page 12. *www.survivorshipguidelines.org.*

7. Children's Oncology Group Long-Term Follow-Up Guidelines, Version 3.0, page 37. *www.survivorshipguidelines.org.*

8. Ingrassia T. S. (1991). Oxygen-exacerbated bleomycin pulmonary toxicity. *Mayo Clin Proc*, 66(2): 173–8.

Chapter 14: Kidneys, Bladder, and Genitals

1. Kapoor, M., et al. Malignancy and renal disease. (2001). *Crit Care Clin*, 17: 571–598.

2. Children's Oncology Group Long-Term Follow-Up Guidelines, Version 3.0, page 105. *www.survivorshipguidelines*.org.

3. Ginsberg, J. P., Hobbie, W. L., et al. (2004). Prevalence of and risk factors for hydrocele in survivors of Wilms Tumor. *Pediatr Blood and Cancer*, 42: 361–363.

Chapter 15: Liver, Stomach, and Intestines

1. U. S. Centers for Disease Control and Prevention, retrieved March 10, 2012, from *www.cdc.gov/hepatitis/HCV/HCVfaq.htm#section4.*

2. Castellino, S., et al. (2010). Hepato-biliary late effects in survivors of childhood and adolescent cancer: a report from the Children's Oncology Group. *Pediatr Blood Canc*, 54(5): 663–669.

3. Children's Oncology Group Long-Term Follow-Up Guidelines, Version 3.0, page 97. *www.survivorshipguidelines.org.*

4. Hutter, R. V. P., et al. (1960). Hepatic fibrosis in children with acute leukemia: a complication of therapy. *Cancer*, 13: 288–307.

5. Castellino, S., et al. (2010). Hepato-biliary late effects in survivors of childhood and adolescent cancer: a report from the Children's Oncology Group. *Pediatr Blood Canc*, 54(5): 663–9.

6. Strasser, S. I., et al. (1999). Cirrhosis of the liver in long-term marrow transplant survivors. *Blood*, 93(10): 3259–66.

7. Children's Oncology Group Long-Term Follow-Up Guidelines, Version 3.0, pages 5 and 6. *www.survivorshipguidelines.org*.

8. National Library of Medicine, retrieved March 10, 2012, from *www.ncbi.nlm. nih.gov/pubmedhealth/PMH0001318*.

Chapter 16: Immune System

1. Children's Oncology Group Long-Term Follow-Up Guidelines, Version 3.0, page 132. *www.survivorshipguidelines.org*.

2. Bisharat, N., et al. (2001). Risk of infection and death among post-splenectomy patients. *J Infect*, 43(3): 182–6.

3. Children's Oncology Group Long-Term Follow-Up Guidelines, Version 3.0, page 162. *www.survivorshipguidelines.org*.

4. Horwitz, T. Z. & Sullivan, K. M. (2006). Chronic graft-versus-host disease. *Blood Reviews*, 20: 15–27.

5. Chisholm, J. C. (2007). Reimmunization after therapy for childhood cancer. *Clinical Infectious Disease*, 44: 643–645.

6. U. S. Centers for Disease Control and Prevention. Human Papillomavirus (HPV). Retrieved April 21, 2012, from *www.cdc.gov/hpv/vaccine.html*.

7. Van Tilburg, C. M., et al. (2006). Loss of antibodies and response to re-vaccination in children after treatment for acute lymphocytic leukemia: a systematic review. *Leukemia*, 20: 1717–1722.

Chapter 17: Muscles and Bones

1. Paulino, A. C. (2004). Late effects of radiotherapy for pediatric extremity sarcomas. *Int J Radiat Oncol Biol Phys*, 60(1): 265–274.

2. Hobbie, W. L., et al. (2008). Late effects in survivors of tandem peripheral blood stem cell transplant for high-risk neuroblastoma. *Pediatric Blood & Cancer*, 51(5): 679–683.

3. Loder, R. T., et al. (1998). Slipped capital femoral epiphysis associated with radiation therapy. *J Pediatr Orthop*, 18(5): 630–636.

Chapter 18: Skin, Breasts, and Hair

1. Furst, J., et al. (1989). Breast hypoplasia following irradiation of the female breast in infancy and early childhood. *Acta Oncology*, 28(4): 519–23.

2. Rosenfield, N. S., et al. (1989). Failure of development of the growing breast after radiation therapy. *Pediatric Radiology*, 19(2): 124–7.

3. Travis, L. B., et al. (2003). Breast cancer following radiotherapy and chemotherapy among young women with Hodgkin disease. *Journal of the American Medical Association*, 290(4): 465–75.

4. Henderson T. O., et al. (2010). Systematic review: Surveillance for breast cancer in women treated with chest radiation for childhood, adolescent, or young adult cancer. *Ann Intern Med,* 152(7): 444–55.

5. Tosti, A., et al. (2005). Permanent alopecia after busulfan chemotherapy. *Br J Dermatol,* 152(5): 1056–8.

Chapter 19: Second Cancers

1. Children's Oncology Group Long-Term Follow-Up Guidelines, Version 3.0, page 101. *www.survivorshipguidelines.org.*

2. Bhatia, S., et al. (2007). Therapy-related myelodysplasia and acute myeloid leukemia after Ewing sarcoma and primitive neuroectodermal tumor of bone: A report from the Children's Oncology Group. *Blood,* 109(1): 46–51.

3. Smith, M. A., et al. (1999). Secondary leukemia or myelodysplastic syndrome after treatment with epipodophyllotoxins. *J Clin Oncol,* 17(2): 569–577.

4. Neglia, J. P., et al. (2001). Second malignant neoplasms in five-year survivors of childhood cancer: childhood cancer survivor study. *J Natl Cancer Inst,* 93(8): 618–629.

5. Bhatia, S., et al. (2003). High risk of subsequent neoplasms continues with extended follow-up of childhood Hodgkin's disease: Report from the Late Effects Study Group. *Journal of Clinical Oncology,* 12(23): 4386–94.

6. Kleinerman, R. A., et al. (2005). Risk of new cancers after radiotherapy in long-term survivors of retinoblastoma: An extended follow-up. *Journal of Clinical Oncology,* 23(10): 2272–9.

7. Breslow, N. E., et al. (1995). Second malignant neoplasms following treatment for Wilms' tumor: A report from the national Wilms' Tumor Study Group. *Journal of Clinical Oncology,* 13(8): 1851–9.

8. Neglia, J. P., et al. (2006). New primary neoplasms of the central nervous system in survivors of childhood cancer: A report from the Childhood Cancer Survivor Study. *J Natl Cancer Inst,* 98(21): 1528–1537.

9. Rimm, I. J. (1987). Brain tumors after cranial irradiation for childhood acute lymphoblastic leukemia. *Cancer,* 59(8): 1506–1508.

10. Goshen, Y. (2007). High incidence of meningioma in cranial irradiated survivors of childhood acute lymphoblastic leukemia. *Pediatr Blood Cancer,* 49(3): 294–297.

11. Forrest, D. L., et al. (2003). Second malignancy following high-dose therapy and autologous stem cell transplantation: Incidence and risk factor analysis. *Bone Marrow Transplant,* 32(9): 915–923.

12. Baker, K. S., et al. (2003). New malignancies after blood or marrow stem-cell transplantation in children and adults: incidence and risk factors. *J Clin Oncol,* 21(7): 1352–1358.

Index

and skin, 382
and radiation, 345
Decadron. *See* dexamethasone (Decadron)
dental problems, 152, 155, 171
depression, 33, 37–39, 57, 135, 141, 145, 200, 246
dexamethasone (Decadron),
    and acute lymphoblastic leukemia, 150
    and cataracts, 264
    and tests needed after treatment with, 194
    and GVHD, 191
    and osteonecrosis, 372
    and osteoporosis, 371
    and stretch marks, 384
diabetes insipidus, 176, 177
diet, 133–136, 198, 205, 207, 298, 300, 347, 365
digestion, 342
doxorubicin (Adriamycin)
    and acute lymphoblastic leukemia, 150
    and heart damage, 290–293
    and Hodgkin lymphoma, 163
    and liver cancers, 178
    and liver damage, 338
    and neuroblastoma, 167
    and non-Hodgkin lymphoma, 169
    and osteosarcoma, 173
    and lung problems, 310
    and rhabdomyosarcoma, 184
    and second tumors, 401, 402
    and tests needed after treatment with, 193, 306
    and Wilms tumor, 187
dry eyes, 182, 264, 268–269
dry mouth, 164, 191, 282–283, 285
dysmotility, 344
DTIC (dacarbazine), 163

E

ears, 269–276
edema, 293, 312, 322
education,
    Canadian laws, 91
    financial aid for college, 103–104
    individualized education program (IEP), 92, 94–97

in Canada, 91
    individualized transition plan (ITP), 97–98
    post-high school, 98–102
    college, 101–102
    financial aid, 103
    for disabled survivors, 101
    vocational training, 98
    specific U.S. laws, 90–91
    Americans with Disabilities Act, 87, 115, 118
    Individuals with Disabilities Education Act (IDEA), 90
    Section 504, Federal Rehabilitation Act, 91, 98, 119–120, 125
emotions and feelings
    about teens leaving home, 13
    anger, 22, 33, 36
    anniversary reactions, 30, 32
    anxiety, 5, 27, 33, 37–39, 41, 145
    depression, 33, 37–39, 57, 135, 141, 145, 200, 246
    at end of treatment, 6
    fears of recurrence/late effects, 27–30
    grief and loss, 33–35
    guilt because of survival, 39–40
    not releasing as cause of problems, 45
    nurturing the spirit, 144–146
    post-traumatic stress, 40–42
    relief, 49
    responses to infertility, 81
    sadness, 34, 38, 201,
    of siblings, 57
    writing about, 145
Employee Retirement and Income Security Act (ERISA), 112
employment. *See* jobs
ending treatment, 6–10
endoprosthesis, 287, 377
energy, low level of. *See* fatigue
enteritis, 346,
enucleation, 181, 182, 197, 262
ependymomas, 156, 271
epipodophyllotoxins, 400
epirubicin, 193, 290, 306
Equal Employment Opportunity Commission (EEOC), 116, 118, 119, 121
ERISA (Employee Retirement and Income Security Act), 112
ESFT. *See* Ewing's sarcoma family of tumors (ESFT)

K

Kennedy-Kassebaum law, 112
kidneys, 235, 317–323
Klausner, Richard, 21
kyphosis, 195, 196, 369, 370, 375, 377

L

Langerhans' cell histiocytosis, 176–177
large cell lymphoma, 169
laser therapy, 181
learning disabilities, 213–215, 89–102
leg length discrepancy, 196, 373–374
leiomyosarcoma, 179
leukemia
    ALL, 149–153 *See also* acute
      lymphoblastic leukemia
    AML, 153–155 *See also* acute
      myelogenous leukemia
    chronic myelocytic leukemia (CML),
      174–176
    juvenile CML, 174
leukoencephalopathy, 213
Leydig cells, 248–252
life insurance, 104–106
limb radiation, 368
limb salvage procedures, 159, 367
liposarcoma, 179
liver, 335–341
liver tumors, 177–178
lomustine (CCNU), 78, 141, 193, 311, 398
loss. See grief and loss
lungs, 307–317
lymphatic system. See lymph nodes; spleen
lymphedema, 184, 354–355
lymph nodes, 162, 167, 169, 185, 330,
    349–355
lymphocytes, 149, 162, 169, 353

M

maintenance therapy, 150, 151, 153
malabsorption, 342, 345, 364
malignant fibrous histiocytoma, 179
malignant peripheral nerve sheath tumor,
    179
mandible, 278
mantle radiation, 243, 245, 278, 284, 294,
    302, 303, 309, 310, 390, 401, 404
marriage, 76

Matulane. See procarbazine
mechlorethamine (Mustargen), 163, 193,
    249, 398
medical follow-up,
    See follow-up programs
medical history, 15
    and adoption, 87
    and insurance, 104, 111, 112,
    and jobs, 116
    and second cancers, 404
Medicare/Medicaid, 110–111
medulloblastoma, 15–157, 271, 392
melphalan (Alkeran), 78, 190, 249, 398,
    400
mercaptopurine (Purinethol, 6-MP), 150,
    170, 194, 378
methotrexate,
    and acute lymphoblastic leukemia,
      150–151
    and acute myelogenous leukemia, 154
    and learning disabilities, 210–211,
      213–214
    and liver damage, 338
    and Hodgkin lymphoma, 163
    and neuroblastoma,
    and non-Hodgkin lymphoma, 170
    and osteoporosis, 371
    and osteosarcoma, 173
    and tests needed after treatment with,
      194
military service, 122–123
moles, 144, 383, 388
MOPP, 79, 163, 165, 229, 249, 250, 256
mouth, dry, 164, 191, 282–283, 358
mouth, damage to, 285, 287
Mullan, Fitzhugh, 17
muscles, 361–364
Mustargen. See mechlorethamine
    (Mustargen)
Myleran. See busulfan (Myleran)
myelosuppression, 349
myelodysplastic syndromes, 400

N

nasopharyngeal carcinoma, 271, 278
nephrectomy, 186, 197
nephritis, 185, 319
nerves, 225–232, 329, 330, 351, 354
networking for support, 42–44

Hodgkin lymphoma, 162
neuroblastoma, 167
non-rhabdomyosarcoma soft tissue
    sarcomas, 180
osteosarcoma, 172
retinoblastoma, 181
rhabdomyosarcoma, 183
Wilms tumor, 186–187
survivor guilt, 39–40
survivor sketches, 409–418
sweat and sebaceous glands, 381, 386, 388
syngeneic transplants, 189
sympathetic nervous system, 166
synovial sarcoma, 179

T

taste, 283
teeth, 285–287
teniposide, 194, 400
testes, 78, 151, 165, 170, 185, 196,
    248–254, 327–329,
testicles, 240, 248–249, 330
tests,
    annual, 346
    following chemotherapy, 193–194
        (table)
    following other treatments, 198
        (table)
    following radiation, 194–197 (table)
    following surgery, 197 (table)
thioguanine (6-TG), 150, 170, 194, 338
thyroid gland, 243–248
thyroglobulin, 248
tinnitus, 271, 275
topoisomerase inhibitors, 402
topotecan, 167
transitions as part of survivorship, 5
treatment teams for follow-up care, 19–22

U

U.S. government healthcare plans, 106,
    110–111
uterus, 85, 256, 327–329

V

vagina. *See* genitals
valves, heart, 290
Velban. *See* vinblastine (Velban)
Vepesid. *See* etoposide (VP-16, Vepesid)
vertigo, 271
vinblastine (Velban), 163, 165, 229, 250
vincristine (Oncovin),
    and acute lymphoblastic leukemia,
        150
    and Ewing sarcoma family of tumors,
        160
    and decrease in the number of sperm,
        249
    and Hodgkin lymphoma, 163
    and liver tumors, 178
    and neuroblastoma, 167
    and non-Hodgkin lymphoma, 169
    and peripheral neuropathies, 226, 229
    and retinoblastoma, 181
    and rhabdomyosarcoma, 184
    and Wilms tumor, 187
    and tests needed after treatment with,
        194
vision problems, 89, 213–215
vocal cords, 285,
vocational training, 98–100
VP-16 (etoposide). *See* etoposide (VP-16,
    Vepesid)

W

warts, 142
wax buildup in ears, 272, 274
weight, 135, 142, 213, 246, 298, 323, 345
weight lifting, 296, 298
Wilms tumor, 186–189
working with health professionals, 23–26

X

x-rays and reports, copies of, 25

About the Authors

Nancy Keene, a well-known advocate and writer, is the parent of a 20-year survivor of childhood cancer. Nancy has written several books about childhood cancer including *Childhood Leukemia: A Guide for Families, Friends & Caregivers* (now in its fourth edition); *Childhood Cancer: A Parent's Guide to Solid Tumor Cancers* (now in its second edition); *Chemo, Craziness & Comfort; Working with Your Doctor*; and *Your Child in the Hospital* (now in its second edition and translated into Spanish). She has edited many books, including *Educating the Child with Cancer* and *Childhood Brain and Spinal Cord Tumors*.

Nancy spends considerable time talking in person, on the telephone, and online with parents of children with cancer and survivors. She was the first chair of the Children's Cancer Group Patient Advocacy Committee, and then the first chair of the Children's Oncology Group (consortium of approximately 230 institutions that care for children with cancer) Patient Advocacy Committee. She is one of the original members of the online support groups sponsored by the Association of Online Cancer Resources (*www.acor.org*) that provide resources and emotional support to families and survivors.

Nancy lives in Washington State and works to keep the pediatric oncology books in print through the nonprofit Childhood Cancer Guides (*www.childhoodcancerguides.org*).

Wendy Hobbie is Associate Director of the Cancer Survivorship Program at Children's Hospital of Philadelphia, one of the first comprehensive follow-up clinics in the United States. In addition to co-authoring *Childhood Cancer Survivors*, Wendy is one of the editors and chapter authors of the textbook for professionals, *Survivors of Childhood Cancer: Assessment and Management* (now in its second edition). She has published numerous articles in peer-reviewed journals on topics such as the late effects of treatment for childhood cancer, the role of the nurse practitioner in follow-up care, and risk taking and decision making by survivors of childhood cancer. She is frequently invited to present lectures to healthcare professionals, cancer survivors, and their families on a variety of cancer survivorship issues.

For 29 years, Wendy has devoted her professional life to the research and clinical care of survivors of childhood cancer and their families. Through education, Wendy has empowered survivors with the knowledge to advocate for themselves in the healthcare system and society. Wendy lives with her husband Dan and two children, Jonathan and Sarah, in Philadelphia.

Kathy Ruccione is Co-Director of the HOPE (Hematology-Oncology Psychosocial and Education) Program in the Children's Center for Cancer and Blood Diseases at Children's Hospital Los Angeles (CHLA). She has been involved in the areas of late effects and survivorship for more than 25 years. Kathy established the CHLA LIFE Program along with its annual Survivor's Day celebrations and survivor scholarship program. Kathy is one of the editors and chapter authors of the textbook for professionals, *Survivors of Childhood Cancer: Assessment and Management* (now in its second edition). She has published and lectured extensively on topics such as transitions in care, survivorship needs, and the role of nurses in late effects evaluation.

Kathy is the mother of a son, Daniel, who is now 26. Living with Daniel, who is profoundly deaf, has brought new challenges and opened new worlds. Her personal experience as the mother of a young person with a disability has enriched her perspective and deepened her commitment to finding ways to help children and their families survive and transcend the experience with cancer.

Childhood Cancer Guides™

Questions Answered
Experiences Shared

When your life is turned upside down, your need for information is great. You have to make critical medical decisions, often with what seems like little to go on. Plus, you have to break the news to family, quiet your own fears, help your ill child and your other children, figure out how you are going to pay for things, and sometimes get to work or put dinner on the table.

Childhood Cancer Guides provide authoritative information for the families and friends of children with cancer or survivors of childhood cancer. They cover all aspects of how these illnesses affect family life. In each book, there's a mix of:

- **Medical information**
  Dozens of experts on childhood cancer and survivorship contributed to these books to provide state-of-the-art information to help you weigh treatment options. Modern medicine has much to offer. When there are treatment controversies, we present differing points of view.

- **Practical information**
  After making treatment decisions, life focuses on coping with treatment and any late effects that develop. We cover day-to-day practicalities, such as those you'd hear from a helpful nurse or a knowledgeable support group.

- **Emotional support**
  It's normal to have strong reactions to a condition that threatens your life or your child's life. It's normal that the whole family is affected. We cover issues such as the shock of diagnosis, living with uncertainty, and communicating with loved ones.

Each book contains stories from parents, children, and siblings—medical "frequent flyers" who share, in their own words, the lessons they have learned and what truly helped them cope.

We provide information online, including updated listings of some of the resources that are listed in our books. This is freely available for you to print out and share with others, as long as you retain the copyright notice on the printouts.

www.childhoodcancerguides.org

Other Books for Families

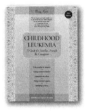

Childhood Leukemia
A Guide for Families, Friends & Caregivers, 4th Edition

By Nancy Keene
ISBN 978-1-4493-8043-4, Paperback, 7" x 9", $29.95,
503 pages

"What's so compelling about Childhood Leukemia is the amount of useful medical information and practical advice it contains. Keene avoids jargon and lays out what's needed to deal with the medical system."

— The Washington Post

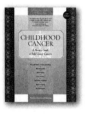

Childhood Cancer
A Parent's Guide to Solid Tumor Cancers, 2nd Edition

By Honna Janes-Hodder & Nancy Keene
ISBN 0-596-50014-9, Paperback, 7" x 9", $29.95, 537 pages

"I recommend [this book] most highly for those in need of high-level, helpful knowledge that will empower and help parents and caregivers to cope."

—Mark Greenberg, M.D.
Professor of Pediatrics, University of Toronto

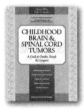

Childhood Brain & Spinal Cord Tumors
A Guide for Families, Friends & Caregivers

By Tania Shiminski-Maher, Patsy Cullen, & Maria Sansalone
ISBN 0-596-50009-2, Paperback, 7" x 9", $29.95, 546 pages

"A must read for both parents and professionals."

—Henry Friedman, M.D.
Co-Director, The Clinical Neuro-Oncology
Center of the Brain Tumor Center at Duke

Childhood Cancer Guides
Our helpful guides are available at
an online bookseller or a bookstore near you.

www.childhoodcancerguides.org
P.O. Box 31937, Bellingham, WA 98228